Abortion Care

Edited by
Sam Rowlands
Dorset HealthCare and the School of Health and Social Care, Bournemouth University, Bournemouth, UK

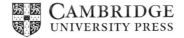

CAMBRIDGE
UNIVERSITY PRESS

University Printing House, Cambridge CB2 8BS, United Kingdom

Cambridge University Press is part of the University of Cambridge.

It furthers the University's mission by disseminating knowledge in the pursuit of
education, learning and research at the highest international levels of excellence.

www.cambridge.org
Information on this title: www.cambridge.org/9781107647381

© Cambridge University Press 2014

First published 2014

Printed in the United Kingdom by Clays, St Ives plc

A catalogue record for this publication is available from the British Library

Library of Congress Cataloguing in Publication data
Abortion care (Rowlands)
Abortion care / edited by Sam Rowlands.
    p. ; cm.
Includes bibliographical references and index.
ISBN 978-1-107-64738-1 (paperback)
I. Rowlands, Sam, editor. II. Title. [DNLM: 1. Abortion, Induced. WA 550.1]
RG734
363.46–dc23
2014022525

ISBN 978-1-107-64738-1 Paperback

....

Abortion Care

This book is due for return on or before the last date shown below.

Contents

Contributors

Edna Astbury-Ward, PhD, MSc, DipHEd, FHEA, RGN, COSRT accredited
Senior Lecturer, Faculty of Health & Social Care, Department of Midwifery & Reproductive Health, University of Chester, Chester, UK

Toni Belfield, HonFFSRH, FRCOG
Specialist in Sexual Health Information, Lyndhurst, Hampshire, UK

Joanna Brien, BA
Sexual Health Counselling Manager, Brook London & South East, UK

Sharon Cameron, MBChB, MD, FRCOG, MFSRH
Consultant Gynaecologist, Chalmers Sexual and Reproductive Health Service, NHS Lothian and Division of Obstetrics and Gynaecology, University of Edinburgh, Royal Infirmary of Edinburgh, Edinburgh, UK

Michael Carrette, MBBS, MRCOG, FRANZCOG
Senior Lecturer in Reproductive and Neonatal Health, James Cook University, Cairns Campus, Queensland and Gynaecologist, Solander Centre, Cairns, Queensland, Australia

Joyce Chai, MBChB, MRCOG, FHKAM(O&G)
Clinical Assistant Professor, University of Hong Kong, Queen Mary Hospital, Hong Kong

Kelly Cleland, MPA, MPH
Research Specialist, Office of Population Research, Princeton University, Princeton, NJ, USA

Rodica Comendant, MD, PhD
Associate Professor, Nicolae Testemiţanu State University of Medicine and Pharmacy, Chişinău and Director, Reproductive Health Training Centre of Moldova, Republic of Moldova

Kelly R. Culwell, MD, MPH, FACOG
Medical Director, Planned Parenthood of the Pacific Southwest; Volunteer Assistant Clinical Professor, Department of Reproductive Medicine, University of California San Diego, San Diego, CA, USA

Caroline de Costa, MBBS, PhD, MPH, FRCOG, FRANZCOG
Professor of Obstetrics and Gynaecology, James Cook University School of Medicine, Townsville City, Queensland, Australia

James Drife, MD, FRCOG, FRCPE, FRCSE, HonFCOGSA, HonFFSRH
Emeritus Professor of Obstetrics and Gynaecology, University of Leeds, Leeds, UK

Joanna N. Erdman, BA, JD, LLM
MacBain Chair of Health Law and Policy and Assistant Professor, Schulich School of Law, Dalhousie University, Halifax, Nova Scotia, Canada

Kristina Gemzell-Danielsson, MD, PhD
Profesor of Obstetrics and Gynaecology, Department of Women's and Children's Health, Division of Obstetrics and Gynaecology, Karolinska Institutet, Stockholm, Sweden

Caitlin Gerdts, PhD, MHS
Epidemiologist, Bixby Center for Global Reproductive Health, University of

California San Francisco, Oakland, CA, USA

Daniel Grossman, MD, FACOG
Assistant Clinical Professor, Department of Obstetrics, Gynecology and Reproductive Sciences, University of California San Francisco and Vice-President for Research, Ibis Reproductive Health, Oakland, CA, USA

Lisa Hallgarten, BA
Specialist in Sexual and Reproductive Health and Rights, London, UK

John Harris, FMedSci, FRSA, FSB, BA, DPhil, HonDLitt
Lord Alliance Professor of Bioethics and Director of the Institute for Science, Ethics and Innovation, Faculty of Life Sciences, University of Manchester, Manchester, UK

Oskari Heikinheimo, MD, PhD
Professor, Department of Obstetrics and Gynaecology, University of Helsinki and Helsinki University Central Hospital, Helsinki, Finland

Pak Chung Ho, MD, FRCOG, FHKAM(O&G)
Chair and Professor, University of Hong Kong, Queen Mary Hospital, Hong Kong

Stelian Hodorogea, MD, PhD
Associate Professor, Nicolae Testemiţanu State University of Medicine and Pharmacy, Chișinău, Republic of Moldova

Roger Ingham, BSc, DPhil
Professor of Health and Community Psychology, University of Southampton, UK and Director of the Centre for Sexual Health Research, Southampton, UK

Helgi Johannsson, BMedSci, MBBS, MRCP, FRCA
Consultant Anaesthetist and Chief of Service, Anaesthesia, Critical Care and Pain, Imperial College Healthcare (St Mary's), London, UK

Anneli Kero, BSW, PhD
Assistant Professor, Department of Social Work, Umeå University, Umeå, Sweden

Helena Kopp Kallner, MD, PhD
Senior Consultant, Danderyd Hospital, Karolinska Institutet, Stockholm, Sweden

Pekka Lähteenmäki, MD, PhD
Adjunct Professor, Department of Obstetrics and Gynaecology, University of Helsinki, Helsinki, Finland

Patricia A. Lohr, MD, MPH, FACOG
Medical Director, British Pregnancy Advisory Service (bpas), Stratford Upon Avon, UK

Richard Lyus, BSc, MBBS
Clinical Lead – London and South East, British Pregnancy Advisory Service (bpas), Middlesex, UK

Wendy Macdowall, BSc, MSc
Lecturer and MSc Public Health Course Director, Centre for Sexual & Reproductive Health Research and the Department of Social & Environmental Health Research, London School of Hygiene & Tropical Medicine, London, UK

Sharon Moses, MSc, MRCOG, MFSRH
Consultant in Sexual and Reproductive Health, Bristol Sexual Health Services, Central Health Clinic, Bristol, UK

Emeka Oloto, FWACS, FRCOG, FFSRH
Consultant in Sexual and Reproductive Health, University Hospitals of Leicester NHS Trust, St. Peters Health Centre, Leicester, UK and Independent Gynaecological Surgeon to bpas

Kate Paterson, MBBS, MRCOG, MFSRH
Consultant in Community Gynaecology and Reproductive Health Care, Imperial College Healthcare (St Mary's), London, UK

Kerry Petersen, LLB, LLM, PhD
Barrister and Solicitor, Supreme Court of
Victoria and Associate Professor, School
of Law, La Trobe University, Melbourne,
Victoria, Australia

Sadie Regmi, BSc, MBChB
Junior Research Fellow, Institute for
Science, Ethics and Innovation, University
of Manchester, Manchester, UK

**Regina-Maria Renner, MD, MPH, FRCSC,
    FACOG**
Clinical Assistant Professor, Department
of Obsterics and Gynecology, University of
British Columbia, BC, Canada

Pascale Roblin, MD
Consultant in Family Planning,
Department of Obstetrics and Gynaecology,
Centre Hospitalier Universitaire Nord,
Assistance Publique-Hôpitaux de Marseille,
Marseille, France

Stephen C. Robson, MBBS, MD, MRCOG
Professor of Fetal Medicine, Institute of
Cellular Medicine, Newcastle University,
Newcastle upon Tyne, UK

**Sam Rowlands, MBBS, MD, LLM, FRCGP,
    FFSRH**
Clinical Lead in Community Sexual and
Reproductive Health, Dorset HealthCare
and Visiting Professor, School of Health
& Social Care, Bournemouth University,
Bournemouth, UK

Irina Sagaidac, MD
Resident Physician in Obstetrics and
Gynaecology, Nicolae Testemiţanu State
University of Medicine and Pharmacy,
Chişinău, Republic of Moldova

Joanna Speedie, MBChB, DFSRH
Community Sexual and Reproductive
Health Trainee, Northern Deanery,
Newcastle upon Tyne, UK

Satu Suhonen, MD, PhD
Adjunct Professor, University of Helsinki,
Centralized Family Planning, Department
of Social Services and Health Care,
Helsinki, Finland

James Trussell, BPhil, PhD
Professor of Economics and Public Affairs,
Princeton University, Princeton, NJ, USA
and Visiting Professor, The Hull York
Medical School, Hull, UK

**Kaye Wellings, MA, MSc, HonFFSRH,
    HonFFPH, FRCOG**
Professor of Sexual & Reproductive Health
Research and Head of the Department of
Social & Environmental Health Research,
London School of Hygiene and Tropical
Medicine, London, UK

Ellen Wiebe, MD, FCFP
Clinical Professor in Reproductive Health,
Department of Family Practice, Faculty of
Medicine, University of British Columbia,
Vancouver and Medical Director, Willow
Women's Clinic, Vancouver, BC, Canada

Preface

This book is designed to be a resource for all those providing abortion care around the world. It is acknowledged that the book has a degree of UK bias. Attempts have been made, however, to give the book an international flavour by inviting contributions from around the world. It is hoped that there will be substantial applicability of the content of all chapters to all readers.

The book can be read from cover to cover or dipped into. It is more than a medical textbook. It deals with human rights, law, ethics and social factors too. It puts abortion into a global context. Those trained in medicine or nursing may find some of the chapters outside their normal sphere of experience, but it is hoped that these will be rewarding, albeit a little more challenging to read. Sociological jargon was rejected by the editor in order to make the text more accessible to a medical readership.

The contributors have been selected because of their excellence and expertise. Each chapter is an authoritative review of the subject. There is considerable innovation. For instance the historical chapter cites online archives of medical journals going as far back as the 1830s. The subject of stigma is newly emerging with respect to abortion and shows how the social sciences can make an important contribution to our understanding. Some readers may view chapters by lawyers with some trepidation, but we should not underestimate how powerful combining forces with other disciplines can be when it comes to reducing the harm of unsafe abortion and improving services for women.

The editor provided a framework for the content of the book. The authors were given suggested topics but were free to develop these as they saw fit. The editor tried to hold back from suggesting too much in the way of alterations.

Although the conception and oversight of the book was down to the editor, many people have supported its coming to fruition. Tracey Masters highlighted the need for the book in the first place and read through the manuscript. Selected chapters were peer reviewed, in particular those with content beyond the editor's knowledge and experience. Thanks to David Horwell, Caroline Moreau, Omi Ohizua and John Spencer for this support. Scan images for the ultrasound chapter were kindly supplied by Trevor Wing.

Shelley Mehigan Raine read every word of the book and provided valuable advice. The publisher never flinched, despite anticipated hesitations on grounds of controversy and stigma. As always, though, the editor takes responsibility for the book in its final form.

Introduction

Sam Rowlands

Abortion can be looked at in many ways ranging from an historical viewpoint from ancient times to the present; from the individual woman and her relationships to society as a whole; from medical and nursing care and counselling through to public health and epidemiology; from basic science such as drug development and ultrasound scan technology through to service delivery to a local population; medical versus surgical techniques; from ethical, human rights and criminal law perspectives. All these interlink. Our understanding and our ability to make improvements depend on integrating all the knowledge and skill accumulated in these many disciplines. For those whose professional lives involve working in abortion care or with the issue of abortion, it is this need for working across the boundaries of various disciplines that is often both the hardest challenge but also the greatest reward.

Global issues

Unsafe abortion has been described as a preventable pandemic [1] and unfortunately this still holds true today predominantly in the developing world. Forty-nine per cent of abortions worldwide are unsafe; this amounts to 22 million unsafe abortions per year [2]. Unsafe abortion accounts for 13% of maternal mortality; it results in 47,000 deaths annually, 98% of these in low-resource countries [3]. As many as five million women in low-resource countries are admitted to hospital each year as a result of complications of unsafe abortion [4]; it has been estimated that in one year (2006) this cost between 460 and 550 million US dollars [5].

It is encouraging that harm-reduction programmes such as the *Initiativas Sanitarias* in Uruguay [6] have been developed which demonstrably reduce morbidity and mortality. It is, however, disappointing that we still see the wealthiest (US) donors (USAID, Bill & Melinda Gates Foundation, for example), who fund reproductive health projects designed to reduce maternal mortality, specifying that not a single dollar can be spent on any activity that could possibly be construed as relating to abortion. This even applies to women who have been raped in zones of conflict. Fortunately some high-resource Western European countries have no such inhibitions: examples are the Swedish International Development Cooperation Agency (Sida) and the UK Department for International Development (DFID) as well as funds from Denmark, Finland, the Netherlands and Norway [7].

Abortion Care, ed. Sam Rowlands. Published by Cambridge University Press. © Cambridge University Press 2014.

Attitudes to abortion

Attitudes play an enormously important part in abortion care – among society in general, politicians, policy makers, health professionals and women themselves. Attitudes to abortion tend to be very polarized in a minority of the population. This is manifest in groups at opposite extremes: for instance those pressing for further liberalization of the law and those organizing anti-abortion protests outside clinics. We should never forget the dedicated healthcare providers who have been subjected to violence (including assassination) by anti-abortion extremists in North America and Australasia [8,9].

Opinion polls consistently show a majority of the population in favour of women's access to abortion on health and socio-economic grounds in most European countries, but politicians are sensitive to extreme anti-abortion views among their constituents and, predominantly in countries in which Roman Catholic doctrine holds sway, to the views of the church. When it comes to voting in Parliaments, politicians can be very conservative.

When women request an abortion, they may come up against hostile attitudes among their family and friends and from healthcare professionals. These pervasive attitudes are based on how society and its laws and policies represent abortion. Women often internalize the stigma which leads to unhealthy self-censorship and secrecy. Those providing abortion care need to be careful that the settings in which they work are, to the greatest extent possible, free from stigmatization of the women coming through their services. It is shocking that the shame and secrecy associated with abortion pushes women into seeking clandestine procedures, thereby contributing to maternal morbidity and mortality especially in the developing world.

Evolution of methods, types of provider and service models

Vacuum aspiration can be traced back as far as the 1860s when it was described by James Young Simpson of Edinburgh [10]. The concept of having an abortion without being admitted to a hospital bed overnight was developed in the 1970s. The development of manual vacuum aspiration has been a big advance, because of its simplicity and cost-effectiveness, although in many settings it has still not been widely adopted.

The concept of medical abortion was not present in medical practice when many countries' current abortion laws were passed. We have seen the development and introduction of drugs (prostaglandins in the 1960s and mifepristone in the 1980s) that have radically changed the face of treatment options. Hence, in countries with less restrictive abortion law, medical abortion under the care of health professionals but at home can be offered; even in countries with highly restrictive abortion laws self-administration of medical abortion drugs without the involvement of health professionals leads to reduced abortion-related morbidity and mortality [11].

In terms of service provision, it seems that criticisms of over-medicalization and over-reliance on doctors have been heeded. Engagement of non-physicians (mid-level providers) is now well-established and such services evaluated as not inferior in terms of safety and acceptability. This kind of multidisciplinary collaboration makes for more holistic and cost-effective care and is highly acceptable to women.

There have been many other valuable developments in models of service delivery.

- Access can be facilitated by use of appointment systems that allow women direct access without referral by a primary healthcare professional.

- Communication and consultations by telephone, fax, email or video-link can reduce delays and long journeys and this can be particularly valuable for women with medical conditions who will need more specialized care, allowing them to be identified at an early stage and directed along an appropriate care pathway.
- When there is no legal imposition of a 'cooling-off period', assessment and treatment can often be combined on the same day thereby further reducing delays and journeys.
- Use of cervical preparation reduces complications of abortion and makes procedures easier and quicker.
- Contraception can be initiated on the day of abortion in most cases.
- Follow-up regimens can be simplified to reduce the number of consultations required without compromising safety and effectiveness and allow women to move on with their lives swiftly after the event.

Regulation by laws and policies

About 26% of all people live in countries in which abortion is generally prohibited: abortion permitted to save the woman's life only or prohibited altogether applies in 69/203 jurisdictions [12]. The most restrictive laws tend to be in the countries of Central and South America, Africa, the Middle East and the Far East.

Regulation by criminal law is still the case in all countries except Canada and three Australian states (Australian Capital Territory, Tasmania and Victoria) [12]. This perpetuates a chilling effect on clinicians taking part in abortion care and on women with unwanted pregnancies who continue to look towards clandestine providers or increasingly nowadays drugs on the internet. For example, in Northern Ireland (part of the UK) doctors feel they cannot offer abortion to a woman with an anencephalic fetus because of uncertainties in interpretation of the law. It is inhumane that women around the world continue to be sent to prison for procuring their own abortion.

Alongside medical advances, we have seen significant shifts in legal and policy approaches to abortion. Following several decades of progressive liberalization of abortion laws in many countries, there has been a backlash in a few European countries (Macedonia, Russia and Slovakia – and threatened in Lithuania and Spain). Those in power who resist liberalization should appreciate not only is it the case that where abortion is legal on broad socio-economic grounds and at a woman's request, both unsafe abortion and abortion-related mortality and morbidity are reduced [13]; but also, that the proportion of women living under liberal abortion laws is inversely related to the abortion rate in the regions of the world [2].

However, a liberal law is not everything. India and Zambia are examples of countries that have had liberal abortion laws since the 1970s but, due to poor services and procedural barriers, safe abortions are hard to come by [14]. Either interpretation of the law or how a country's Health Department/Ministry decides to deal with abortion can to a great degree determine the actual availability of abortion services. Necessary conditions include the dissemination of knowledge about the law to providers and women, the development of guidelines for abortion provision, the willingness of providers to obtain training and provide accessible services and government commitment to provide the resources needed [2]. Obstacles may well be encountered; International Planned Parenthood Federation have developed a tool for assessing procedural barriers to the provision of and access to safe abortion services [15]. On the international stage the influence of the United Nations treaty bodies, with its extension from public health concerns to a dignity-based approach, is increasingly being felt.

Making abortion legal, safe and accessible does not appreciably increase demand for abortion [1]. Rather, the principal effect is to reduce the number of clandestine and unsafe procedures, in favour of legal, safe abortions. By reducing or eliminating the need for unsafe procedures, the liberalization of abortion law increases women's chances of surviving the procedure and improves their subsequent health.

Aims

This book attempts to assemble the main evidence to date on abortion care. The authors sincerely hope that dissemination of this evidence will contribute to improved effectiveness and safety of treatment for women. It is acknowledged that the book does not cover all the practicalities of how to provide a service. Readers are directed to a comprehensive chapter in the World Health Organization guidance on this [13] together with the *Clinical Practice Handbook for Safe Abortion* [16].

The book title is Abortion Care, not Abortion Treatment, to signify the need for clinicians to be concerned, not just with effective treatment, but with quality of care based on compassion, respect and acknowledgement of an individual's autonomy and dignity. It is hoped that the multidisciplinary approach to abortion care reflected in this book will inspire readers and stimulate thought, research and action to provide even better care for women in the future.

References

1. Grimes DA, Benson J, Singh S, *et al.* Unsafe abortion: the preventable pandemic. *Lancet* 2006;368:1908–19.

2. Sedgh G, Singh S, Shah IH, Åhman E, Henshaw SK, Bankole A. Induced abortion: incidence and trends worldwide from 1995 to 2008. *Lancet* 2012;379:625–32.

3. World Health Organization. *Unsafe Abortion: Global and Regional Estimates of the Incidence of Unsafe Abortion and Associated Mortality in 2008.* Geneva: WHO, 2011.

4. Singh S. Hospital admissions resulting from unsafe abortion: estimates from 13 developing countries. *Lancet* 2006;369:1887–92.

5. Singh S, Wulf D, Hussain R, Bankole A, Sedgh G. Abortion worldwide: a decade of uneven progress. www.guttmacher.org/pubs/Abortion-Worldwide.pdf (accessed 17 October 2013). New York: Guttmacher Institute, 2009.

6. Briozzo L, Vidiella G, Rodríguez F, Gorgoroso M, Faúndes A, Pons JE. A risk reduction strategy to prevent maternal deaths associated with unsafe abortion. *Int J Gynecol Obstet* 2006;95:221–6.

7. Barot S. Unsafe abortion: the missing link in global efforts to improve maternal health. *Guttmacher Policy Review* 2011;14:24–8.

8. Wikipedia: Anti-abortion violence. http://en.wikipedia.org/wiki/Anti abortion_violence (accessed 30 November 2013).

9. Joffe C. *Dispatches from the Abortion Wars: The Costs of Fanaticism to Doctors, Patients, and the Rest of Us.* Boston: Beacon Press, 2010.

10. Potts M, Diggory P, Peel J. *Abortion.* Cambridge University Press, 1977.

11. Dzuba HG, Winikoff B, Peña M. Medical abortion: a path to safe, high-quality abortion care in Latin America and the Caribbean. *European Journal of Contraception & Reproductive Health Care* 2013;18:441–50.

12. Rowlands S. Abortion law of jurisdictions around the world. www.fiapac.org/static/media/docs/abortion-law-around-world-sam-rowlands.pdf (accessed 11 March 2014).

13. WHO. *Safe Abortion: Technical and Policy Guidance for Health Systems*, 2nd edn. Geneva: World Health Organization, 2012.

14. Benson J, Andersen K, Samandari G. Reductions in abortion-related mortality following policy reform: evidence from Romania, South Africa and Bangladesh. *Reproductive Health* 2011;8:39.

15. Vekemans M, de Souza U, Hurwitz M. Access to safe abortion: a tool for assessing legal and other obstacles. www.ippf.org/sites/default/files/access_to_safe_abortion.pdf (accessed 17 October 2013). London: IPPF, 2008.

16. WHO. *Clinical Practice Handbook for Safe Abortion*. Geneva: World Health Organization, 2014. www.who.int/reproductivehealth/publications/unsafe_abortion/clinical-practice-safe-abortion/en/ (accessed 8 March 2014).

Chapter

1

An historical perspective

James Drife

There are many possible perspectives on the history of abortion, but this chapter will limit itself to three interlinked questions. Did past generations of women have access to effective methods of abortion? How commonly was abortion practised? And what were society's attitudes towards it? All three questions are hard to answer until we come to the nineteenth century. Up till then historical sources were written mainly by men and tell us little about women's reproductive health. Indeed, until the late twentieth century, abortion was carried out in secret and rarely mentioned in medical texts.

Today abortion is widely debated and the main problem for the internet user is to distinguish fact from misinformation (see Chapter 19). In the past, however, the subject was taboo, which tends to give us the impression that the history of abortion dates from some time in the twentieth century. This idea is swiftly dispelled by a brief search of *The Lancet* and the *British Medical Journal* (BMJ), whose online archives stretch back to the 1830s and 1840s respectively. These have provided much of the information in this chapter, giving it a mainly UK perspective. The chapter will be limited to the time before the British Abortion Act of 1967.

Methods of abortion

Throughout history, drugs taken as abortifacients have ranged from poisons to placebos. Intravaginal honey and crushed dates were mentioned in the Ebers papyrus from ancient Egypt, and herbs and mercury in Chinese texts. The Greek philosopher Plato (428–348 BC) wrote that midwives, 'by means of drugs and incantations are able to … cause abortions at an early stage if they think them desirable' [1]. Methods taught by Hippocrates (*c.* 460–370 BC) and Soranus (second century AD) included physical exercise, massage of the uterus, a tight belt, diuretics, enemas and venesection – all of them ineffective. More than half the surviving medical texts from ancient Rome [2] gave methods for abortion, some of which may have worked. Silphium, an abortifacient plant from North Africa, was harvested to extinction, and hellebore ('Christmas rose'), which was potentially lethal to the pregnant woman, was an ingredient of 'abortion wine'.

The choice between ineffective and harmful medication continued for the next two millennia. In Britain in 1843 the *Provincial Medical Journal (PMJ)*, forerunner of the *BMJ*, recorded that a woman aged 17 almost died after a mid-trimester abortion produced by 'pills of unknown composition'. (Trying to save her life, the doctors treated her with mercury,

---

Abortion Care, ed. Sam Rowlands. Published by Cambridge University Press. © Cambridge University Press 2014.

opium and venesection – a combination probably more dangerous than the original pills.) In 1844, a report of the trial of an abortionist listed fatalities resulting from the use of savine (juniper) or ergot of rye, and counselled against the use of either (for references, see Drife [3]).

Surgical intervention in ancient times was probably limited to late pregnancy. Surgeons' tools included an annular blade and a hook for extracting the fetus, which were used in obstructed labour when the pregnant woman's life was in danger. 'Such apparatus', said one author, 'was possessed by Hippocrates ... and even the milder Soranus.' Instructions for instrumental abortion are contained in Persian texts of the tenth century [4].

After that we have little information about surgical abortion until the nineteenth century. It was specifically outlawed in England in 1803, so it must have been practised before that time. In the 1850s there were reports of the death of a woman after surgical abortion by a 'quack' doctor, and the prosecution of 'two persons calling themselves surgeons'. These cases helped to bring about the establishment of the UK medical register in 1858 [5]. Thereafter surgical abortion was practised by both qualified and unqualified men. In 1869 *The Lancet* recorded a criminal conviction after a non-medical 'abortion-monger ... passed some instrument into the uterus', and in 1885 a Mr Sprow was convicted of procuring abortion: his 'terms were £15 a year for any number of operations required to keep a married woman free from children' [3].

Prosecutions of women were rare, perhaps because they preferred medical methods, although in 1896 a midwife was sentenced to death for procuring an abortion which ended with the death of the woman. Earlier, in 1843, a leading article in the *PMJ* stated: 'We have heard of a French hag, living somewhere near Marylebone Lane, who enjoys no small share of fame for her success, the means which she employs consisting in the daily administration of the oils of pennyroyal and savine, with a violent cathartic at intervals of two or three days' [6].

Self-abortion came to public attention only when it had a fatal outcome. In 1831, for example, *The Lancet* reported a case from Paris in which a woman, pregnant with her fifth child, had injected sulphuric acid into her vagina on the advice of a female neighbour. The pregnancy nonetheless went to term. With the vagina obliterated, caesarean section was attempted (a drastic step in that pre-anaesthetic era) but mother and baby died.

Infanticide was an option for some. In 1837 *The Lancet* recorded that 'bodies of infants are often found in parts of dwelling houses, not infrequently in privies, or in gardens adjoining houses' [7], and in 1869 the *BMJ* reported 'mill-ponds, in the neighbourhood of factories, that have been made the receptacles for many a new born child'. In 1873 the British Medical Association (BMA) lobbied for the legal registration of stillbirth, asserting that 'children killed during birth and after birth are doubtless buried as still-born'. It cited a case 'at Plymouth, where one midwife appeared at a cemetery so constantly with the bodies of children for burial as still-born, that suspicion was excited'. Stillbirth registration, however, was not introduced in England and Wales until 1927 [3].

By the twentieth century most abortions carried out by British doctors were surgical. The royal gynaecologist, writing in 1921, stated that in 35 years of private practice he had carried out only 57 abortions, all of them for life-threatening indications such as placenta praevia, breast cancer and 'mental aberration' leading to intractable vomiting. For late abortion he used a specially made bag to dilate the cervix and induce labour, adding: 'I know of no more difficult vaginal operation than the removal of a 16–20 weeks' pregnancy by means of ovum forceps after rapid dilatation' [8].

Legal attitudes

In the sixteenth century, because a woman with an unwanted pregnancy might keep it secret and dispose of the baby, pregnancy concealment was a classed as a felony. This meant it was punishable by death and in the reign of James I of England an Act was passed by which the jury were obliged to convict on presumptive evidence. In 1809 the law was relaxed slightly: pregnancy concealment became merely a misdemeanour, punishable with imprisonment not exceeding two years, and child murder required the same level of proof as in charges of ordinary homicide [7].

It is sometimes stated that abortion was made illegal in England by an Act of Parliament brought in by Lord Ellenborough in 1803, but his Act merely formalized and extended the existing common law. Attempting to procure medical abortion after quickening was already a capital offence and remained so, but the Act extended the law to cover medical or surgical abortion before quickening. It specified that 'the person so offending, their counsellors, aiders, and abetters, … shall be liable to be fined, imprisoned, set in and upon the pillory, public or privately whipped, or transported beyond the sea for any term not exceeding fourteen years' [7].

In 1837, section 58 of the Offences Against the Person Act removed the distinction between pre- and post-quickening abortions and replaced the death penalty with life imprisonment for abortion at any stage of pregnancy. This applied to anyone procuring abortion, including the woman herself. In 1861 the Act was modified by adding the words 'whether she be or be not with child'. Thus the intention to procure an abortion became a crime. This law is still in force today, amended by the Abortion Act of 1967.

Public attitudes

Public attitudes to abortion are linked to society's attitudes to women, whose status declined during and after the Dark Ages. Contraception and abortion were contained within a women's culture and midwives providing such services were periodically persecuted as 'witches'. During the thirteenth century, the medical profession in Western Europe became entirely male (like the church and the law) and women were excluded from universities. The University of Cambridge, for example, did not award degrees to women until 1947.

The perspectives of the day are seen in nineteenth-century descriptions of attitudes to abortion. In 1843 the *PMJ* asserted that many a young girl requested abortion 'with as much coolness and naivete as if she wished to be relieved of a troublesome tooth' and concluded: 'The opinion that the fetus, for the first two or three months, is an insensate vegetable mass, but that it becomes quick at a definite period, was once held true in medicine, and adopted as the principle of legislation, and, although discarded, it still lingers, like a threadbare garment, amongst the lower orders of society; and it serves, perhaps, to quiet the scruples of some few of the less hardened offenders' [6]. Aside from the phraseology, this sums up one strand of public and professional opinion that has remained more or less unchanged to this day.

Doctors' attitudes

For other doctors, however, their attitude to abortion depended on whether or not they were in control of the process. In 1852 the French Academy debated the differences between criminal abortion and abortion induced under medical supervision. Medical indications included pelvic deformity so severe as to make the death of the pregnant woman inevitable if the pregnancy went to term, as caesarean section had a high mortality at that time. Some members argued, however, from moral and religious principles that abortion was still murder, and that the parents of deformed girls should not allow them to marry [3].

In Britain, midwives' involvement with abortion was a concern for doctors in the nineteenth century. In 1895 the British Medical Association (BMA) stated: 'whilst a few years ago … all the practice which tended towards the production of Abortion was written in Latin, it is now customary to teach pupil midwives … the symptoms and treatment of abortion and miscarriage … this practice is unsound and directly leads to the practice of Criminal Abortion'. Despite the BMA's opposition, the Midwives Act, which established midwifery as a profession, was passed in 1902.

For many years, although abortion was illegal, it was widely accepted that a doctor acting in good faith would not be prosecuted. Nevertheless doctors were still at risk, and eventually this hypocrisy began to be questioned. In 1927 *The Lancet* pointed out that the law prohibiting abortion was 90 years old and suggested that if it were 're-enacted again today an express proviso would be inserted to exempt from criminal liability the fully qualified practitioner who terminates a pregnancy for the bona fide purpose of preserving the mother from special danger to life or health' [18].

The Infant Life Preservation Act of 1929, which punished the killing of a fetus after 28 weeks' gestation, exempted acts 'done in good faith for the purpose only of preserving the life of the mother', but still left doctors at risk of prosecution. In 1932 *The Lancet* reported that, at a meeting of the Medico-Legal Society of London, 'legal opinion was universally in favour of a modification of the law in this country or even of legalization of abortion, while with few exceptions the medical members present supported the present position'. *The Lancet* called for 'new legislation appropriate to the outlook and habits of our times', and repeated this call in 1936, stating 'Feminine opinion, never so well organised or so articulate as today, will no doubt be heard' (see Drife [3]).

In 1938 a test case involving a gynaecologist, Mr Aleck Bourne, of St Mary's Hospital, London, attracted much media attention. He had carried out an abortion on a 14-year-old girl pregnant after rape by two soldiers. The judge summed up sympathetically (pointing out that the girl was 'not of the prostitute class but an ordinary decent girl') and the jury took only 40 minutes to return a verdict of not guilty [19]. After the case, leading members of the Eugenics Society called for facilities for voluntary termination. Dr Joan Malleson, who had referred the patient to Mr Bourne, wrote: 'it is the working-class mother, particularly the most ill-nourished, exhausted, and sick, who most readily resorts to criminal abortion and who takes the gravest risks to achieve it'. She suggested a network of centres providing pregnancy tests, abortion referral and such contraceptive work as was allowed at that time by the Ministry of Health [20].

The Second World War interrupted the debate, but in the post-war era there was, as mentioned above, increasing evidence that criminal abortion was 'sufficiently widespread to constitute a grave social evil', as the *BMJ* put it. The 1967 Abortion Act, sometimes perceived to be the result of 1960s permissiveness, was in fact the outcome of a steady change in public and professional opinion over many years. Nevertheless it polarized the medical profession. In Scotland, for example, Professor Dugald Baird of Aberdeen had implemented a liberal abortion policy (with the support of the local police) long before the law changed, but in Glasgow Professor Ian Donald (the pioneer of ultrasound) was an outspoken opponent of the Act. Across Britain, divergences of view among influential doctors meant that after 1967 there were marked regional differences in the availability of National Health Service abortion, and these continued for many years after abortion law had been liberalized [3].

Conclusion

The three questions at the beginning of this chapter might be answered as follows. (1) Past generations of women had illicit access to medical methods of abortion which were of dubious effectiveness. Surgical intervention was documented in the nineteenth century and carried out in risky circumstances until the 1970s. (2) Data on the frequency of abortion are scanty until the twentieth century. In Britain the annual number of illegal abortions was officially estimated at 100,000 per year in early 1960s, and seems likely to have been around this figure for many years before that. (3) Society's attitudes towards abortion can best be characterized as 'turning a blind eye'. Doctors were involved in only a small proportion of cases and were rarely prosecuted. Attitudes slowly changed and the liberalization of abortion law in Britain in 1967 was the result of a shift in public and professional opinion that had begun in the 1920s.

References

1. Riddle JM. *Contraception and Abortion from the Ancient World to the Renaissance.* Cambridge, MA: Harvard University Press, 1992.

2. Hopkins K. Contraception in the Roman Empire. *Comparative Studies in Society and History* 1965;8:124–51.

3. Drife JO. Historical perspective on induced abortion through the ages and its links with maternal mortality. *Best Pract Res Clin Obstet Gynaecol* 2010;24:431–41.

4. Joffe C. Abortion and medicine: a socio-political history. In M Paul *et al.* (eds.) *Management of Unintended and Abnormal Pregnancy: Comprehensive Abortion Care.* Oxford: Wiley-Blackwell, 2009: 1–9.

5. Leading article. The criminal production of abortion by persons calling themselves surgeons shows that a medical reform act is required as a measure of public safety. *Association Medical Journal* 1853;19:410.

6. Leading article. On the frequency of criminal abortion. *Provincial Medical Journal* 1843;ii:471–2.

7. Thomson AT. Lectures on medical jurisprudence now in the course of delivery at the University of London: Lectures XVII and XVIII. *Lancet* 1837;27:625–30 and 657–63.

8. Philips J. The induction of abortion. *Lancet* 1921;197;266–8.

9. Grace WH. Pathology of criminal abortion. *BMJ* 1937;i:727.

10. Davis A. 2,665 cases of abortion: a clinical survey. *BMJ* 1950;ii:123–30.

11. Teare RD. The medico-legal significance of death following abortion. *BMJ* 1951;i:1388–9.

12. Chapple JAV, Pollard A (eds.). *The Letters of Mrs Gaskell.* Letter no. 233, to John Greenwood of Haworth, 12th April 1855. Manchester University Press, 1966.

13. Whitehouse B. The indications for the induction of abortion. *BMJ* 1932;ii:337–41.

14. Ministry of Health. Investigation of maternal mortality. *BMJ* 1937;i:972–6.

15. Ministry of Health. Reports on Public Health and Medical Subjects No 97. *Report on Confidential Enquiries into Maternal Deaths in England and Wales 1952–1954.* London: Her Majesty's Stationery Office, 1957.

16. McFarlane A. In G Lewis (ed.) *The Confidential Enquiry into Maternal and Child Health (CEMACH). Why Mothers Die 2000–2002.* The Sixth Report on Confidential Enquiries into Maternal Deaths in the United Kingdom. London: CEMACH, 2004.

17. Leading article. The increase of criminal abortion. *Lancet* 1920;195:268.

18. Leading article. Abortion: lawful and unlawful. *Lancet* 1927;209:237–8.

19. Anonymous. A charge of illegal abortion: Rex v. Bourne. *Lancet* 1938;232:220–6.

20. Malleson J. Criminal abortion: a suggestion for lessening its incidence. *Lancet* 1939;233:366–7.

Chapter

2

Ethics

Sadie Regmi and John Harris

Attempts to terminate pregnancies are probably as old as attempts to originate them; carrying them to term is not necessarily always less traumatic than abortion. For various reasons, abortion continues to be the subject of much ethical, philosophical and religious debate. This chapter will discuss the moral issues surrounding the deliberate and premature ending of a pregnancy in a way that entails the death of the embryo or fetus, and touch upon policy considerations. No attempt will be made to address religious objections to abortion. The reason for this, perhaps surprising, exclusion is that all religious views are particular to followers of that faith, and are unlikely to be appealing or persuasive to followers of other religions or of none. In a democracy, we must base principles and policies on moral considerations that are in principle open, and potentially persuasive to all. Religious positions, depending as they do not on quality and force of evidence or argument, but on authority exclusive to the adherents of that religion, are decidedly not of this kind. Of course religious texts do contain arguments and compelling analogies and thought experiments, and can be read as philosophical texts. The problem is, as far as evidence goes, they are usually pre-scientific and woefully out of date.

The pregnant woman and her rights and interests

The rights of the pregnant woman have often evoked the 'choice' argument: the claim that it is a woman's right to choose. The argument involves the claim that the unborn fetus is inhabiting the woman's body, and she has the right to do as she pleases with her body, and if necessary 'defend herself' against the threats posed by the embryo or fetus [1]. It relies on the assumption that the woman's autonomy, which involves both rights and responsibilities relating to choice, allows and obliges her to choose what to do with her body. The free exercise of autonomy is of course constrained in many ways. To paraphrase John Stuart Mill: my liberty to extend my arm stops somewhere short of your nose [2]. As we shall see, however, the autonomy argument is not directly relevant to the abortion debate. The women's rights or pro-choice argument depends on first settling the question as to whether or not the rights/ interests of the fetus are comparable in strength to those of the woman's right to choose – if they are then it is a matter of competing rights and a new argument would be required to show which right holder (if any) takes preference [3]. This will be true even in the case of a self-defence argument since, absent guilty intent by the fetus or convincing arguments

---

Abortion Care, ed. Sam Rowlands. Published by Cambridge University Press. © Cambridge University Press 2014.

as to the different moral, political or legal status of the parties, the appeal to self-defence is available to both the fetus and the pregnant woman.

Some see this issue not merely as a question of autonomy but one of ownership. However, to imply that abortion is based on the ownership of the embryo or fetus is even more problematic than basing it on autonomy. Property rights are constrained and limited in most societies by, for example, licensing (firearms, cars and animals), and taxation, product and ownership liability. Property rights when applied to the status of the embryo or fetus are also inappropriate because, if it is a person not a thing, abortion under any circumstances would be problematic, whereas if it is a thing not a person, normal ownership rights would, because of its location, be un-exercisable by anyone but the pregnant woman. Perhaps the way of thinking about our relationship to the fetus can be likened more to the concept of custodianship rather than to ownership? But again the scope and limits of the powers of the custodian would be determined by independent arguments concerning the nature and value of the item in custody.

If the unborn fetus was valuable in its own right, the arguments based on autonomy or ownership would not hold. The woman's right to choose is, therefore, intrinsically tied to the value of the unborn fetus. As has previously been argued by one of the authors:

> [E]ven if the fetus were beyond a peradventure the property of the mother, she would only be entitled to do with it what she chose (and even end its life) if there were no independent grounds for valuing it more than as an item of her property. If the life of the fetus is valuable, then it should not be ended unless the reasons for doing so are more important than its life. The fact that someone has a claim to ownership is not a feature of comparable importance to the value of life. If a woman is right to choose, she is right not because she has a claim to ownership of the fetus, or because it is in her body, she is right because the moral reasons for respecting its life are less important than the moral reasons for respecting her decision to end its life. [4]

Thus, to decide whether or not the woman does in fact have the right to choose, we must examine what, if any, rights and interests the unborn fetus may possess. In order to do this, we must first discuss the concept of the person and what it means to be human. Whether or not we regard the embryo or fetus as a person is likely to significantly alter our assessment of its entitlements.

What does it mean to be human?

> What a piece of work is a man, how noble in reason, how infinite in faculties, in form and moving how express and admirable, in action how like an angel, in apprehension how like a god: the beauty of the world, the paragon of animals – and yet, to me, what is this quintessence of dust? [5]
> That is the question: [6]

Consider, the hospital is on fire. It contains an assisted reproduction unit with refrigerated trays of embryos awaiting either implantation or disposal. The fire officers arrive and have time to carry to safety either two unconscious human technicians or two trays of embryos containing five hundred embryos per tray. If there is a decision to make here it involves judgements about the relative moral importance of the alternative acts. Judgements that are the subject of this chapter.

Suppose, in another scenario, extraterrestrials who look considerably different to us, but are intelligent, articulate and empathetic, arrive on earth. Despite their membership of a different 'species', we would hold certain qualities they may possess in high enough regard for them to qualify as 'persons'. It is also interesting to explore how we might go about explaining to the aliens why we are worthy of more moral consideration than cabbages, chickens or bananas. We may borrow from the philosopher John Locke and answer thus:

> We must consider what person stands for; which I think is a thinking intelligent being, that has reason and reflection, and can consider itself the same thinking thing, in different times and places; which it does only by that consciousness which is inseparable from thinking and seems to me essential to it; by being impossible for anyone to perceive without perceiving that he does perceive. [7]

Locke's 'forensic' definition identifies the concept of a person in a species-neutral way, and in a way that attempts to account for the peculiar value of beings that are persons. On such an account, it is possible to distinguish persons from non-persons based on the traits possessed by individuals. This does not mean that we value different persons on the basis of these traits or that someone with an exceptional ability to solve mathematical problems or a gift for music is somehow worthy of more moral consideration than a person without those abilities. It would be more accurate to think of Locke as offering the minimum criteria for personhood, criteria which constitute a threshold beyond which all qualifiers are entitled to equal moral consideration. Locke's definition of person relies on the ability of that individual to have a sense of itself. This is sometimes summed up as the capacity to value its own life and existence, not on some external objective measure of its worth [4]. On such a view, the wrong of ending the life of a person is the wrong of taking from that individual something that he or she does not wish us to take. Non-persons such as fetuses and embryos and most animals cannot be harmed in this way, which is one way of explaining why abortion is, in the moral systems of most societies and cultures, sometimes permissible.

Potentiality

It is exactly this perspective on the special moral importance of persons that causes many to argue against abortion. Many of those who value an emerging human individual argue that, while not yet a person, it has the potential to become a person. It is important first of all to note here that it is the moral worth of the person that is so valuable that some believe it accords moral worth to anything that has the potential to become that thing. It is interesting, therefore, that in some extreme circumstances, so-called 'pro-life' activists who do reject abortion have been known to murder actual persons worthy of moral consideration because of their belief in the potential moral worth of the emerging human individual [8]. In less extreme circumstances, those who argue against a woman's right to choose must value the potential moral worth of the emerging human individual over the freedoms of a female individual who unquestionably already has that moral worth.

A major drawback of the argument from potentiality is, of course, that many things have the potential to become something else, but never actually end up achieving that potential. Ears of wheat are not loaves of bread, nor piles of stones houses. Although all seeds and indeed all stones have the potential to become something else, if placed in the right environment or combined in the right way, they are not in fact the same as the end product. As one of the present authors has previously argued, it does not follow from the fact that we are all potentially dead, that it might be legitimate to treat any of us still living as though we were already dead.

Applying this argument to the embryo, it is undeniable that given the right environment and good luck, embryos do in fact have the potential to become persons. However, given the appropriate environment, any cell from a human body has the potential through cloning by nuclear transfer, or probably reprogramming the cell to become an 'induced pluripotent cell' (iPC), stem cells that may demonstrate the same key properties of regeneration and unrestricted differentiation that human embryonic stem cells (hESCs) possess, to become a new human [9]. Embryos also have the potential to become hydatidiform moles, and because of the up to 80% failure rate of human reproduction between three and five embryos are lost for every live human birth, washed out in the monthly menstrual flow, unnoticed and unmourned by the women whose bodies they were temporarily inhabiting. The obligation to actualize potential leads us to an ethic of maximal procreation since in every fertile man and woman there is for the woman every month and the man every minute, the possibility to actualize that potential. Monty Python takes this idea seriously in a famous song: 'Every sperm is sacred, every sperm is great. If a sperm is wasted, God gets quite irate' [10]. It may seem facetious to suggest that proponents of the potentiality argument believe every sperm and every egg is sacred, but that does seem to be the logical conclusion of this line of reasoning.

The emerging human individual, at all stages of development from embryonic status to birth (and, as noted, beyond), has the potential to some day become a person. However, this does not mean the unborn human individual is in fact a person or entitled to the same moral consideration as a person. It is of course difficult to determine when exactly in the process of development the embryo or fetus becomes a person and here, we believe, it is right to 'err on the safe side', and treat them as we would persons even if they are, as infants, incapable of fulfilling the minimum criteria required for personhood: namely the ability to be self-conscious and value one's own existence. However, to err so far on the side of caution as to accord equal moral worth to an embryo or fetus as one would to a person, seems problematic.

Postnatal abortion, more commonly referred to as infanticide, has been the subject of recent philosophical discussion [11]. Whether and in what circumstances infanticide might be justifiable is an extensive topic, and beyond the purview of this chapter.

Abortion and sex selection

A recent controversy about abortion on the grounds of sex selection in the UK, initiated by stories in the newspaper the *Daily Telegraph*, provoked a response from the UK Director of Public Prosecutions [12]. While the idea that mothers or parents might wish to select for gender may be considered distasteful by some [13,14], it is important to distinguish (and the UK law clearly distinguishes) the reasons a mother might have for wishing to terminate a pregnancy (which are likely to be complex) and the legal justifications for an abortion.

As the UK Director of Public Prosecutions has clearly stated recently:

> Procuring a miscarriage is an offence contrary to section 58 of the Offences Against the Person Act 1861. However, section 1 of the Abortion Act 1967 provides that a person should not be guilty of an offence when a pregnancy is terminated by a registered medical practitioner if two registered medical practitioners are of the opinion, formed in good faith, inter alia, that 'the pregnancy has not exceeded its 24th week and that the continuance of the pregnancy would involve risk, greater than if the pregnancy were terminated, of injury to the physical or mental health of the pregnant woman or any existing children of her family'.
>
> Thus the law does not, in terms, expressly prohibit gender-specific abortions; rather, it prohibits any abortion carried out without two medical practitioners having formed a view, in good faith, that the health risks (mental or physical) of continuance outweigh those of termination. This gives a wide discretion to doctors in assessing the health risks of a pregnant patient. [15]

The UK thus puts the life and health of the pregnant woman, and even of her other children, considerably ahead of any interest of a pre-24 week embryo in existence. This low importance to the life of the early embryo is also to be found in nature, and for those who believe God to be responsible for nature, presumably also in God's will. Sexual reproduction with an up to 80% failure rate creates, uses and destroys between three to five sibling embryos for every live birth.

In certain societies, women are not held in the same regard as men, and sex-selective abortion can be seen to be a symptom of such prejudices. The issue of women's subjugation and position in society certainly deserves attention and recent efforts in global health to tackle these issues are to be welcomed [16,17]. The resulting excess of heterosexual men without partners in those societies creates other problems. However, it must be noted that it is the prejudiced views of individuals and not the regulatory regime surrounding abortion that is the problem here.

Society's interests in abortion: policy dimensions

Policies are not always based on clear-cut moral arguments. It is not illegitimate for societies to have social policy, even backed by legislation, on almost anything that they deem sufficiently important. For example, in the UK we drive on the left and we stop at traffic lights and the government takes our money in taxation and forces our children to attend schools. It doesn't have to be immoral to do what is forbidden by law or more moral to do what is permitted or required by law. However, while it is possible to legislate on almost anything, we must recognize that many laws respond to social and political, and not moral, imperatives. But on the whole, laws that are backed by strong moral reasons are regarded as more serious than are those backed by social convenience reasons. Murder and assault are regarded as serious crimes in a way that the use of drugs which do not harm anyone but the user is not.

On the assumption that the developing embryo or fetus does not have a moral status that protects its life at any time before birth (a position which incidentally is taken by UK law [18]), then the method of preventing birth is entirely a matter for the pregnant woman. A combination of common sense, prudence and economy would suggest that contraception is preferable to abortion and early abortion preferable to late abortion for obvious reasons. In fact, in the UK, around 90% of abortions are carried out before 13 weeks of pregnancy and 98% before 20 weeks [19]. Although, as noted, early abortions are preferable to late abortion, there are many circumstances in which abortions at more advanced gestations will continue to be required to protect the life and health of the pregnant woman.

An important issue that is worthy of mention is whether or not women's mental health is affected by undergoing abortion. Chapter 18 discusses this in greater length, with the author concluding that denying women abortion has greater adverse consequences for women psychosocially. It is important to note that even if women were found to have long-term mental health problems as a consequence of abortion, it is unclear whether those after-effects would continue to be present in a world in which abortion was more widely accepted.

Rights and interests of male progenitors

The law in the UK gives no say to male progenitors on whether or not their impregnated partner should have an abortion. Nevertheless, in the past two decades, about two dozen men have approached courts in an attempt to stop their partners from getting an abortion [20]. Given that the fetus usually [21] receives half of its genes from the father, it is worth considering the rights of the father. While the 'ownership' arguments relating to women's choice may imply that men ought to be given an equal say in the fate of their creation, it is harder to justify the claims of the father based on the custodianship approaches mentioned above. A woman is free to decide the fate of the fetus due to the relative lesser moral status of the fetus, and because the fetus affects her health, wellbeing and at least nine months of her life – not because she has any claim to *ownership*. As the ownership argument is not relevant to the right of the woman to choose it cannot be relevant to the man's right to choose.

Even if would-be fathers cannot use arguments relating to ownership, could they deploy arguments regarding the right to father a child? It is difficult to justify this line of reasoning as there cannot be a right to father a child per se – that depends on a willing partner. A willing partner cannot merely mean a willing sexual partner, but must relate to the whole enterprise of childbearing. As the consequences of pregnancy will have to be borne largely, if not solely, by the woman her willingness to enter the enterprise of childbirth can be withdrawn without the consent of her partner. Whatever the contractual nature of partnerships in or outside of marriage, in a world where there is choice at every stage, partnerships cannot be contracts to have children. Even if that were the nature of certain partnerships, the contracts would be unenforceable. A woman's prior agreement to have sexual intercourse with a man on a particular day in the future would not mean that if she were to change her mind in the interim, the man would be within his rights to force her to have sex. Similarly, pregnancy and childbirth involve compromises and are potentially dangerous undertakings. Even if a woman may have agreed to go ahead with a pregnancy, she is within her rights to change her mind before undergoing the dangers of childbirth.

Viability does not alter or create moral status

Many use the viability argument as a compromise argument, because they are comfortable with its policy conclusions, not necessarily because it is what they really believe. As it stands, it is a useful tool for both pro- and anti-abortion lobbies. In his seminal paper on abortion, Roger Wertheimer characterizes what he calls the liberal view on abortion in terms of viability. 'According to the liberal, the fetus should be disposable upon the mother's request until it is viable' [22]. Here we follow the second 1828 definition of 'viability' in the *Shorter Oxford English Dictionary* viz: 'Capable of living, able to maintain a separate existence' [23]. In the context of abortion this means capable of maintaining an existence independent of the pregnant woman. Since the age at which a fetus can survive after premature delivery has been reducing over the years and may reduce further, many think this indicates that the age at which abortion may be legitimate also reduces.

One problem here is that a purported moral watershed seems to be technology dependent. Another is that we may be on the verge of seeing the perfection of so-called *ectogenesis*, the ability to gestate a human individual from conception to 'birth' entirely outside a human body. This may also be linked to the possibility, still only theoretical, of transferring the embryo or the fetus to an artificial womb, thus protecting it from maternal choice to abort and also liberating the mother from the necessity of giving birth. If and when these possibilities become actual we will face a difficult question: will this also mean that the life of a zygote, embryo or fetus may never be ended during its progress from conception to neonate? Certainly, without an acceptable account of when the emerging human individual acquires a moral (and perhaps legal) status comparable to that of normal, fully conscious, adult humans, we will have no coherent reason to protect its life in ways comparable to those in which our own lives are currently protected by law, morality and custom in most jurisdictions.

Indeed viability does not start with conception, with formation of the zygote. Viability as the capacity 'to maintain a separate existence' from the mother covers all stages of human development because the 'emerging' will not need ever to have been in a human womb [24–26]. Pressure will continue to regard as viable not only the zygote but whatever has the existing capacity to become a zygote. This is almost certain to be the case with any human cell appropriately treated and of course with gametes of both genders, stored [27,28] or in vivo.

What is now the 'moral problem of abortion' will inevitably become the moral problem of coping with all the human cells that will be viable precursors of human persons. This we will not be able to do by drawing arbitrary lines in the sand, lines like birth, viability or conception, but by trying to understand what really matters, what really confers the sort of moral status that we must protect and about which we should care. This chapter has been an attempt to explore the difficulties of achieving this understanding.

References

1. Thomson JJ. A defense of abortion. *Philosophy & Public Affairs* 1971;1:47–66.

2. Mill JS. On liberty. In M Warnock (ed.) *Utilitarianism*. Collins/Fontana, 1972: 135 ff.

3. Harris J. Human beings, persons and conjoined twins: an ethical analysis of the judgment in *Re A. Medical Law Review* 2002; 9: 221–36.

4. Harris J. *The Value of Life*. London: Routledge, 1985: Chapter 1.

5. Shakespeare W. Hamlet Act II, Scene 2 Line 305ff. *The Arden Shakespeare* Richard Proudfoot, Ann Thompson and David Scott Kasten (eds.). Walton-on-Thames: Thomas Nelson and Sons Ltd, 1998.

6. Shakespeare W. Hamlet Act III Scene 1 Line 56. *The Arden Shakespeare* Richard Proudfoot, Ann Thompson and David Scott Kasten (eds.). Walton-on-Thames: Thomas Nelson and Sons Ltd, 1998.

7. Locke J. *An Essay Concerning Human Understanding*. Oxford University Press, 1964: Bk II, Chapter 27.

8. Huffington Post. George Tiller Killed: Abortion Doctor Shot At Church. 7 January 2009.

9. Chan S, Harris J. Adam's fibroblast? The (pluri)potential of iPCs. *Journal of Medical Ethics* 2008;34:64.

10. Monty Python. The Meaning of Life. Every Sperm is Sacred. www.youtube.com/watch?v=fUspLVStPbk (accessed 30 October 2013).

11. Giubilini A, Minerva F. After-birth abortion: why should the baby live? *Journal of Medical Ethics* 2013;39: 261–3.

12. Watt H, Newell C. Ministers in new row over abortion ruling. www.telegraph.co.uk/health/healthnews/10365070/Ministers-in-new-row-over-abortion-ruling.html (accessed 12 November 2013).

13. Harris J. No sex selection please – we're British! *Journal of Medical Ethics* 2005;31:286–8.

14. Harris J. Sex selection and regulated hatred. *Journal of Medical Ethics* 2005; 31: 291–5.

15. Statement from Director of Public Prosecutions, Keir Starmer QC, on abortion related cases, 7 October 2013. The Director of Public Prosecutions has written to the Attorney General, Dominic Grieve QC MP, to introduce the statement above. www.cps.gov.uk/news/assets/uploads/files/07_10_13_letter_dominic_grieve_mp.pdf (accessed 3 March 2014).

16. Harvard School of Public Health. Women and Health Initiative. www.hsph.harvard.edu/women-and-health-initiative/ (accessed 31 October 2013).

17. Every Woman Every Child. www.everywomaneverychild.org (accessed 31 October 2013).

18. *Re F (in utero)* [1988] 2 All ER 193.

19. Department of Health. *Abortion Statistics, England and Wales:* 2012. www.gov.uk/government/uploads/system/uploads/attachment_data/file/211790/2012_Abortion_Statistics.pdf (accessed 14 November 2013).

20. Nolan D. Abortion: a man's right to choose? 22 March 2011. www.spiked-online.com/newsite/article/11775#. UnKphhbWba4 (accessed 31 October 2013).

21. Easley CA, Phillips BT, McGuire MM, *et al.* Direct differentiation of human pluripotent stem cells into haploid spermatogenic cells. *Cell Reports* 2012;2:440–6.

22. Wertheimer R. Understanding the abortion argument. *Philosophy & Public Affairs* 1971;1:67–95.

23. *Shorter Oxford English Dictionary*, Volume II. Oxford: Clarendon Press, 1968: 2352.

24. Alghrani A. Viability and abortion: lessons from ectogenesis. *Expert Review of Obstetrics and Gynecology* 2009;4:625–34.

25. Alghrani A, Brazier M. What is it? Whose is it? Repositioning the fetus in the context of research. *Cambridge Law Journal* 2011;70:51–82.

26. Alghrani A. Regulating the reproductive revolution: ectogenesis – a regulatory minefield. In M Freeman (ed.) *Law and Bioethics: Current Legal Issues*. Oxford University Press, 2008; 11: 303–29.

27. Harris J (19 September 2012). *Misleading talk of 'three parent babies' helps no one.* www.guardian.co.uk/commentisfree/2012/sep/19/misleading-three-parent-babies-gene-therapy (accessed 8 May 2013).

28. Bourne H, Douglas T, Savulescu J. Procreative beneficence and in vitro gametogenesis. *Monash Bioethics Review* 2012;30:29–48.

Chapter 3

Epidemiology

Wendy Macdowall and Kaye Wellings

Overview

Globally, there are approximately 210 million pregnancies each year. Of these, around one in five end in induced abortion, some half of which are unsafe [1]. The circumstances under which abortion is legally permitted vary from country to country. The evidence, however, suggests that the legal status of abortion has little effect on abortion rates, but it is associated with the safety of the procedure [1, 2]. Generally, where abortion laws are the least restrictive there is little evidence of unsafe abortion. Conversely, where abortion laws are the most restrictive the proportion of unsafe procedures increases [1, 2]. The risk of complications is low for abortions that conform to medical guidelines. Unsafe abortions, on the other hand, are major contributors to maternal morbidity and mortality [1]. Hence, information on abortion is not only an important indicator of unplanned pregnancies and unmet need for contraception but is also important in measuring progress towards Millennium Development Goal 5 (MDG 5) which seeks to reduce maternal mortality and achieve universal access to reproductive health [3].

Measurement of abortion

Estimating the incidence of abortion globally is extremely complex, as information in many parts of the world is either unavailable or incomplete [2]. In the majority of countries with liberal abortion laws, data on the number of abortions performed are either routinely collected or can be estimated from other sources (such as survey data) [4]. However, the completeness of the data available varies and this variability depends on a number of factors, including whether abortion reporting is voluntary or mandatory, whether medical abortions are reliably reported and whether reporting systems include private providers [5]. Estimating incidence in countries in which abortion is highly restricted is particularly challenging, as by their very nature illegal abortions are performed covertly and are not recorded by providers, and women are, understandably, reticent to report them in surveys or face-to-face interviews. Under-reporting of abortion in population surveys is an issue in all parts of the world, but is particularly acute where laws relating to access are most restrictive [6]. In settings where abortion cannot be measured directly, indirect approaches are used to derive estimates. A number of such approaches exist [6]; see Box 3.1 for two examples.

In order to make meaningful comparisons between countries and regions, it is important to take account of the size of the population; hence rather than absolute numbers,

Abortion Care, ed. Sam Rowlands. Published by Cambridge University Press. © Cambridge University Press 2014.

rates (relative to women of reproductive age) and ratios (relative to live births) are usually calculated [1].

Box 3.1 Examples of methods of estimating the abortion rate in countries where it cannot be measured directly

1. The abortion incidence complications method (AICM)

The AICM has been used widely to estimate incidence of abortion. Two pieces of information are required for the calculation:

A. *The number of women who receive treatment for induced abortion complications in health facilities.* The source of these data depends on the country. Where official health statistics are known to be of high quality, these can be used with greater confidence. Alternatively, the data come from nationally representative sample surveys of health facilities that provide postabortion care.

B. *The proportion of all women having induced abortions who receive treatment for complications in health facilities.* This proportion is obtained by surveying experts in abortion provision in the country in question, who estimate the proportion of women who develop complications and receive treatment for them. This proportion is used to calculate an 'inflation factor' that is applied to the number of women treated for abortion complications to give an estimated total number of induced abortions.

2. A regression equation approach to the estimation of abortion rates

The regression equation approach uses data on contraception use and fertility to predict abortion rates. The equation is based on the strong association seen between modern contraceptive use and the number of lifetime abortions in countries where more complete data are available. The appeal of this approach is that it does not require the collection of new data; the limitation is the lack of data, especially in developing countries, with which to validate results of the models.

Adapted from Singh *et al.* [7] and Westoff [8].

Prevalence of abortion

To date, global estimates of abortions, categorized into those that are safe and unsafe, have been made for 1995 [9], 2003 [10] and 2008 [2]. In total, there were an estimated 43.8 million abortions worldwide in 2008, compared with 41.6 million in 2003 and 45.6 million in 1995. The abortion rate was 28 per 1,000 women aged 15–44 years in 2008 and 29 in 2003, having dropped substantially from 35 abortions per 1,000 women in 1995 (Table 3.1).

While abortion rates are surprisingly similar between developed and developing countries (24 and 29 respectively per 1,000 women of reproductive age), there are large variations between and within regions (Table 3.1) though caution should be exercised when making such comparisons, given differences in how the estimates are derived and the accuracy of the data on which they are based. For example, the abortion rate is 12 per 1,000 women aged 15–44 years in Western Europe (which has the lowest sub-regional rate worldwide), compared with 43 in Eastern Europe (which has the highest sub-regional rate, despite the rate having more than halved from 90 per 1,000 in 1995). Similar variation is seen within Africa, where the abortion rate is 15 per 1,000 women aged 15–44 years in southern Africa compared with 38 in the east of the continent.

Prevalence of unsafe abortion

The World Health Organization defines unsafe abortion as a 'procedure for terminating pregnancy carried out by attendants without appropriate skills, or in an environment that does not meet minimum standards for the procedure, or both' [1]. Such abortions may be self-induced, obtained covertly from medical – or paramedical – practitioners, or provided by traditional healers [11]. The main factor influencing whether a woman has an unsafe abortion is real or perceived legal restriction on safe abortion [12]. Where abortion law is restrictive, it is usually unsafe [1] but women may resort to unsafe abortion in countries where termination of pregnancy is permitted by law for many reasons, chief amongst which are availability and accessibility of services providing safe abortion and the ability to pay for the service [1]. In Eastern Europe where abortion laws are generally liberal, abortion still contributes to 11% of maternal mortality in the region [1].

The 2008 estimates suggest that, worldwide, nearly half (49%) of all abortions were unsafe, an increase from 44% in 2003 (Table 3.1). The absolute number of unsafe abortions also increased to 21.6 million in 2008 from 19.7 million in 2003, and virtually all of these occurred in developing countries [1]. However, the rate remained unchanged at around 14 unsafe abortions per 1,000 women (Table 3.1), as the population of women of reproductive age increased during the period [1].

Rates of unsafe abortion are highest in Latin America, where there are an estimated 31 unsafe abortions per 1,000 women of reproductive age, followed by Africa (28 per 1,000 women of reproductive age) and Asia (11 per 1,000 women of reproductive age) [2] (Table 3.1). Rates are very low in Europe, North America and Oceania. Almost all of the unsafe abortions in Europe take place in Eastern European countries (Table 3.1).

Prevalence of abortion by legality

In 28% of the 193 countries in the world, abortion is permitted on request and in 34% it is available on social or economic grounds [1]. Elsewhere abortion is restricted, for example to cases where the mother's life is threatened by continuing the pregnancy, where the pregnancy is as a result of rape or incest or to instances where there is a fetal impairment. While abortion is allowed to preserve a woman's physical health in 90% of developed countries, in only 60% of developing countries is this permitted [1]. In four countries abortion is not allowed on any grounds (Chile, El Salvador, Malta and Nicaragua). Around the world, nearly one in five women of reproductive age live in countries where abortion is not legally permitted under any circumstances or it is restricted to saving the woman's life [1].

The evidence suggests that laws restricting access to abortion do not translate into lower abortion rates. In fact the reverse may be true: the abortion estimates from 2008 indicate that abortion rates were higher in parts of the world where larger proportions of the female population lived under restrictive abortion laws than in those where liberal laws existed (Figure 3.1) [2].

Abortion ratio

The abortion ratio is the number of abortions performed for every 100 live births (as a proxy for pregnancies). It is an indicator of the likelihood that a pregnancy will end in abortion as opposed to being taken to term. Abortion ratios are high where the incidence of abortion is high, or where fertility rates are low, or both.

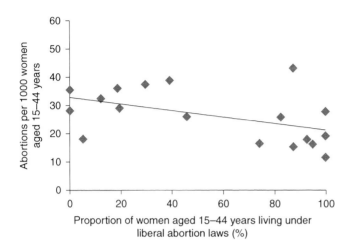

Figure 3.1 Association of abortion rate with prevalence of liberal abortion laws by sub-region in 2008. Source: *The Lancet* 2012; 379:625–32 [2].

Worldwide, 32 abortions were performed for every 100 live births in 2008 [13]; that is, nearly three births occurred for every one abortion performed [13]. The abortion ratio is lower in developing countries (at 31 abortions per 100 live births) than in developed countries (at 44 abortions per 100 live births) because the birth rates are higher. Worldwide, it is highest in Eastern Europe (at 93 per 100 live births), where the incidence of abortion is high and fertility rates are low. It is lowest in Africa, where although abortion rates are relatively high, so too are fertility rates which contribute to the low ratio [13].

Although globally the abortion ratio has remained relatively stable in recent years [13], it declined in developed countries between 2003 and 2008, from 50 to 44; the decline was most marked in Eastern Europe (where it fell from 105 to 93 abortions per 100 live births), reflecting a small increase in the annual number of births and a small decrease in the number of abortions [13].

Factors associated with abortion

Most abortions, over 90%, result from unintended pregnancies [14]. Marital status is the strongest predictor of unplanned pregnancy, more than doubling the risk for single women. Assessments of the age-specific rate of legal abortions (in 41 countries where such calculations are possible) suggest abortion rates show 'an inverted U-shape' distribution [4]. In 23 out of the 41 countries, the age-specific rate was highest in women aged 20–24 years and in 10 countries it was amongst those aged 25–29 years. In seven countries (all former Soviet Bloc, except for Portugal) it was highest (but only just) among women aged 30–34 years. Only in Cuba was the highest age-specific rate in the youngest women (aged 15–19 years) [4]. Young women (aged 15–19 years) accounted for a disproportionate share of the total number of abortions (relative to their share of the population) in 11 countries and was highest in Cuba, New Zealand, Scotland and England and Wales [4].

The age profile of women having unsafe abortion is less easily obtained but is also thought to vary considerably by region [11]. In Africa, unsafe abortion is predominately an experience of younger age; with close to 60% of the estimated number of unsafe abortions occurring among those aged under 25 years. Conversely, in Asia and Latin America a higher proportion of women are older; with 42% and 33% of unsafe abortions respectively be unsafe where clinicians are poorly trained or facilities are inadequate. Some countries in which abortion is legal for most indications continue to have high rates of unsafe abortion. India and South Africa are countries where high rates of unsafe abortion persist despite changes in the law that should make safe abortion readily available [11]. Contributing factors include cost, procedural and bureaucratic delays, inadequate numbers of trained practitioners to meet demand and concerns about confidentiality for women below the age of majority.

References

1. World Health Organization. *Unsafe Abortion: Global and Regional Estimates of the Incidence of Unsafe Abortion and Associated Mortality in 2008*, 6th edn. Geneva: WHO, 2011.

2. Sedgh G, Singh S, Shah IH, Åhman E, Henshaw SK, Bankole A. Induced abortion: incidence and trends worldwide from 1995 to 2008. *Lancet* 2012;379:625–32.

3. United Nations. Millennium Development Goals. www.un.org/millenniumgoals/maternal.shtml (accessed 25 October 2013).

4. Sedgh G, Bankole A, Singh S, Eilers M. Legal abortion levels and trends by woman's age at termination. *International Perspectives on Sexual and Reproductive Health* 2012;38:143–53.

5. Sedgh G, Singh S, Henshaw SK, Bankole A. Legal abortion worldwide in 2008: levels and recent trends. *International Perspectives on Sexual and Reproductive Health* 2011;37:84–94.

6. Rossier C. Estimating induced abortion rates: a review. *Studies in Family Planning* 2003;34:87–102.

7. Singh S, Prada E, Juarez F. The abortion incidence complications method: a quantitative technique. In S Singh, L Remez, A Tartaglione (eds.) *Methodologies for Estimating Abortion Incidence and Abortion-related Morbidity: A Review*. New York: Guttmacher Institute, 2010: 71–97.

8. Westoff CF. *A New Approach to Estimating Abortion Rates*. Calverton, MD: Macro International Inc., 2008.

9. Henshaw SK, Singh S, Haas T. The incidence of abortion worldwide. *International Family Planning Perspectives and Digest* 1999;25(Suppl):S30–8.

10. Sedgh G, Henshaw S, Singh S, Åhman E, Shah IH. Induced abortion: estimated rates and trends worldwide. *Lancet* 2007;370:1338–45.

11. Grimes DA, Benson J, Singh S, *et al.* Unsafe abortion: the preventable pandemic. *Lancet* 2006;368:1908–19.

12. Berer M. Making abortions safe: a matter of good public health policy and practice. *Bulletin of the World Health Organization* 2000;78:580–92.

13. Guttmacher Institute. Abortion ratios worldwide in 2008. June 2012. www.guttmacher.org/media/resources/abortion-ratios.pdf (accessed 3 March 2014).

14. Finer LB, Frohwirth LF, Dauphinee LA, Singh S, Moore AM. Reasons U.S. women have abortions: quantitative and qualitative perspectives. *Perspectives on Sexual and Reproductive Health* 2005;37:110–18.

15. Shah IH, Åhman E. Unsafe abortion differentials in 2008 by age and developing country region: high burden among young women. *Reproductive Health Matters* 2012;20:169–73.

16. Finer LB, Zolna MR. Unintended pregnancy in the United States: incidence and disparities, 2006. *Contraception* 2011;84:478–85.

17. Ikamari L, Izugbara C, Ochako R. Prevalence and determinants of unintended pregnancy among women in Nairobi, Kenya. *BMC Pregnancy and Childbirth* 2013;13:69.

18. Adler AJ, Filippi V, Thomas SL, Ronsmans C. Incidence of severe acute maternal morbidity associated with abortion: a systematic review. *Tropical Medicine & International Health* 2012;17:177–90.

19. Singh S. Hospital admissions resulting from unsafe abortion: estimates

from 13 developing countries. *Lancet* 2006;368:1887–92.

20. Adler AJ, Filippi V, Thomas SL, Ronsmans C. Quantifying the global burden of morbidity due to unsafe abortion: magnitude in hospital-based studies and methodological issues. *International Journal of Gynecology and Obstetrics* 2012;118(Suppl 2):S65–77.

21. Shah I, Åhman E. Age patterns of unsafe abortion in developing country regions. *Reproductive Health Matters* 2004;12(24 Suppl):9–17.

22. Briozzo L, Rodriguez F, Leon I, Vidiella G, Ferreiro G, Pons JE. Unsafe abortion in Uruguay. *International Journal of Gynecology and Obstetrics* 2004;85:70–3.

23. Gasman N, Blandon MM, Crane BB. Abortion, social inequity, and women's health: obstetrician-gynecologists as agents of change. *International Journal of Gynecology and Obstetrics* 2006;94:310–16.

24. UNFPA. *Motherhood in Childhood*. New York, 2013.

25. Benson J, Andersen K, Samandari G. Reductions in abortion-related mortality following policy reform: evidence from Romania, South Africa and Bangladesh. *Reproductive Health* 2011;8:39.

26. Henderson JT, Puri M, Blum M, *et al.* Effects of abortion legalization in Nepal, 2001–2010. *PloS One* 2013;8:e64775.

Psychosocial factors in women requesting abortion

Anneli Kero

Introduction

Abortion is a common phenomenon worldwide and throughout the ages women in most societies have terminated pregnancies, regardless of legislation or prevailing official views on abortion. Most often the underlying attitude to pregnancy in society is to presume that the only natural thing is to continue a pregnancy to term. However, it could be said that it is not unnatural for women to want to terminate a pregnancy that is unwanted or unintended. Every fourth pregnancy, for example, is terminated in Sweden, every fifth in the UK and every sixth in Denmark.

Research shows that many women make decisions about pregnancy in principle as an abstract concept before they find themselves in that position [1]. A Swedish study showed that nearly half of women (42%) had considered abortion as a possible solution at an earlier time and 30% reported that before the present pregnancy they knew that they would have an abortion if they did get pregnant [2]. Other studies show that between about two-fifths and four-fifths of women know before conception that they would terminate a potential pregnancy [3–5]. A study among Swedish male partners of women undergoing abortion showed that every second man had talked to the woman before she became pregnant about what they would do in the event of pregnancy [6]. More than half of these said that they, together with their partner, had decided to have an abortion.

Family planning is a part of women's (and men's) reproductive lives today and abortion is for many an acceptable and integral back-up option when the pregnancy is unwanted. The abortion decision is, for most European women, made in a societal context where abortion is legal but also questioned and/or regarded as ethically problematic. Governments' efforts to reduce the number of abortions indicates ambivalence (albeit unspoken) in relation to abortion while the universality of women's need for abortion, when faced with an unplanned pregnancy, is seldom regarded as self-evident. We know that many regard abortion as 'an act of shame' or as a highly taboo and potentially stigmatizing event [7,8] (see Chapter 20). Prevailing societal attitudes to abortion make it hard for many women to share their experiences – this is particularly true if women want to share positive experiences while remaining respectable.

This chapter is primarily based on research from Scandinavia where abortion has been available without restriction as to reason (or on socio-economic grounds in the case of Finland) since the 1970s. The aim is to highlight some aspects of the complexity of abortion

Abortion Care, ed. Sam Rowlands. Published by Cambridge University Press. © Cambridge University Press 2014.

by describing motives, reasoning and experiences in relation to an unintended pregnancy and the ensuing abortion.

Women resort to abortion in all kinds of psychosocial contexts

As might be expected, many abortions are performed among women lacking socio-economic resources: young women, single women or women living in poor psychosocial conditions. However, abortions also exist among women who can be considered to be in a life situation that is suitable for childbirth [9]. Studies show that many women are married/cohabiting or in a relatively long-term relationship with the man by whom they became pregnant [2,4,10–12]. A study of 211 Swedish women showed that more than half were not only married/cohabiting but most were also satisfied with their partner relationship and their finances [2]. Thus, good finances and a well-functioning relationship do not ensure that a pregnancy will be welcomed. Furthermore every fourth woman had completed university studies and half of the women had children. A study of male partners showed similar results [6].

Abortion is associated with poverty and an underprivileged social background even if research shows that many abortions are performed among stable and well-functioning families. It could be said that there is a tendency for women in higher socio-economic groups to become invisible in this context as the abortion request might be harder to legitimize if it is not associated with psychosocial necessity. However, making the 'abortion couple' invisible perpetuates the picture of abortion as a taboo and a deviant act among special risk groups. Furthermore, male partners remain invisible which, in turn, reinforces and maintains attitudes that unwanted pregnancy is the woman's issue and responsibility.

The male partner's involvement

Behind every unplanned, unexpected, unintended or unwanted pregnancy there are two people: a woman and a man. Not all men are aware of the pregnancy but most are and they are involved in the decision-making process as well [2,6,10–14]. It is also known that men greatly influence their partner in her decision and one of the most frequently stated reasons for terminating a pregnancy is related to the partner. Women have the formal right to decide whether or not a pregnancy should be terminated but in the relationship with the pregnant woman the man can influence her in many ways, e.g. exercising power, taking a stand, supporting or threatening her in her decision-making process. He can also avoid any participation whatsoever or even abandon her.

Indeed, the man's living conditions and experiences related to the pregnancy influence the woman's choice and experiences related to the abortion process. A woman's socio-economic and psychosocial situation is, for example, affected by a partner's employment status as life circumstances are shared within a relationship. His unemployment may interfere with both women's and men's intentions and wishes to carry a pregnancy to term; although this appears obvious it emphasizes the need to address men's needs in abortion care and the prevention of unwanted pregnancies.

In existential terms the woman has to make the decision alone, irrespective of whether or not she has discussed it with the man, but we do know that women want their partner or other intimates to validate and support their decision-making [13]. Most women who had informed their male partner about the pregnancy perceived them to be supportive [10–12]. Male knowledge and support for the abortion is also positively associated with women's postabortion wellbeing and adjustment [15,16]. The results of studies of men indicate that counselling efforts that incorporate male partners may increase support for women obtaining an abortion. Furthermore, sharing abortion experiences, as with sharing other important life events, could be of fundamental importance to the couple's future in general and to reproductive issues specifically. However, having a partner involved will not be appropriate for all women, especially those who have a violent relationship or when the male partner is opposed to the abortion [10].

A Swedish study showed that men generally support an abortion law that gives women the right to decide themselves about the pregnancy but they want to participate in the decision-making process [6]. Men also support women in their decision to terminate a pregnancy by medical abortion at home as this gives them the possibility of being near and of attending to the women's needs during the day of the passage of the pregnancy [14]. However, many men who accompanied their partners to the clinic were not satisfied with the attention they received [11]. Some felt they were neglected within abortion care. Treating male partners with empathy and providing information tailored to their needs is a challenge for abortion care.

Motives for abortion reflect women's need for planned parenthood

Women's decisions to have an abortion are typically motivated by diverse and often interrelated reasons taking into account their own needs, a sense of responsibility to existing children and the potential child, and the contribution of significant others, including the man by whom they have become pregnant [2,17–19]. The dominant reasons behind the abortion described from different parts of the world are 'not ready for a child', 'wrong timing', 'already having the number of children wished for' and/or poor partner relationship with the contemplation of single motherhood. Women often prefer not to raise a child alone. Apart from family planning and partner-related motives, other factors known to be associated with abortion are feelings of being either too young or too old to take on the responsibility of raising a child, poor education, unemployment and low income [1].

Among married/cohabiting Scandinavian women with children most stated that either they already had all the children they wanted and now wished to give priority to work or studies or that they did not have enough time, space or energy for an extra child [2]. Some had problems combining work and parenthood and limiting the number of children was regarded as a necessity with respect to the need to be a 'good' parent and at the same time have a career [2,19]. Among those without children, whether married/cohabiting or with a partner relationship, most wanted to postpone childbirth until they had finished their studies or got a job and an income. Financial security, a completed education and a safe partner relationship were prerequisites that needed to be met before having a family. A characteristic of these women was that they did not describe themselves as 'victims' who were forced to have an abortion because of bad conditions etc., but as active individuals who underlined their need for planned parenthood and the right to decide about and control their fertility [2]. Overall, their motives and reasoning are in line with findings from studies about prerequisites that should be in place before women and men in general want to become parents.

Women's motives for abortion, whether they experience it as a choice or as something they are more or less forced to do, are synonymous with an urge to create functioning and good living conditions for themselves, the family and the presumptive family. A study of male partners shows that their motives and reasoning are more or less identical with those of their partners [6].

Contradictory feelings in relation to the pregnancy and the abortion

Most women make their decision to have an abortion early in the pregnancy and they are usually sure about their decision [1]. A majority (56–92%) of Scandinavian women had, for example, made the decision as soon as the pregnancy was confirmed or before they went to the clinic for the first time [2,4]. In a British study nearly half (48%) said that they had never considered continuing the pregnancy and 58% had made their final decision before they first saw a doctor [1].

Although the decision is made early on, many women experience the time before abortion as the hardest part of the abortion process. An unwanted pregnancy is usually regarded as a stressful event or even a crisis and having an abortion is a multifaceted, emotionally charged event even for women who do not have any doubts about their decision [2,12]. Most women experience the pregnancy as a catastrophe as its consequences would disturb their existence and disrupt their future plans. A study of 211 women showed that 65% felt only painful initial feelings with the current pregnancy such as unreality, despair, panic, grief, guilt, anger, dread, shame and deceit [2]. On the other hand, one-third, in addition to painful feelings, also experienced positive initial feelings such as wonder, joy, happiness and pride about the pregnancy. Besides despair over being pregnant some women described discovering maternal feelings for the first time, as well as the confirmation of fertility and womanhood, as good and positive reactions to the actual pregnancy. Finally, four women with a desire for children expressed only positive feelings in relation to the pregnancy.

This underlines the importance of being open also to possible positive feelings associated with the pregnancy in women seeking abortion. Although the pregnancy is unwanted, and the woman wants to have an abortion, it is important not to trivialize the experience of being pregnant since it concerns life itself and as such touches upon deep and vital emotional levels in human beings. Awareness of these aspects is crucial, especially as abortion as a life event is often women's first experience of their reproductive capability. Despite the fact that an unwanted pregnancy is experienced as a catastrophe, it may also be an important life event for a woman.

Some studies which have examined experiences facing women requesting abortion show that, when the decision-making process is over, the predominant feelings among most women and men are relief and release [2,6]. Abortion is regarded as an act of responsibility and as the best solution to the critical situation that the unintended pregnancy caused [2]. Nevertheless, most found it also sad or more or less painful to go through with the decision, which reveals the complexity of abortion. Besides feelings of relief and release more than half (56%) also felt painful feelings such as anxiety, grief, guilt, anguish, emptiness and shame [2]. One third (33%) felt only painful feelings about the abortion while the remaining 13% felt only positive feelings. On the question of whether ideas about terminating the pregnancy implied any conflict of conscience, more than half stated that they had had 'none' (14%) or 'not much' (40%) while 31% had had 'some' and 15% 'a lot'. In spite of painful feelings, only 9% described their situation as a crisis [2]; 68% also stated that nothing could make them change their mind.

Contradictory feelings in relation to both pregnancy and abortion are common in this situation. It is important to stress that positive feelings in relation to the pregnancy and painful or ambivalent/contradictory feelings about abortion are not synonymous with ambivalence about making the decision itself [2,8,12]. This complexity is seldom apparent in abortion studies, which often focus exclusively on motives for the final choice to terminate or to continue the pregnancy or on the abortion debate that is highly politicized. Abortion is a controversial issue: positive feelings about the pregnancy and painful and ambivalent feelings in connection with abortion can be perceived as risky to elucidate since they could also be used as an argument against legal abortion. As long as these ambivalent/contradictory feelings are not emphasized or legitimized, analyses of abortion will remain incomplete and women's multifaceted experiences hidden.

The complex abortion decision – contradictory feelings reflect divergent coexisting perspectives

Abortion motives show that social perspectives concerning living conditions and expectations about lifestyle, interwoven with aspects linked to care and responsibility for all concerned (the fetus included), legitimize the abortion. Both women and men in Sweden, for example, are expected to be economically self-supporting and the paid parental leave system is based on previous income from employment which leads to a lifestyle where a job before parenthood becomes a necessity. Swedish women and men also stress that they find it important that both parents should desire a child and that they should be able to practise satisfactory parenthood in parallel with having a job or career. To become a teenage parent is more or less regarded as breaking the norm in a country where only 20% of teenage pregnancies continue to term. Thus, abortion is not only a last resort among special risk groups but also a phenomenon reflecting reproductive expectations among all groups in society. When societal norms and expectations about lifestyle are not met, abortion becomes synonymous with not breaking prevailing guiding cultural principles; abortion is experienced as a 'right', a 'best' decision and as an act of responsibility [2,15]. Being saved from unwanted parenthood is then experienced as a relief.

However, ethical and religious perspectives, which imply that the fetus also could be regarded as a person with rights of its own, may question and complicate the decision. Having children and becoming a parent is highly valued in most societies while legal abortion is often a controversial issue. The fact that women in many countries have the legal right to abortion does not imply absence of ethical conflicts or moral reasoning as to whether one has the right to decide about life and death [2,8]. While abortion is experienced as a relief and an act of responsibility, at the same time it can be regarded as 'a violation of nature'. Thus, abortion becomes synonymous with denying a child its life and existing children a sister or a brother. This kind of reasoning may result in feelings of guilt and of having contravened one's personal codes of behaviour.

The complexity increases further when abortion is experienced as a relief and simultaneously as a loss coupled with feelings of sadness, grief and/or emptiness [2,6,15]. The relief at being saved from unwanted parenthood does not always have to exclude feelings of giving up having a child. To terminate a pregnancy is an existential choice which usually is emotionally loaded, especially among women who have a desire for children [2,15]. Some women describe a conflict between 'heart and mind' that is simultaneously wanting to have a child and regarding abortion as a necessity. Feelings of loss and guilt do not necessarily indicate that women will later regret their decision or regard it as wrong. Contradictory feelings are an indication that abortion has a price, which implies that it is a more or less painful solution to an unwanted pregnancy.

Even if the cultural context sanctions abortion as a legal right and even if women are supportive of abortion as a legal right and as an acceptable back-up method they can, at the same time, regard abortion as 'shameful', 'degrading' or as 'a failure' on their part [7,8] (see Chapter 20). Perceived social unacceptability of abortion may result in feelings of shame and reticence to disclose personal information about an abortion because of fear of disapproval from others [7]. This must be considered in the light of history which has regarded female sexuality as well as inappropriate pregnancies as shameful and blameworthy. Abortion also challenges the image of womanhood which in a cultural context may be strongly associated with caring and motherhood. From this point of view, abortion becomes a denial of the essence of motherhood and therefore, in spite of the legal position, might be difficult to integrate into the concept of womanhood. Probably the taboo and the burden of shame on women might be reduced if the men involved were to become more visible. In turn, this might also contribute to a wider focus putting abortion into its socio-cultural context according to the prevailing demands for planned parenthood.

Consequently, since abortion is a phenomenon where divergent perspectives and incompatible values clash, experiences of contradictory/ambivalent feelings become both logical and understandable. A person can simultaneously view abortion as an act that is both 'right' and 'wrong' dependent on what perspective is in focus. Painful and contradictory feelings should therefore not automatically be regarded as problematic but as an unavoidable consequence when coexisting, divergent aspects are mixed in with the decision to have an abortion. This underlines the necessity of being open to contradictory/ambivalent feelings and paradoxes. Otherwise, the impact of abortion will remain hidden and unknown.

There is a strong consensus in research that women in general are mostly able to make the complex decision to have an abortion without suffering any regret or negative effects [15,20,21]. In spite of contradictory feelings about pregnancy and abortion most women 4 and 12 months postabortion considered their ability to cope with the abortion as 'very good' or 'good' [15]. Furthermore, more than half the women reported only positive experiences such as maturity, deeper self-knowledge, strengthened self-esteem and identity, something that is characteristic of successful crisis processing.

The most important factors that have been identified as predictors of poor psychological outcome following abortion include a history of mental health problems, lack of support and suspected coercion [1]. If the decision to have an abortion is not primarily the woman's own or is made under pressure, there is a risk of emotional difficulties [15,18].

Abortion – a taboo right

Although abortion is a highly prevalent phenomenon in our societies it remains a controversial and hidden event. In the public debate abortion is usually discussed only as a moral or human rights issue while women's and men's experiences remain in a sense both concealed and private. Fear of disapproval from others makes many people afraid of disclosing their experiences of abortion, which contributes to isolation, loneliness and vulnerability [7]. The absence of a frank and overt discussion of this issue, and of a frame of reference in this regard, perpetuates myths about abortion and contributes to women's burden of shame.

In a study at one year after abortion many women frequently reflected on the fact that they had not experienced having an abortion as very distressing and that they had felt better than they had expected [15]. It was found that many women are reluctant to admit that they experience relief as they thought that others and society expect them to regard their abortion as a difficult and horrible thing to do. Some even wondered if they would appear to be inhuman, as they had not felt any regret, guilt or grief. Others found it difficult to talk about having painful feelings such as sadness and grief as they did not regret the abortion. Due to taboos, shame and stigma most women keep silent about their abortions and even clinicians and researchers need to be aware of the risk that women will feel obliged to give 'suitable' and 'expected' answers.

In this context it is of interest that women today share abortion experiences with others on internet sites. At one of these sites, Women on Web [22], people can upload their portraits and share their stories to break the taboo and shame surrounding abortion.

Finally, as long as abortion, which should be regarded as a life event, has its image of taboo, most women, regardless of their circumstances, are more or less vulnerable in relation to termination of a pregnancy. This is particularly true for women with a religious, cultural or societal background with anti-abortion or strongly held moral views [1]. To create conditions where women feel safe to talk about their individual experiences in relation to the present pregnancy and abortion requires staff who are open to contradictory feelings and reasoning without automatically associating it with ambivalence about the decision. An approach when seeing the woman that is based on the knowledge that women seldom experience abortion as a trauma or an extremely dramatic event, but not as a small or trivial event either, may create possibilities to identify the small minority of women who are ambivalent about their decision and so at risk of negative postabortion sequelae.

References

1. Rowlands S. The decision to opt for abortion. *J Fam Plann Reprod Health Care* 2008;34:175–80.

2. Kero A, Högberg U, Jacobsson L, *et al.* Legal abortion: a painful necessity. *Soc Sci Med* 2001;53:1481–90.

3. Husfeldt C, Hansen SK, Lyngberg A, *et al.* Ambivalence among women applying for abortion. *Acta Obstet Gynecol Scand* 1995;74:813–17.

4. Holmgren K. Time of decision to undergo an abortion. *Gynecol Obstet Invest* 1988;26:289–95.

5. Cohan CL, Dunkel-Schetter C, Lydon J. Pregnancy decision making: predictors of early stress and adjustment. *Psychol Women Q* 1993;17:223–39.

6. Kero A, Lalos A, Högberg U, *et al.* The male partner involved in legal abortion. *Hum Reprod* 1999;14:2669–75.

7. Astbury-Ward E, Parry O, Carnwell R. Stigma, abortion, and disclosure – findings from a qualitative study. *J Sex Med* 2012;9:3137–47.

8. Kero A, Lalos A. Ambivalence – a logical response to legal abortion: a prospective study among women and men. *J Psychosom Obstet Gynecol* 2000;21: 81–91.

9. Rasch V, Wielandt H, Knudsen LB. Living conditions, contraceptive use and the choice of induced abortion among pregnant women in Denmark. *Scand J Public Health* 2002;30:293–9.

10. Jones RK, Moore AM, Frohwirth LF. Perceptions of male knowledge and support among US women obtaining abortions. *Women's Health Issues* 2011;21:117–23.

11. Makenzius M, Tydén T, Darj E, *et al.* Women and men's satisfaction with care related to induced abortion. *Eur J Contracept Reprod Health Care* 2012;17:260–9.

12. Kero A, Wulff M, Lalos A. Home abortion implies radical changes for women. *Eur J Contracept Reprod Health Care* 2009;14:324–33.

13. Kimport K, Forster K, Weitz TA. Social sources of women's emotional difficulty after abortion: lessons from women's abortion narratives. *Perspect Sex Reprod Health* 2011;43:103–9.

14. Kero A, Lalos A, Wulff M. Home abortion – experiences of male

involvement. *Eur J Contracept Reprod Health Care* 2010;15:264–70.

15. Kero A, Högberg U, Lalos A. Wellbeing and mental growth – long-term effects of legal abortion. *Soc Sci Med* 2004; 58: 2559–69.

16. Major B, Zubek J, Cooper LM, *et al.* Mixed messages: implications of social conflict and social support within close relationships for adjustment to a stressful life event. *Journal of Personality and Social Psychology* 2007;72:1349–63.

17. Finer LB, Frohwirth LF, Dauphinee LA *et al.* Reasons US women have abortions: quantitative and qualitative perspectives. *Perspect Sex Reprod Health* 2005;37:110–18.

18. Kirkman M, Rowe H, Hardiman A, *et al.* Reasons women give for abortion: a review of the literature. *Arch Womens Health* 2009;12:365–78.

19. Knudsen LB. Induced abortions in Denmark. *Acta Obstet Gynecol Scand Suppl.* 1997;164:54–9.

20. Adler NE, David HP, Major BN, *et al.* Psychological responses after abortion. *Science* 1990;6:41–4.

21. Major B, Cozzarelli C, Cooper ML, *et al.* Psychological responses of women after first-trimester abortion. *Arch Gen Psychiatry* 2000;57:777–84.

22. Women on Web. Available at: www. womenonweb.org (accessed 30 August 2013).

Chapter 5

Support and counselling

Joanna Brien and Lisa Hallgarten

Policy context

Even in countries where legal abortion is accessible, there are a range of laws and policies governing the decision-making process. These often owe more to the politics of abortion than to evidence. Laws may include mandatory counselling for all women seeking abortion; provision of mandated quasi-medical information; compulsory viewing of ultrasound images; mandatory waiting periods from decision to abortion procedure; and more. Such laws are commonplace across Western and Eastern Europe [1] and in the USA [2].

As mentioned in Chapter 19, these policies may be indicative of a range of negative ideas and intentions regarding women and abortion, from the paternalistic to the punitive: anxiety that women cannot be trusted to make good decisions; hope that women will change their mind about abortion if given sufficient time; a desire to make the process of accessing abortion difficult, in order to denote the moral enormity of the decision; an attempt to create an onerous process to deter women from accessing abortion; or a way to imply that negative outcomes are likely and thereby increase women's anxiety, resistance to and/or remorse about abortion.

There is no evidence to support these practices, which are not proven to improve a woman's experience of abortion, to reduce adverse psychological sequelae or to reduce the likelihood of a woman experiencing subsequent unintended pregnancy or abortion. On the contrary, these practices are likely to be harmful.

A recent study of women seeking abortion in the UK found that 'subjecting women to compulsory counselling about their decision to have an abortion is in conflict with their wishes and wastes resources … whilst it may be claimed that such policies are intended to ensure that women are certain of their decision, they could be counterproductive as they may introduce delay and so prolong distress for women' [3]. In its evidence-based guideline on women seeking induced abortion the UK's Royal College of Obstetricians and Gynaecologists (RCOG) states that 'women who are certain of their decision to have an abortion should not be subjected to compulsory counselling' [4].

Studies suggest that women are well able to judge the likely impact of a pregnancy on their lives, and predict outcomes for their own and their child's opportunities and wellbeing. 'Based on a substantial volume of reasonable evidence, denial of abortion has a negative psychosocial effect on both a woman and a child born' (see Chapter 18). Early findings from a long-term prospective study in the USA [5] suggest that women 'turned away' from abortion

Abortion Care, ed. Sam Rowlands. Published by Cambridge University Press. © Cambridge University Press 2014.

services experience 'significant negative outcomes in their physical health' and 'economically, the results are even more striking'. Adjusting for any previous differences between the two groups, women denied abortion were three times as likely to be below the federal poverty line two years later [6].

Support with the decision-making process

Serious psychological problems following abortion are rare, though studies have identified predictors of more negative outcomes [7]. There is good evidence to suggest that outcomes are best when a woman has made an *informed decision*, i.e. understands all the different pregnancy options available; has assessed the relative benefits and disadvantages of those options in the context of her unique circumstances, feelings, aspirations and beliefs; has acknowledged and addressed any ambivalence she feels; has come to the decision of her own free will without pressure or coercion; and is confident in her decision. 'The more effort put into considering the various influential factors, the less likelihood there is of post-decisional regret' [8]. These facts should help inform approaches to decision-making support and counselling.

Even if there is no legal requirement for a woman accessing abortion to be provided with or to participate in a pregnancy options discussion, all women should have had the opportunity to discuss their choices at some point before consenting to abortion. This should be a universal service, which may be provided by a referring doctor, contraception clinic or an abortion provider. Offering this is a vital aspect of good practice: 'all women attending an abortion service will require a discussion to determine the degree of certainty of their decision and their understanding of its implications' [4].

Informed pregnancy decision-making and support

Any appropriate professional can facilitate this process. This support should be 'confidential, non-directive, non-judgemental, supportive and understood by the woman to be independent of any assessment for legal approval for abortion' [8]. At its most basic, it provides an opportunity for a woman to consider and discuss her feelings and options confidentially with a non-judgemental professional. It is not counselling, and need not be provided by a counsellor, but entails providing the information and type of discussion a woman thinks is relevant to her.

This is not a one-size-fits-all model. Women seek information about, and referral for, abortion at very different points in their decision-making process. Some have already weighed up their options and many have decided to have an abortion before accessing any service [9,10] (see Chapter 4). Others are undecided, struggling to decide or experiencing conflict between their values and their circumstances; some need additional information to complete their decision; others need an opportunity to talk to someone who is not part of their life because having to take others' views or values into account can obscure their own feelings. Any service that is not flexible and responsive to the needs and stage of decision-making of individuals 'is likely to result in some women finding the level of intervention invasive or obstructive and others finding it inadequate to meet their needs' [11,12].

When it is truly responsive to the woman's own needs, this discussion can help her to make a confident, informed decision. It can address 'messages that stigmatize women who have abortions (which) may directly contribute to negative psychological experiences post abortion' [7] and may help to create an environment in which she is better able to choose and use an effective contraceptive method following abortion [13].

Crucially, the discussion can help to identify women who may be feeling ambivalent about their decision, or experiencing coercion (both of which are associated with poorer mental health outcomes); or who have more complex issues in their lives that are outside of the scope or expertise of those working in general practice, sexual and reproductive health or abortion provision. In that sense decision-making support can provide a 'triage' process – identifying and referring those who need additional support to counselling and other appropriate specialist services to address issues such as substance use and intimate partner violence. 'Clinic staff must be sensitive to the different stages of decision-making that individual women have reached and must be able to identify those who may require additional support and counselling' [4].

Box 5.1 Key aspects of decision-making support

Women need:

- to be seen as quickly as possible
- to be reassured of the confidentiality of the service
- to be seen alone for at least some part of the consultation
- to feel confident that the information they are given is impartial, evidence-based, accurate and taken from reputable sources
- to be listened to by people who are respectful and non-judgemental
- to be offered sufficient information about all their options
- to be able to ask questions
- to be informed about 'what next' depending on the pathway they choose
- an opportunity to establish their confidence in their decision
- an experience of decision-making which is free from stigma or negativity associated with abortion
- an opportunity to think about contraceptive options post-pregnancy.

In addition they may need or want:

- an opportunity to discuss the pros and cons/risks and benefits of all the options
- an opportunity to think about which people (professional and personal) can offer them effective support in relation to their different options
- to be signposted/referred to specialist services to help with other issues in their lives
- to be offered counselling to address more complex feelings.

Not all consultations – even those that take place within an abortion service – will result in the woman having an abortion. Abortion providers expect a proportion of women to leave their service without having an abortion, following further discussion. Women who attend the initial assessment may subsequently change their mind about proceeding with an abortion, miscarry, be too late for a legal abortion or may require additional time or an additional consultation. Women should be reassured that they will not be penalized for changing their minds, or be pressured to have an abortion if they no longer believe it is the right choice for them.

More intensive counselling

Research has identified groups of women who might be more at risk of adverse psychological sequelae and might benefit from a more intensive level of support in advance of abortion. The universal provision of decision-making support provides an opportunity for professionals to identify women who may want to take up an offer of counselling.

It is for the woman herself to decide if she would benefit from counselling having understood what this entails. However, it is helpful for those working with women seeking abortion to be alert to those who may be more vulnerable to negative outcomes after abortion. Offering them support before abortion could reduce their needs subsequently. This may include women:

- with a history of mental health problems
- undergoing abortions on medical grounds
- presenting later in pregnancy
- with limited social support
- with feelings of extreme ambivalence towards the abortion
- experiencing pressure from partners or family to have, or not to have, an abortion
- belonging to a religious, social or cultural group which is antagonistic towards abortion
- who have been adopted or brought up in the public care system
- adolescents, especially under-16s
- choosing to end a wanted pregnancy because of a dramatic change in circumstances, adverse health diagnosis or diagnosis of fetal anomaly
- with experience of neglect or abuse
- experiencing repeated pregnancy scares, unintended pregnancies or abortions which are not attributable to high fertility and may be an indication of an inability to negotiate contraception use within a coercive relationship.

It should not be assumed that all women in these categories will have difficulty with the decision to have an abortion, nor that women outside of these categories will not need additional support. Those providing basic support should be alert to the expressed desires of the woman for counselling, as well as verbal and non-verbal signs of extreme ambivalence, and distress. Taking into account this caveat, the following checklists may provide a useful indication of appropriate actions to meet women's needs during the decision-making process:

1. Provide pregnancy decision-making support if the woman:

    - says that her pregnancy was unintended [3]
    - understands her options and has reliable external support from friends, family or partner
    - has no overwhelming/significant moral objections to abortion and no past pregnancy losses
    - has an absence of other serious risk factors (see list above).

2. Refer for counselling at the woman's request or with her agreement if the woman:

    - has one or more of the serious risk factors (see list above)
    - is displaying withdrawn or other unusual behaviour, or signs of extreme distress
    - says that the pregnancy was initially intended or wanted
    - is completely undecided about her pregnancy
    - says she is certain of her decision, but is clearly very conflicted about the decision
    - has past pregnancy losses
    - is pregnant as a result of rape or abuse

- is thinking about adoption – refer client to specialist adoption social care worker/ counsellor.
3. Work closely with the medical team if the woman:
   - is considering ending a wanted pregnancy because of her own health or diagnosis of fetal anomaly
   - has a complex medical history or has medical complications
   - presents with or has a history of serious mental health issues
   - has been subjected to female genital mutilation (FGM).

Counselling and its relevance to the abortion decision

Counselling is a collaborative activity voluntarily entered into by a person who wants to explore and understand issues in their lives which may be causing them difficulty, pain and/ or confusion. Counselling in the context of pregnancy decision-making establishes that this is protected time free from interruptions, which allows women the opportunity to talk through and clarify feelings, values, concerns and options about their pregnancy. Any factual information that the client requests is also provided.

The counsellor will not steer the woman in any particular direction. The woman is helped to weigh up the likely consequences of all the possible options so that she can feel that any decision she makes (continuing, adoption or abortion) is made carefully and with due deliberation. The counsellor recognizes that the enormous physiological changes that occur as the body adapts to its pregnant state are accompanied by emotional and psychological changes, which can make thinking and acting more difficult [14]. The counsellor makes a careful assessment, and if longer-term help is needed a referral to other services is made. Providing a simple explanation of this process to women who are considering counselling or those who professionals believe would benefit from counselling may serve to allay any resistance they have to the process.

Resistance to counselling

Those with no prior knowledge or experience of counselling may expect counselling to be didactic, that is 'telling them what to do' – to continue or to end the pregnancy – or provide an admonishment – 'telling them off'. People can see counselling as only for the 'bad, sad or mad', a pathologizing event associated with mental illness or something that implies that abortion per se is traumatic and a woman having one will necessarily require psychological help. Women can perceive any counselling or talking about a decision that has been arrived at as providing a barrier to getting an abortion, or delaying a referral.

Time is of the essence

While many counselling processes take place over an extended period, for a woman seeking or considering abortion, counselling is, by necessity, short-term and counsellors must have the skills to work within a brief time frame.

What is addressed in abortion counselling?

Useful counselling interventions are those that help to facilitate decision-making and acknowledge and facilitate grieving for a loss. Time-limited counselling can provide gentle encouragement and empathic listening by using open-ended questions exploring the specific surrounding circumstances and the meaning of loss to the individual in their culture and context [15]. This may uncover extra vulnerability (such as abuse, addictions, depression, self-harm or family problems). It may touch on the circumstances and feelings surrounding previous pregnancies and pregnancy losses. Women can find that their pregnancy is a trigger for deeply embedded semi-conscious conflicts that they struggle to make sense of for the first time.

The counsellor can help the woman to express what she has constructed as symbolizing her pregnancy (anything from a blob of cells to a baby), and address the meaning for the woman herself of voluntarily ending this pregnancy as she has imagined it. There is also the opportunity in pregnancy counselling to look at why the woman has been unable to protect herself from this and perhaps previous unintended pregnancies, the part her sexual partners have played in decision-making about contraception and personal barriers to negotiating and using contraception effectively.

Counselling techniques

The counsellor needs to establish a rapid engagement with the woman, as much through approach and tone of voice as what is actually said: to demonstrate that the counsellor understands fully her dilemma and recognizes the nub of the problem as the woman sees it. The counsellor needs to be responsive to her style of communication and mirror her preferred ways of relating. The counsellor can use praise, be direct, validate her beliefs, encourage trust and demonstrate understanding of the individual's perceptions.

Box 5.2 Case study

Michelle was 16. She came in tense, anxious and trembling slightly.

She had carried out multiple pregnancy tests, all of which were positive. She knew in her heart that she was pregnant but she found the truth unbearable and hoped that subsequent tests would show a different result.

She had been living with a foster carer, was under the care of a therapist, and had already made a suicide attempt before discovering she was pregnant.

She said that she could not continue with her pregnancy, and had chosen to have an abortion; but also stated that she didn't want to have an abortion, feeling it would be 'cruel', and that an abortion was abandoning and abusing her own child. This information was blurted out rapidly – an indication of how conflicted she was about this choice.

The counsellor helped Michelle to acknowledge her feelings of attachment to a pregnancy she experienced as innocent and in need of protection, but that she knew she had no resources to cope with. She helped her to explore whether an abortion would cause her to feel guilty afterwards and increase the likelihood of a serious reactive depression or suicide, or return to other self-harming behaviour. Conversely would continuing with the pregnancy lead to increased anxiety and depression affecting her and her pregnancy?

Michelle was relieved to find out that she would not have to pay if she had an abortion and was reassured to know that her carer would not automatically be informed and that she could be in control of the information about herself, i.e. that confidentiality would be maintained.

After she decided she would have an abortion, Michelle was given follow-up appointments, numbers to ring for support and the offer of postabortion counselling.

Though this case was complex, it was not exceptional. The woman presented with several risk factors: youth, lack of partner support, current mental health problems and extreme ambivalence about the best option. The key concern of the counsellor was to allow the woman the space to articulate her contradictory thoughts and feelings – and having acknowledged this conflict to decide, on balance, the best option.

Counselling with individuals and those important to them

Counsellors can work with significant others. The presence of a neutral professional might help the woman talk to an accompanying partner, parent or friend about her decision. Relationships may end during decision-making or shortly afterwards and men and significant others can benefit from space to talk about their own feelings. If not given this chance they can prevent the woman from being able to concentrate on her own decision-making. Sometimes a woman might bring another person with her with the conscious or unconscious intention of demonstrating to the counsellor what she is experiencing, in terms of support or lack of support for her decision.

A counsellor should be sensitive to how far someone accompanying the woman is able to create the space for the woman to feel she can freely express her own wishes. Counsellors need to be alert to signs of coercion and to be aware of safeguarding concerns (such as incest or sexual abuse of a minor, suicidal ideation). While acknowledging the significance of other people's views and opinions (see Chapter 4), the counsellor should state categorically that it is, ultimately, the woman's choice. The counsellor should clarify that doctors will not authorize an abortion for a woman who is acting under duress and so cannot, by definition, give valid consent.

It is good practice to see all women alone at some point to ensure that there is no coercion and encourage them to explore and express their own feelings. However, counsellors will be aware that control is often exerted or can be experienced by the woman even if the person is not in the room or on the premises.

Postabortion support

Women commonly report relief following abortion and can gain further self-awareness and develop more confidence in their own decisions after having elected to have an abortion. While many feel a mixture of positive and negative feelings following abortion, serious adverse psychological sequelae are rare. Some women make a poor adjustment after an abortion but it may well be that continuing the pregnancy would lead to similar symptoms, and the poor adjustment is not caused by the abortion per se but by the surrounding circumstances.

However, when there is significant guilt and self-blame, women may benefit from open-ended counselling or therapy. Women and men can suffer the full impact of perinatal bereavement after an abortion. The unique aspect of grief connected with abortion is that there is no tangible person to mourn. It is dreams and fantasies that are lost with the pregnancy. Therapists can find that buried feelings from past negative experience of miscarriage or abortion may surface years later and therapy might enable the client to revive and mourn their losses. It can be helpful to eschew reassurance or sympathy and allow the person to revisit their initial reaction to their pregnancy and the unfolding circumstances, pressures, reactions and feelings of others that led to them actually having an abortion.

Who needs counselling?

It can be difficult to identify who will benefit from counselling, so it is good practice to offer pre- and postabortion counselling to all women. Some women recognize a need for postabortion counselling prior to the abortion. Others may feel that they do not deserve any support, as they have been responsible for 'taking' a life and may not return for postabortion follow-up of any sort.

Women need to know that they can go for counselling days, weeks, months or years after the abortion. Some will feel numb afterwards and only begin to question their decision or feel unhappy when they reach a significant milestone, e.g. anniversary of the abortion, or the due date had the pregnancy continued.

Training, information, the principles of professional care and counselling qualifications

Core principles of professional care

Those providing decision-making support and/or counselling should be committed to:

- the principle of reproductive control and the right of women to be able to choose the number and spacing of their children; to choose a form of contraception that suits them and to choose whether or not to continue a pregnancy
- providing impartial, evidence-based support and information
- expediting access to appropriate services
- providing an opportunity to discuss options for post-pregnancy contraception
- learning about and meeting the diverse needs of the population

and should reflect the duty to:

- provide services within an equalities framework
- mitigate potential delays caused by conscientious objectors
- protect women from inappropriate medical interventions
- create an environment free from pressure or coercion
- reduce stigma.

Practitioners should have participated in good practice training, which addresses personal values, professional boundaries and impartiality. Training should ensure that practitioners are confident about answering women's basic questions regarding their pregnancy options, and that they can signpost them into the appropriate pregnancy service for antenatal care or abortion.

Practitioners must be able to provide accurate, up-to-date and evidence-based information including patient literature on antenatal care and abortion referral processes, legal and service time-limits, counselling options and requirements, abortion methods, and options for contraceptive provision at the time of and after abortion.

Additional qualifications for counsellors

Counselling needs to be provided by suitably trained, qualified (e.g. in the UK to Diploma level) and experienced people who have a particular interest in this area. Counselling should be available locally for those women who need or request it before or after an abortion [9].

Professional boundaries and personal feelings

A non-directive approach is essential as even an implicit bias can be construed by the woman as disapproval, which can block her working on her own feelings. Counsellors need to demonstrate neutrality. It is important for the individual who is counselling to have explored their own motivations and consciously examined their own losses, ideas and religious or cultural views; and any ambivalence to conception, especially personal experiences, or unresolved feelings surrounding abortion or pregnancy. This helps to contain or set aside their own assumptions and prejudices to be able to follow the woman's own thoughts and feelings about her pregnancy, which can be illogical, fragmentary or punitive.

These moral dilemmas and ambivalences may touch on painful areas for professionals such as their own inability to conceive, or moral or religious values and attitudes around conception and about those women who appear reckless or feckless. These feelings can, if not contained, lead to a suppression of empathy. A hardening of sensitivity can develop that serves to protect the practitioner. It is important for counsellors to have regular case supervision in order to understand these enmeshed feelings.

Unethical counselling practice

As mentioned in Chapter 19, there is widespread evidence from around the world of organizations offering abortion counselling with the intention of deterring or obstructing women from accessing abortion [16]. Health professionals should ensure they do not refer women to agencies, sometimes called Crisis Pregnancy Centres, which do not work to core principles of professional care.

Box 5.3 Caveat for legally restricted jurisdictions

In jurisdictions where abortion is prohibited or severely restricted, women face the same dilemmas and require the same support, but the additional risks (legal and clinical) will affect the information that can be provided and the information that is needed in order to minimize these risks. In these contexts it is likely that abortion is highly stigmatized and women will face additional stress and fear in relation to the procedure itself and possible distress in relation to the decision.

References

1. International Planned Parenthood Federation. *Abortion Legislation in Europe.* 2012. www.ippfen.org/NR/rdonlyres/ED17CA78-43A8-4A49-ABE7-64A836C0413E/0/Abortionlegislation_May2012corr.pdf (accessed 19 September 2013).

2. Guttmacher Institute. *State Policies in Brief: An Overview of Abortion Laws.* 2013. www.guttmacher.org/statecenter/spibs/spib_OAL.pdf (accessed 19 September 2013).

3. Cameron S, Glasier A. Identifying women in need of further discussion about the decision to have an abortion and eventual outcome. *Contraception* 2013;88:128–32.

4. Royal College of Obstetricians and Gynaecologists. *The Care of Women Requesting Induced Abortion – Evidence-based Clinical Guideline Number 7.* 2011. www.rcog.org.uk/files/rcog-corp/Abortion%20guideline_web_1.pdf (accessed 19 September 2013).

5. Advancing New Standards in Reproductive Health. *Turnaway Study.* www.ansirh.org/research/turnaway.php (accessed 19 September 2013).

6. Lang J. *What Happens to Women Who are Denied Abortions?* The New York Times Magazine. www.nytimes.com/2013/06/16/magazine/study-women-denied-abortions.html?pagewanted=4&tntemail0=y&r=2&emc=tnt (accessed 19 September 2013).

7. American Psychological Association Task Force on Mental Health and Abortion. *Report of the Task Force on Mental Health and Abortion*. 2008. www.apa.org/pi/women/programs/abortion/mental-health.pdf (accessed 19 September 2013).

8. Rowlands S. The decision to opt for abortion. *J Fam Plann Reprod Health Care* 2008;34:175–80.

9. Hunton RB, Spicer J. An evaluation of the counselling given to patients having a therapeutic abortion. *Australian and New Zealand Journal of Obstetrics and Gynaecology* 1979;19:169–73.

10. Brown S. Is counselling necessary? Making the decision to have an abortion. A qualitative interview study. *European Journal of Contraception and Reproductive Health Care* 2013;18:44–8.

11. Hallgarten L. *Decision-making Support within the Integrated Care Pathway for Women Considering or Seeking Abortion*. London: Brook and FPA, 2014. www.brook.org.uk.

12. Allen I. *Counselling Services for Sterilisation, Vasectomy and Termination of Pregnancy*. Policy Studies Institute No 641, 1985.

13. Hoggart L, Phillips J, Birch A, Koffman O. *Young People in London. Abortion and Repeat Abortion*. Government Office for London, DCSF, 2010. www.bpas.org/js/filemanager/files/tpyoungpeopleinlondonabortionandrepeatabortion.pdf (accessed 19 September 2013).

14. Brien J, Fairbairn I. *Pregnancy and Abortion Counselling*. London: Routledge, 1996.

15. Leon IG. Perinatal loss. In DE Stewart, NC Stotland, MD Herz (eds.) *Psychological Aspects of Women's Health Care. The Interface between Psychiatry and Obstetrics and Gynaecology*, 2nd edn. Washington, DC: American Psychiatric Press, 2000: 141–76.

16. Education for Choice. *Crisis Pregnancy Centres*. London: EFC at Brook, 2014. www.brook.org.uk/images/brook/professionals/documents/page_content/EFC/CPCreport/crisis_preg_centres_rept_10.2.14-2hiFINAL.pdf (accessed 1 May 2014).

Chapter

6

Ultrasound scanning in early pregnancy

Emeka Oloto and Sharon Moses

Introduction

Ultrasound scanning has been used for diagnostic purposes since the 1960s with the first demonstration of an intrauterine pregnancy by transvaginal (TV) ultrasound in 1967 by Kratochwil and Eisenhut [1]. Improvements in ultrasound technology such as higher frequency transducers and increased use of TV sonography have led to a greater understanding of early pregnancy development and transformed the role of ultrasound scanning in early pregnancy assessment.

The majority of women with an unplanned, or planned but unwanted, pregnancy will present to services in the first trimester and early stages of pregnancy. This chapter will cover normal findings in early pregnancy and an overview of the ultrasound diagnosis of early pregnancy failure. Detailed description of ectopic pregnancy, gestational trophoblastic disease, uterine or adnexal abnormalities and scanning in the second and third trimester are outside the scope of this chapter.

Ultrasound scanning in early pregnancy can achieve the following objectives:

- To confirm the presence of an intrauterine pregnancy (IUP)
- To estimate gestational age
- To confirm cardiac activity
- To confirm the number of embryos
- To evaluate uterine abnormalities
- To evaluate abnormal pregnancy
- To evaluate the adnexa.

Early pregnancy ultrasound is usually performed using either the transabdominal (TA) or TV route. TA and TV sonography require the use of different transducers. TA sonography will be adequate to identify an IUP and estimate gestational age but TV sonography allows for a more detailed assessment. The TV transducer is placed closer to the target structures and the higher frequency means that the image's spatial resolution and near-field focus are improved. TV sonography is particularly useful in women with a high body mass index and in very early pregnancy. TA sonography will still have a role depending on patient preference and is the imaging of choice for an enlarged uterus or where other pelvic pathology, including large fibroids or ovarian cysts, are suspected.

Abortion Care, ed. Sam Rowlands. Published by Cambridge University Press. © Cambridge University Press 2014.

When performing an ultrasound scan in early pregnancy it is recommended that the following should be thoroughly evaluated and reported [2]:

- Uterus and adnexa for presence of a gestation sac
- If a gestation sac is seen whether a yolk sac (YS) or embryo is present
- Gestational age estimation by measuring the embryo or, if absent, the mean sac diameter (MSD)
- Whether cardiac activity is present
- Number of embryos (for multiple amnionicity and chorionicity)
- Any abnormalities of the uterus and adnexa
- Fluid in the pouch of Douglas.

A consistent and systematic approach to early pregnancy ultrasound scanning will reduce the likelihood of missing abnormalities, particularly ectopic pregnancy, which can be difficult to diagnose.

Normal ultrasound findings in the first trimester

The first trimester is the best time to estimate gestational age of a pregnancy, as normal pregnancies develop in a defined and predictable way. A thorough understanding of the growth milestones in the first trimester is essential to using ultrasound successfully in the assessment of early pregnancy. With serial scans failure to meet the expected milestones indicates a failed pregnancy. The milestones described in this chapter will consistently be imaged earlier with a TV compared to a TA approach [3]. The majority of women requesting an abortion will only have a single scan and once an IUP is confirmed further scans are usually not required.

Gestation sac

This is the first unequivocal sign of an early IUP. A normal gestation sac will be located in the upper portion of the uterine cavity towards the fundus. The sac is implanted just below the surface of the endometrium (midline echo) and has an anechoic centre with an echogenic rim (representing the developing chorionic villi). The shape of the sac is usually round or oval in all views, appearing more elliptical as it grows. An irregular gestation sac is usually due to an abnormality of the uterine cavity such as fibroids or haematoma [4].

Between 5 and 11 weeks the MSD can be used to calculate the gestational age in days. To do this the MSD is first obtained by measuring the anechoic portion of the sac in three planes and dividing by three: in the sagittal or longitudinal view of the uterus the anteroposterior and craniocaudal diameters are measured and the transverse diameter is measured in the transverse view. It is important not to include the echogenic ring in the measurement. The MSD in mm added to 30 gives the gestational age in days [5]. An MSD of 2–3 mm can be seen with TV sonography corresponding to four weeks' gestation. Using TA sonography a sac will not be seen consistently until five weeks when the MSD is 5 mm.

Double decidual sac sign

The double decidual sac sign (DDSS) was first described by Bradley *et al.* in 1982 [6]. As the gestation sac grows it deforms the central cavity echo, resulting in two concentric echogenic rings that surround a portion of the gestation sac (Figure 6.1). This finding may be the earliest sign of an IUP using TA ultrasound and may be seen at five weeks from last

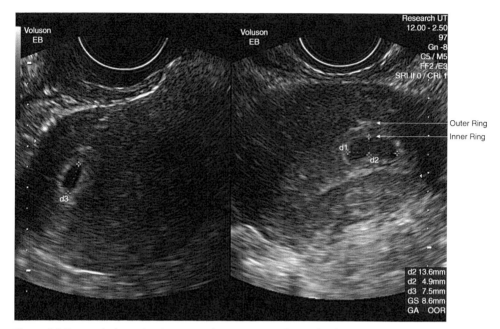

Figure 6.1 Transvaginal scan showing a normal gestation sac at five weeks. The sac is eccentric in location and surrounded by two echogenic (white) rings – the double decidual sac sign. Courtesy of Dr Trevor Wing.

menstrual period (LMP). The inner ring represents the decidua capsularis and the outer ring the decidua parietalis. There may be a space between the rings containing a small amount of endometrial fluid. The DDSS may be helpful if the YS is not yet visible. Using TV ultrasound, however, a YS can usually be seen at the same gestational age as the DDSS, which limits its usefulness to TA examinations [7]. It is important to differentiate between a true gestation sac and intrauterine fluid collections that look like a gestation sac (pseudosac). Unlike the true gestation sac that is eccentric in location, a pseudosac is centrally located and may be a sign of an extrauterine pregnancy.

Yolk sac

The presence of a YS is diagnostic of a true gestation sac and IUP. The YS is a round structure with an echogenic rim and anechoic centre (amnion) visualized within the gestation sac (Figure 6.2). It is usually seen by 5 to 5.5 weeks. The YS grows to a maximum diameter of 6 mm at 10 weeks' gestation and then gradually decreases, disappearing at about 14 weeks. The earliest sonographic evidence of the embryo can be seen as a small thickening over part of the circumference on the YS sometimes referred to as the 'diamond ring' sign where the embryo is the diamond.

Embryo/fetus

The terms embryo and fetus appear to be used interchangeably in the literature. However, strictly, the product of conception is called an embryo until 8 weeks after fertilization (10 weeks after the LMP) and from then it is called the fetus. The embryonic or fetal pole is the echogenic thickening on the margin of the yolk sac of an embryo or fetus. The embryonic

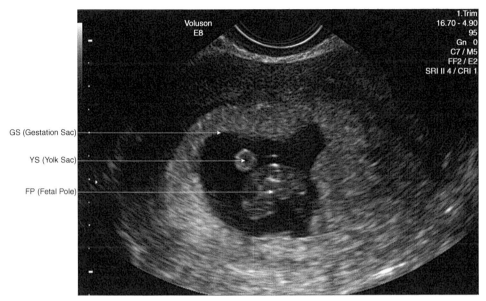

Figure 6.2 Transabdominal scan showing a normal pregnancy (GS, YS and FP) at seven to eight weeks. Courtesy of Dr Trevor Wing.

pole can first be visualized on TV ultrasound at five to six weeks' gestation. Cardiac activity can be detected from 6 to 6.5 weeks (MSD 13–18 mm). With TA ultrasound cardiac activity may not be seen until 8 weeks (MSD 25 mm). At 6 to 7 weeks the appearance of the embryo changes from being a straight line at the top of the YS to more of a kidney bean shape (Figure 6.2). As the embryo develops it moves away from the YS, but remains attached by the vitelline duct [5].

At 6 to 12 weeks measuring the crown–rump length (CRL) is the most accurate method of dating a pregnancy (Figure 6.3). The now classic study by Robinson and Fleming [8] regarding CRL is still the main reference for the assessment of gestational age in early pregnancy, although due to increased TV sonography new charts have had to be devised for gestations of less than seven weeks [9].

CRL measurements can be carried out using the TA or TV approach. A midline sagittal section of the whole embryo or fetus should be obtained, ideally with the embryo or fetus horizontal on the screen so that the line between crown and rump is at 90 degrees to the ultrasound beam. Linear calipers should be used to measure the maximum unflexed length, in which the end points of crown and rump are clearly defined. The best of three measurements should be taken.

In very early gestations, care must be taken to avoid inclusion of the YS in the measurement of CRL, as this will overestimate the gestational age [10].

Other sonoembryological development

By eight weeks the rhombencephalon becomes distinguishable as a diamond-shaped cavity, enabling distinction of cephalad and caudal. The amniotic membrane and umbilical cord can also be seen. By nine weeks limb buds are visible. The forebrain, midbrain, hindbrain

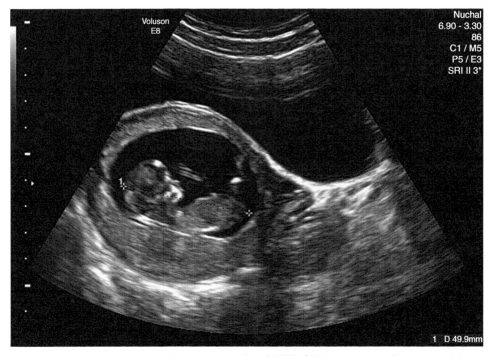

Figure 6.3 Transabdominal scan showing crown–rump length (CRL) of 49.9 mm corresponding to 11 weeks' gestation. Note that the measurement (calipers) was obtained in an unflexed fetus. Courtesy of Dr Trevor Wing.

and skull are distinguishable. Physiological herniation of the midgut is present, the bowel rotates 270 degrees and returns to the abdomen by 11 weeks. The hands and feet are fully formed by 13 weeks [11].

After 12 weeks' gestation the head, the femur and the abdomen are used to determine the gestational age. The head measurements include the biparietal diameter (BPD) and the head circumference (HC), both measured in the same plane. The correct plane for measuring the BPD and HC should demonstrate the following landmarks: the thalamus, the cavum septum pellucidum, the falx and the ventricles (Figure 6.4). This is also called the transthalamic plane. The BPD is measured from the outer fetal skull edge nearest to the transducer to the inner fetal skull edge farthest from the transducer, commonly referred to as 'outer to inner' measurement.

Multiple gestations

Understanding of the detailed anatomy of multiple-order pregnancy is important when it is necessary to carry out selective fetal reduction for medical or non-medical reasons. The reduction procedure is generally carried out in the first trimester. A decision to terminate or continue with the pregnancy may be influenced by the knowledge of the number of fetuses and the associated risks. The knowledge may be positive for some but negative for others. It is therefore good practice to inform women about multiple-order pregnancy when diagnosed by ultrasound as part of pre-abortion assessment.

Twins are either monozygotic (fertilization of one ovum) or dizygotic (fertilization of two ova). The majority, approximately two-thirds of spontaneously conceived pregnancies,

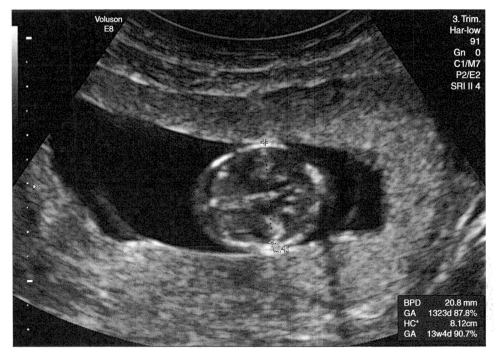

Figure 6.4 Transabdominal scan showing a biparietal diameter (BPD) of 20.8 mm corresponding to 14 weeks' gestation. Note that the measurement is from the outer to the inner fetal skull edge nearest and farthest to the transducer respectively. Courtesy of Dr Trevor Wing.

are dizygotic with their own placentas and amniotic sacs. All dizygotic pregnancies will be dichorionic and diamniotic (DCDA). With monozygotic twins the number of placentas and amniotic sacs depends on the timing of when the zygote divides: 25% will be DCDA, 75% monochorionic diamniotic (MCDA) and less than 1% monochorionic and monoamniotic (MCMA). Chorionicity is important for continuing pregnancies as the perinatal mortality is two to three times higher in monochorionic than in dichorionic twin pregnancies. In the first trimester between 6 and 10 weeks chorionicity can be determined by counting the number of gestation sacs and amnionicity can be assigned based on the number of YSs [12].

The optimal time to distinguish between dichorionic, monochorionic and monoamniotic twin pairs is between 10 and 14 weeks' gestation. A dichorionic twin pregnancy will always have two separate sacs each with its own placenta. Two placentas implanted adjacently can look like a single placenta so chorionicity should be established by locating insertion of the chorional membranes into the placenta. The 'delta' or 'lambda' sign signifies a DCDA pregnancy with the amniotic and chorionic membranes separated by a tongue of placental tissue. The 'T sign' is found in MCDA pregnancies, where the fused amniotic membranes surrounding each fetus insert into the shared placenta. If no dividing membrane is seen then an MCMA pregnancy is likely and should be confirmed in the second trimester [13].

Ultrasound findings in failed pregnancy

The failure to meet expected milestones and follow the predictable pattern of development suggests a potential problem. In some cases a single scan will be definitive but serial scans may be required for confirmation. Current guidelines from the UK National Institute for

Health and Care Excellence (NICE) [14] discuss the use of ultrasound to determine viability of an early IUP. Abnormal findings using TV sonography would be a CRL of 7 mm or more with no visible heartbeat or an MSD of 25 mm or more and no visible fetal pole. NICE suggests that with these findings a diagnosis of miscarriage can be confirmed by a second sonographer or by performing a second scan seven or more days later.

Ultrasound is the most accurate way to triage women presenting with pain and bleeding in the first trimester. It is, however, important to consider indicators from the clinical history and physical examination in conjunction with ultrasound images and serum hormonal measurements; progesterone and human chorionic gonadotrophin (hCG) are often used for triage and further assessment. In the UK the majority of women with these symptoms will be managed in dedicated early pregnancy units.

Ultrasound scanning in abortion care

In abortion care ultrasound examination will often complement clinical assessment in determination of gestational age. Clinical assessment by use of the LMP and/or pelvic examination can estimate gestational age; the latter, even for experienced clinicians, may be difficult in obese women, multiple pregnancy, pelvic mass and when the uterus is retroverted. Some doctors and most nurses do not have sufficient skills to carry out the required pelvic assessment to date pregnancy. There is a serious capacity issue in most Radiology Departments to support abortion care in most National Health Service hospitals in the UK. Therefore most UK abortion providers have embarked on targeted training for nurses and doctors to carry out ultrasound scanning, which has revolutionized abortion care in the UK. This initiative was made possible by the availability of different low-cost, portable and fit-for-purpose ultrasound scan machines.

Ultrasound scanning is used in three aspects of abortion care: preabortion, intraoperative and postabortion assessment.

Preabortion assessment

The primary role of ultrasound in preabortion assessment is to confirm that the pregnancy is intrauterine and to estimate gestational age. It may also be useful in the assessment of viability in cases of suspected miscarriage and in the identification of missing intrauterine devices. A two-dimensional ultrasound is a good screening tool for the detection of placenta accreta in those at risk – placenta praevia, previous caesarean delivery or other uterine surgery, age greater than 35 and multiparity [15]. Incidental findings may include ovarian cysts or fibroids. Medical abortion, when first introduced, had a strict upper limit of nine weeks for eligibility which has led to increased utilization and now routine use of preabortion ultrasound assessment. Disadvantages of routine ultrasound are the additional cost to the service and a potential reduction in the number of available appointments for assessment depending on service organization. Internationally, local resources and training will determine the feasibility of ultrasound in different abortion care settings.

There is some evidence to suggest that women who choose to view the ultrasound scan images preabortion find it a positive experience. Wiebe and Adams [16] reported that when women were offered the choice to view the images, 73% accepted, of whom 86% found it a positive experience. None of the women who accepted viewing the images changed their minds about having the abortion. In a systematic review, Kulier and Kapp [17] also reported similar findings. However, Gatter *et al.* analysed the data in over 15,000 patients and reported that only 43% chose to view the images and that viewing may contribute to a small number of women with a medium or low decision certainty deciding to continue with the pregnancy [18]. They also found that choosing to view the images was associated with non-white ethnicity, young age (less than 25 years), lower socio-economic status and lower certainty of decision to terminate. Choosing not to view the images, on the other hand, was associated with being older than 30, being multiparous or having a greater gestational age (more than nine weeks).

Intraoperative assessment

Intraoperative ultrasound scan guidance can be helpful during surgical abortions in cases of acutely anteverted or retroverted uterus, fibroid uterus and bicornuate uterus. It also assists in the correct placement and location of instruments during an intrauterine procedure to remove an early gestation sac or fetal parts in mid-trimester abortion. It is also useful to avoid or identify perforation of the uterus. Furthermore, at the end of a procedure it can be helpful to confirm that the pregnancy has been completely evacuated.

Postabortion assessment

Ultrasound scanning can be useful for assessment in the immediate postoperative period where there is concern about retained products of conception (RPOC), haematometra or other complications. Ultrasound scanning can also be useful to detect a continuing pregnancy after surgical or early medical abortion; to confirm expulsion of the gestation sac after early medical abortion; to assist in a clinical diagnosis of RPOC; and to assess concern about retained placenta after a late medical abortion.

The above uses of ultrasound in abortion care notwithstanding, the UK national evidence-based guidelines from the Royal College of Obstetricians and Gynaecologists (RCOG) make the following recommendations for ultrasound scanning in abortion care [19]:

- Use of preabortion ultrasound scanning in every woman undergoing abortion is unnecessary
- Ultrasound scanning must be available to all services as it may be required as part of the assessment
- Ultrasound scanning should be provided in a setting and manner sensitive to the woman's situation
- Before ultrasound is undertaken, women should be asked whether they would wish to see the image or not.

The rationale for not requiring routine preabortion ultrasound assessment is based on the fact that there is no direct evidence that ultrasound improves either the safety or efficacy of abortion procedures. The World Health Organization also recommends that use of routine preabortion ultrasound scanning is not necessary but commented that the quality of the evidence, based on a randomized controlled trial and observational studies, is very low [20]. In settings in which resources do not allow routine use of ultrasound it should be reserved for cases where there is a discrepancy between LMP and uterine size, bleeding or symptoms of an ectopic pregnancy.

In addition to the use of sonography in preabortion assessment the RCOG guideline [19] discusses other uses of ultrasound for women requesting abortion. Continuous ultrasound scanning is recommended for late abortions over $21+^6$ weeks when performing feticide (see Chapter 16). Ultrasound may also have a role during vacuum aspiration procedures to minimize risk of uterine perforation and ensure that the procedure is complete, but is not advised routinely. For later surgical procedures requiring dilatation and evacuation (D&E) continuous ultrasound during the procedure is recommended to reduce the risk of surgical complications (see Chapter 10). For medical abortion ultrasound can be used in the assessment of retained products of conception following treatment; it is essential, however, that clinical signs and symptoms are taken into account. The guideline also identifies the need for further research regarding the role of ultrasound in preabortion assessment and postabortion complications.

Conclusion

Ultrasound technology is constantly improving, higher frequency probes will improve image resolution and newer technologies such as three- and four-dimensional scanning may improve the ability to assess early pregnancies. Worldwide access to ultrasound machines, and the skills to use them, may still be restricted but the role of early pregnancy scanning in abortion care services will continue to be defined and developed.

References

1. Kratochwil E, Eisenhut L. Der früheste nachweis der fetalen herzaktion durch ultraschall. *Geburtshilfe Frauenheilkunde* 1967;27:176–80.

2. American College of Obstetricians and Gynecologists. Ultrasonography in pregnancy. ACOG Practice Bulletin No. 58. *Obstet Gynecol* 2004;104:1449–58.

3. Ferrazzi E, Garbo P, Sulpizio L, Setti L, Buscaglia M. Miscarriage diagnosis and gestational age estimation in the early first trimester of pregnancy: transabdominal versus transvaginal sonography. *Ultrasound Obstet Gynecol* 1993;3:36–41.

4. Graham GM. Ultrasound evaluation of pregnancy in the first trimester. *Donald School Journal of Ultrasound in O & G* 2010;4:17–28.

5. Laing FC, Frates MC. Ultrasound evaluation during the first trimester of pregnancy. In PW Callen (ed.) *Ultrasonography in Obstetrics and Gynaecology*, 4th edn. Philadelphia: WB Saunders, 2000: 105–45.

6. Bradley WG, Fiske CE, Filly RA. The double sac sign of early intrauterine pregnancy: use in exclusion of ectopic pregnancy. *Radiology* 1982;143:223–6.

7. Yeh HS. Efficacy of the intradecidual sign and fallacy of the double decidual sac sign in the diagnosis of early intrauterine pregnancy. *Radiology* 1999;210:579–81.

8. Robinson HP, Fleming JEE. A critical evaluation of sonar 'crown rump length' measurements. *Br J Obstet Gynaecol* 1975;82:702–10.

9. Hadlock FP, Shah YP, Kanon DJ, Lindsey JV. Fetal crown rump length: re-evaluation of relation to menstrual age (5–28 weeks) with high resolution real time US. *Radiology* 1992;182:501–5.

10. Loughna P, Chitty L, Evans T, Chudleigh T. Fetal size and dating: charts recommended for clinical obstetric practice. *Ultrasound* 2009;17:161–7.

11. Blaas H-G K, Eik-Nes S. Sonoembryology: ultrasound examination of early pregnancy. In D Jukovic, L Valentin, S Vyas (eds.) *Gynaecological Ultrasound in Clinical Practice*. London: RCOG Press, 2009: 143–58.

12. Hall JG. Twinning. *Lancet* 2003;362:735–43.

13. Chudleigh T, Thilaganathan B (eds.) *Obstetric Ultrasound How: Why and When*, 3rd edn. London: Elsevier, Churchill Livingtone, 2004.

14. National Institute for Health and Care Excellence. Ectopic pregnancy and miscarriage. Diagnosis and initial management in early pregnancy of ectopic pregnancy and miscarriage. NICE Clinical Guideline 154. December 2012. www.nice.org.uk/nicemedia/live/14000/61854/61854.pdf (accessed 1 August 2013).

15. Berkley EM, Abuhamad AZ. Prenatal diagnosis of placenta accreta: is sonography all we need? *J Ultrasound in Medicine* 2013;32:1345–50.

16. Wiebe ER, Adams L. Women's perceptions about seeing the ultrasound picture before an abortion. *Eur J Contracept Reprod Health Care* 2009;14:97–102.

17. Kulier R, Kapp N. Comprehensive analysis of the use of pre-procedure ultrasound for first- and second-trimester abortion. *Contraception* 2011;83:30–3.

18. Gatter M, Kimport K, Foster D, *et al.* Viewing the pre-abortion ultrasound image. *Contraception* 2013;88:440–1.

19. Royal College of Obstetricians and Gynaecologists. The management of women requesting induced abortion. November 2011. www.rcog.org.uk/womens-health/clinical-guidance/care-women-requesting-induced-abortion (accessed 23 July 2013).

20. World Health Organization, Department of Reproductive Health and Research. *Safe Abortion: Technical and Policy Guideline for Health Systems*, 2nd edn. 2012. www.who.int/reproductivehealth/publications/unsafe_abortion/9789241548434/en/ (accessed 24 November 2013).

Chapter

7

Early medical abortion

Caroline de Costa and Michael Carrette

Records of early human civilization make it clear that women have always attempted to end unwelcome pregnancies with various herbs and potions. There is no reason to believe that any of these ancient measures were very successful, and it is likely that the effects on women were often fatal.

As recently as the last century various folk remedies, referred to in British abortion law as 'noxious substances', were still being used in attempts at abortion and again they were more likely to damage the woman than her pregnancy. Examples are lead compounds, purgatives, liberal amounts of alcohol and proprietary medicines such as Beecham's Pills (see Chapter 1).

All this has changed since the 1980s. The discovery of anti-progesterones, and very specifically their use sequentially with prostaglandins, has meant that medical abortion has become a practical reality, with reliability and safety comparable to that of surgical abortion.

Early medical abortion (EMA) is rapidly becoming available worldwide, allowing women in developed countries the choice between medical and surgical methods of abortion. Furthermore, EMA puts safe abortion within reach of women in poor communities, remote communities, and societies where surgical facilities are primitive, dangerous or forbidden for religious or cultural reasons.

The history of mifepristone

Progesterone, as the name would suggest, is the sex steroid that acts for and on behalf of pregnancy. Secreted immediately after ovulation by the corpus luteum of the ovary, its production is continued after conception by the corpus luteum of pregnancy, with production eventually taken over by the placenta. Progesterone produces maturation, thickening and increased vascularity of the endometrium, prevents myometrial contractions, and reduces the sensitivity of the myometrium to prostaglandins. This effectively causes the feto-maternal allograft/host reaction to be suppressed – which is a unique biological situation.

From the above it could be expected that any substance which opposes progesterone would make an efficient routine contraceptive, a postcoital contraceptive and an interrupter of pregnancy at any stage from implantation to full term. The clinical result and management of such interruption depends crucially on the stage of gestation.

In 1980 the research laboratory of the French pharmaceutical company Roussel-Uclaf was investigating numerous synthetic steroids and identified the first anti-progesterone, a

Abortion Care, ed. Sam Rowlands. Published by Cambridge University Press. © Cambridge University Press 2014.

drug that occupies the progesterone receptors in the genital tract and blocks the action of progesterone. The compound under investigation was called steroid number 38,486; hence RU-486. Although it has since been formally named mifepristone, to the public it is often still known and quickly recognized as RU-486 [1,2]. Initially Roussel's scientists did not appreciate the importance of anti-progesterones; it was the intervention of Dr Etienne-Emile Baulieu, and his strong support of the necessary preclinical studies and early trials, that allowed the development of the drug [2]. Mifepristone was lab-tested in France in 1981 before undergoing trials in women volunteers in France and Switzerland in 1981/82. Roussel's management at the time was concerned about public and church opposition to the development of an anti-abortion drug, and there were attempts at political interference in France. However, research and trials continued, partly owing to the French government having a financial stake in Roussel. In 1989 that government licensed the use of mifepristone in France, the French Health Minister famously declaring: 'I could not permit the abortion debate to deprive women of a product that represents medical progress' [2].

The drug is currently the only commercially available anti-progesterone for use in medical abortion, at any gestation. It is widely used in many parts of the world, its efficacy and safety firmly established [1,3–6]. Used alone, mifepristone will bring about abortion in around 70% of early pregnancies, although this can take some time [1,2].

The Chinese were the first to use mifepristone outside of clinical trials, in 1988, relying not on the French suppliers, but rather on their own domestic product. It was first prescribed in clinics in France in 1989 and in the UK in 1991. It was released in the United States in 2000. Its acceptance has become almost universal in Western Europe over the past twenty years: only in Ireland and Malta is the drug still unavailable through legal channels. However it is still unavailable in much of Eastern Europe [1–6].

Mifepristone was introduced in New Zealand in 2001 [7]. In Australia it was another matter. In 1996 the Australian government needed just one extra vote in the upper house to pass an unrelated financial bill. An independent senator with strong anti-abortion views agreed to vote with the government in exchange for effectively banning the import of mifepristone. It was clearly thought that setting women's rights back a decade was a trivial price to pay for political expediency. This ban was not overturned until 2006 [8].

The acceptance of mifepristone by various other countries has been complicated by politics, religion and the belief that easier, cheaper or safer abortion would lead to raised abortion rates. This last concern has proved to be unfounded; it has been clearly demonstrated that women make the decision for abortion before, and independently of, their decisions about abortion methods [1–5,7].

The history of misoprostol

The history of misoprostol is longer and less controversial. A prostaglandin E_1 analogue, for over three decades misoprostol has been widely used in the treatment of gastric ulcers, especially those caused by non-steroidal anti-inflammatory drugs (NSAIDs). It also softens the cervix and promotes myometrial contractions, and the anomalous position has been reached where other and better drugs have largely taken over its role in the prevention and treatment of gastric ulcers, while its role in gynaecology is almost universal despite often being used 'off-label' in this regard [5,9,10]. There are other and more powerful prostaglandin E_1 analogues such as gemeprost, but misoprostol is cheap to produce, stable, metabolically resistant and can be given by many routes. Used alone, misoprostol will abort 80% of early pregnancies, although this may take some time and may involve multiple doses [9].

The abortion process

An early medical abortion (EMA) consists of the administration of the two drugs in sequence; ideally mifepristone then misoprostol. Put simply, mifepristone causes the uterus to reject the conceptus after which misoprostol causes it to be expelled. Together they will successfully abort 95–98% of pregnancies up to 63 days (menstrual age); successful use to 70 days in outpatient medical abortion has also been reported [1,3–7,10].

This process is clinically indistinguishable from a miscarriage. Abortion or miscarriage will involve pain and bleeding to an unpredictable degree, but related primarily to the length of gestation. A very early miscarriage can mimic a heavy and late menstrual period. Up to nine weeks' gestation, an abortion can be well tolerated outside hospital, the degree of tolerance depending on the medical supervision available, the supply of pain relief, and not least the preparedness and fortitude of the woman and those supporting her. Bleeding and cramping will usually occur within a few hours of taking the misoprostol; nearly all women will have finished expelling the pregnancy within 24 hours [3–6].

Since miscarriages are common, occurring in some 25% of early pregnancies, it is recognized that they will rarely present a great risk to the patient, that many women will have experienced one or know someone who has, and that most medical personnel involved in women's reproductive healthcare will be experienced at managing miscarriage. Women and healthcare personnel should then in general be well equipped to manage EMA.

Medical abortion in the clinic, at home and in general practice

Originally in both France and the UK, EMA was offered in clinics that were also offering surgical abortion. The woman took the mifepristone orally on day one, went home and returned to the clinic 24–48 h later, when misoprostol was administered. The woman remained in the clinic until the abortion process was complete. Where the process was incomplete it could be completed surgically in the same facility [3,6].

More recent studies have demonstrated the safety and acceptability to women of either administering both mifepristone and misoprostol in the clinic or doctor's surgery, then allowing the woman to undergo the abortion process at home, or administering mifepristone in the clinic and supplying the misoprostol, to be taken at home, by either the oral, buccal or vaginal routes by the woman herself. The woman has been required to have a support person to accompany her home and stay with her until the abortion process is complete; she also needs to be easily able to access emergency care close to home if she needs it. Abortion at home has been the most common way EMA is provided since mifepristone first became available in Australia, as well as being widely practised in the USA and many developing nations; it is also increasingly practised in Europe [5,8,11–13].

The choice between medical and surgical abortion

When both surgical and medical early abortion are available, the consultation with the woman should include a discussion of both options; it is important that the arguments for and against each are explained clearly [3,4,14]. Both abortion methods are so safe that comparison of safety generally has little role in this discussion. Mortality rates are around 1 per 100,000 for both methods in appropriate clinical environments in countries where abortion is legal [4,5]. Home EMA in general has only been practised up to 63 days (and more recently to 70 days, as noted above); at later gestations it should be performed in a hospital

Table 7.1 Rates of complete abortion and complications for medical and surgical abortion [5,25]

	Medical	Surgical
Complete abortion	95–98%	96–98%
Continuing pregnancy	1–3%	0.2%
Incomplete abortion	2–5%	2–3%
Haemorrhage (with transfusion or with uterine evacuation)	0–0.3% (transfusion) 0.4–2.6% (evacuation)	0.15%
Infection	<0.3%	0.1–5%
Time taken to abort	A few hours to several days post misoprostol	Duration of surgery and anaesthetic

or similar clinical environment, rather than in the home (see Chapter 9), and surgical abortion at 9–14 weeks is widely considered more practical as the medical abortion process may be more prolonged and more painful than at earlier gestations. Both methods carry a small risk of failure and hence the need for a further procedure (around 1% although studies vary in the figures reported); both also carry a small risk of complications during and following the procedure (see Table 7.1) [5]. Surgical abortion involves some form of anaesthetic which carries its own small risk, and there will be also a slightly higher risk of damage to the uterus, namely uterine perforation, cervical trauma or intrauterine adhesion formation (Asherman's syndrome), than with medical abortion [14]. Surgical abortion will be more expensive than medical in most countries.

There are some women with concurrent medical or surgical risks for whom the medical abortion process would be safer conducted in hospital. Examples are severe anaemia, heart disease and uncontrolled diabetes. There are also women whose social circumstances or whose emotional or psychological state would make outpatient abortion inappropriate.

Apart from these exceptions (and pregnancy generally occurs in healthy young women) in nearly every case where both medical and surgical options are available it becomes a matter of the woman's choice. There are some women who will strenuously avoid being admitted to hospital and all that this implies. It has also been found that having the opportunity for the abortion process to take place in a situation where she can safely enjoy both privacy and a degree of control can be a valuable way for a woman to reassert ownership of her life and put behind her the failure of a relationship or a failure of contraception, if these have been factors leading to her decision to terminate the pregnancy. Other women know they would not cope in any other way than by placing themselves under direct medical supervision and anaesthesia. Although in some countries matters of cost and availability will arise, the preference of the woman should be the main deciding factor between early medical and early surgical abortion.

However, it is also reasonable that the decision regarding the suitability of the woman for outpatient abortion be assessed by the doctor or other health professional in charge as well as the woman herself, bearing in mind her home circumstances, safety and the need for privacy. If the abortion process is to occur outside hospital, there must be an appropriate support person nominated who ideally should be involved from the initial consultation forward until the process is complete, and adequate well-understood arrangements for emergency care if needed [8,14].

Protocols to be followed before EMA

Work-up for EMA will be essentially the same as for a surgical abortion. That is, medical, surgical, obstetric and social history will be taken, a physical examination conducted, information sheets given, consent obtained, pelvic ultrasound performed in many cases, and haemoglobin level and blood group determined (Rh-negative women undergoing EMA should have anti-D immunoglobulin administered). The recommendation of the UK Royal College of Obstetricians and Gynaecologists (RCOG) is that all women undergoing abortion should be screened for *Chlamydia trachomatis*, undergo a risk assessment for other sexually transmitted infections (STIs) including gonorrhoea and syphilis and be tested for these where appropriate [3]. In situations where multiple clinic visits or follow-up in person are problematic, or patient adherence a concern, then an acceptable alternative is to give antibiotics immediately after the abortion process including those suitable for treating chlamydia and anaerobes, for example doxycycline or azithromycin and metronidazole [3,14]. All appropriate methods of contraception should be discussed at the initial preabortion visit to the healthcare provider and a plan agreed upon for postabortion contraception that is realistic and accessible for the woman concerned. There should also be discussion about safe sex practices.

There are, however, some important differences in the preparation for medical and surgical early abortion. Allergy to mifepristone and misoprostol should be excluded. The local legality of medical and surgical abortions may be different, in particular in regard to where the two may be performed. There must be evidence of an intrauterine gestation at the appropriate stage, which is why pelvic ultrasound plays an important role in preparation for EMA [5]. An intrauterine gestation sac should be visible at 5+ weeks and/or hCG of >1,500 mIU/mL. The continuing pregnancy rate following EMA before a sac is seen is 7.5% in contrast to 0.2% when a sac has been seen [15]. Where the abortion process is to take place at home ultrasound confirmation of intrauterine pregnancy of the expected gestation is mandatory unless the products passed are to be inspected by appropriate medical personnel. Where medical abortion takes place in a clinic the combination of physical examination and inspection of the products may be sufficient to confirm the abortion has taken place. The gestational window of opportunity is relatively small for an EMA. If the gestation is too early there is the risk of an undiagnosed ectopic pregnancy; too late (>63 days) and a surgical abortion is the method of choice.

There is Level A evidence (from randomized controlled trials (RCTs)) to confirm that the use of prophylactic antibiotics reduces the risk of infection following surgical abortion even in the absence of any established preabortion vaginal or cervical infection [3]. There is insufficient Level A evidence to demonstrate similar advantage after EMA, but this is due to RCTs having not yet been conducted; currently evidence to support the use of prophylactic antibiotics for EMA is Level C [3]. There is no evidence to suggest that the use of such prophylaxis is *inappropriate* in EMA.

A woman undergoing an EMA should not have a low haemoglobin nor be in a state of hypocoagulation. Likewise she should not be on high-dose corticosteroids, nor in adrenal failure, because of the antiglucocorticoid effect of mifepristone. Severe asthma and chronic renal disease are also contraindications [3,4,6,13,15]. A woman presenting for EMA with a history of multiple caesarean sections should be treated with caution as with increasing numbers of caesareans there is an increasing risk of placental ingrowth into the uterine scar, which can lead to incomplete separation of placental tissue at the time of the abortion and resultant heavy bleeding [16].

In general women undergoing EMA require some form of analgesia. This is considered in more detail in Chapter 11. Paracetamol has been shown in well-conducted trials to be ineffective; NSAIDs are most frequently used and are generally effective and well tolerated, in particular ibuprofen 400 mg [3]. Codeine preparations have been used with good effect. Where a woman is undergoing EMA at home it is important to ensure that she has a supply of analgesics prior to administering the misoprostol. Metoclopramide 10 mg, domperidone 10 mg or the more expensive ondansetron 4–8 mg may be given for nausea.

In all cases of EMA at home the suitability of the home environment regarding privacy, communications and available care should be assessed [13]. There must be a plan in place to allow for the occurrence of immediate complications. Infection, excess bleeding and unacceptable pain are all possible and the woman must have information in writing on how to access a telephone advice centre, the nearest appropriate doctor and the nearest hospital or clinic [1,3]. It is also important that the woman will feel comfortable accessing these services if they are needed; this is particularly relevant for women who have travelled away from home, often from small rural or remote areas, in order to access abortion without the knowledge of family, friends or local medical personnel. To ensure the safety of EMA at home for such a woman, arrangements must be in place for emergency care if needed that are acceptable to her.

It is also essential to impress on the woman undergoing EMA at home the importance of following instructions. Once the mifepristone has been taken then the misoprostol must follow as instructed, as the teratogenic potential of mifepristone is not yet fully determined.

EMA management

There is consensus concerning the administration of mifepristone. One 200 mg tablet is given orally. In many health services this must take place in view of the doctor or a health professional delegated by the doctor [5]. Following this, the woman may go home. Only occasionally (<1%) will the abortion process follow the administration of mifepristone alone [5].

The misoprostol is ideally taken 24–48 h later and there are various options [3–6]. Studies in which misoprostol is given at the same time as mifepristone have shown higher rates of failure. The initial dose of misoprostol in the authors' practice is 800 μg and it may be given in a hospital, a clinic or taken by the woman at home. The RCOG recommendation is 400 μg misoprostol to 49 days' gestation and 800 μg at 49–63 days. Misoprostol is absorbed when taken by the vaginal, oral, sublingual or buccal routes [14–16]. Vaginal insertion causes fewer gastrointestinal side-effects, namely nausea, diarrhoea and vomiting. When misoprostol is used vaginally, administration should be followed by half an hour of bed-rest to prevent the tablets from slipping out of the vagina or by use of a tampon. Buccal tablets are absorbed quickly and are easier for the woman to self-administer [6,13]. Any residual tablet remaining in the mouth after half an hour should be swallowed. However it is given or taken, expulsion will start within four hours, and the conceptus will be expelled within 24 hours [3–6,13]. Contractions will then become less painful. If there is neither bleeding nor pain, a further 400–800 μg of misoprostol can be taken either after four hours or as late as the following day [3]. If, with or without a repeated dose, there is no response surgical abortion must be arranged, although in some situations a further attempt at EMA may be more appropriate. A recent systematic review showed higher failure rates associated with oral administration of misoprostol and 400 μg as compared to 800 μg for the initial dose [5].

Follow-up within two weeks is essential, particularly for women undergoing home abortion [8,13]. Several large studies have confirmed the safety of telephone follow-up in most cases, with the opportunity for a personal consultation if indicated [11–13] (see also Chapter 12). Abortion providers should be aware of the appreciable risk of failed abortion and the absence of histopathology in EMA. Any doubt in this regard can be resolved with hCG tests or ultrasound. The possibility of infection, retained products of conception or excess blood loss must also be assessed at follow-up. In the uncommon situation of continuing pregnancy, a surgical procedure is mandatory in view of the risk of fetal abnormality, although if the pregnancy is <63 days one further attempt at EMA may be made [5,6,15]. If there are clinical signs of infection bacteriological examination is required followed by appropriate antibiotics. The presence of retained products and prolonged bleeding may sometimes be treated successfully with further misoprostol but may require surgical removal. In addition to being aware of the need to return for a formal follow-up appointment, women should be informed about the need to present earlier with any concerns – particularly excessive vaginal bleeding (bleeding greater than that on day one of the woman's normal cycle and occurring for more than seven days following EMA), fever, abdominal pain and/or vaginal discharge at any time postabortion.

Further discussion about safe sex and ongoing contraception is very appropriate at the time of follow-up, and this is an opportunity to ensure that the plan for contraception from the initial visit is being followed. Women undergoing EMA should be aware that ovulatory cycles resume very quickly, ovulation occurring on average 20 days following the abortion process [15]. Combined oral contraception, the etonogestrel rod, the progestogen-only pill and depot medroxyprogesterone acetate injections may all be commenced on the day of misoprostol administration; intrauterine devices can be inserted two to four weeks following EMA [15]. See Chapter 13 for further discussion of contraception following EMA.

Women presenting with signs of infection following EMA should be appropriately investigated and treatment instituted as early as possible. Though mortality rates from EMA are vanishingly low, infection is a major cause of those deaths that have occurred [15]. Since 2001 eight deaths have been reported following EMA in North America and one in Portugal due to infection with *Clostridium sordellii*, an organism also known as the rare cause of infection following caesarean section, normal birth and various forms of surgery in women and men [15,17,18]. This topic is discussed further in Chapter 14.

Methotrexate

Mifepristone is expensive and not universally available. Where it has been, or remains, unavailable methotrexate has been used for EMA and there is good evidence to support its use in these circumstances. Methotrexate alone does not have a high success rate in inducing an abortion but methotrexate followed by misoprostol will cause abortion in around 95% of early pregnancies [19,20].

Methotrexate has long been used as a chemotherapeutic agent and to treat autoimmune disease. It is a folic acid antagonist which acts specifically during DNA and RNA synthesis and thus has a toxic effect on rapidly dividing cells such as those in malignant tissue or involved in embryogenesis. When used in chemotherapeutic doses there is a risk of serious side-effects such as gastrointestinal mucosal damage, leukopenia and cerebral toxicity but given in the low doses, and for the short duration required for EMA, it is safe and well tolerated. Methotrexate is cheap and widely available. Whether given alone or in combination, its use in EMA is 'off-label' [19,20].

Various protocols with methotrexate have been employed in EMA, but all are similar to those used with mifepristone. The initial dose of methotrexate can be given orally or intramuscularly, or a combination of the two; 25 mg to 75 mg orally would be typical, followed three to seven days later by misoprostol in very similar fashion to the mifepristone/misoprostol regimen described above [19,20]. One especially important precaution with methotrexate is awareness of its serious teratogenic potential; failed EMA in these cases presents an even greater imperative to terminate the pregnancy surgically and successfully.

Misoprostol as a single agent

Misoprostol has also been used as a single agent for EMA, in doses of 400–800 µg. Its effectiveness in this situation is around 80%. Where it is ineffective recourse to surgical abortion is indicated [9,19,21].

Clandestine use of misoprostol in countries where abortion law is restrictive has significantly reduced the maternal mortality from abortion [9,22,23]. While it is recommended that all women undergoing EMA have input and oversight from a trained health professional, in regions of the world where this cannot occur it is clear that self-administration of misoprostol is safer than the use by untrained practitioners of unsterile implements to try to bring about 'surgical' abortion.

The internet and early medical abortion

All drugs effective for medical abortion can be obtained relatively easily on the internet although this process carries potential risks if a medically trained person is not involved in assessing the woman. Aspects of a woman's history or physical condition may make her unsuitable for the procedure, as discussed above. Moreover drugs obtained via the internet may not be what they are purported to be, and may in fact be toxic [9,24]. Nevertheless there are several reputable organizations advertising medical abortion on the internet directed at women unable to easily access abortion in their own countries (see Chapter 25). Governments and healthcare providers, both individually and in professional organizations, need to realize that the long history of abortion shows that where women cannot easily access abortion legally and safely they will do so illegally and potentially less safely.

Conclusion

Since its introduction, early medical abortion has greatly increased the reproductive health choices for women in most developed nations and in many developing ones. In England and Wales more than 50% of all early abortions are now performed using mifepristone and misoprostol; in Scotland this is close to 90%. This trend is likely to continue elsewhere, improving the options for women to control their fertility, with all the positive consequences, for their own health and that of their families, that flow from this.

References

1. Hapangama DK. Mifepristone – the multifaceted hormone. *Journal of Drug Evaluation* 2003;1:149–75.

2. Ulmann A. The development of mifepristone: a pharmaceutical drama in three Acts. *Journal of the American Medical Women's Association* 2000;55:117–20.

3. The Royal College of Obstetricians and Gynaecologists, London. *The Care of Women Requesting Induced Abortion*, 2011. www.rcog.org.uk/files/rcog-corp/ Abortion%20guideline_web_1.pdf (accessed 3 March 2014).

4. World Health Organization. *Safe Abortion: Technical and Policy Guidance for Health Systems.* Geneva: WHO, 2012.

5. Raymond EG, Shannon C, Weaver MA, Winikoff B. First-trimester abortion with mifepristone 200mg and misoprostol: a systematic review. *Contraception* 2013;87:26–37.

6. Faúndes A. The combination of mifepristone and misoprostol for the termination of pregnancy. *Int J Gynecol Obstet* 2011;115:1–4.

7. Sparrow M. The introduction of mifepristone in New Zealand. *Venereology* 2001;14:143–7.

8. de Costa CM, Russell DB, de Costa NR, Carrette M, McNamee HM. Introducing early medical abortion in Australia: there is a need to update abortion laws. *Sex Health* 2007;4:223–6.

9. Chong YS, Su L-L, Arulkumaran S. Misoprostol: a quarter century of use, abuse and creative misuse. *Obstetric and Gynecological Survey* 2004; 59:128–40.

10. Winikoff B, Dzuba I, Chong E, *et al.* Extending outpatient medical abortion services through 70 days of gestational age. *Obstet Gynecol* 2012;120:1070–6.

11. Gaudu S, Crost M, Esterle L. Results of a 4-year study on 15,447 medical abortions provided by privately practicing general practitioners and gynecologists in France. *Contraception* 2013;87:45–50.

12. McKay RJ, Rutherford L. Women's satisfaction with early home abortion with telephone follow-up: a questionnaire based study in the UK. *J Obstet Gynaecol* 2013;33:601–4.

13. Goldstone P, Michelson J, Williamson E. Early medical abortion using low-dose mifepristone followed by buccal misoprostol: a large Australian observational study. *Med J Aust* 2012;197:282–6.

14. Say L, Kulier R, Gülmezoglu M, Campana A. Medical versus surgical methods for first trimester termination of pregnancy. *Cochrane Database Syst Rev* 2005;(1):CD003037.

15. Government of South Australia. *South Australian Perinatal Practice Guidelines. 1st trimester medical and surgical termination of pregnancy.* Adelaide: Department of Health, Government of South Australia, 2013.

16. Centre for Maternal and Child Enquiries. Saving mothers' lives. Eighth Report of the Confidential Enquiries into Maternal Deaths in the United Kingdom. *BJOG* 2011;118(Suppl 1):81.

17. Meites E, Zane S, Gould C. Fatal *Clostridium sordellii* infections after medical abortions. *NEJM* 2010;363:1382–3.

18. US Food and Drug Administration Center for Drug Evaluation and Research. Question and Answers on Mifeprex (Mifepristone). www.fda.gov/cder/drug/infopage/mifepristone (accessed 9 March 2014).

19. Pymar HC, Creinin MD. Alternatives to mifepristone regimens for medical abortion. *Am J Obstet Gynecol* 2000;183(2 Suppl):S54–64.

20. Downing S, McNamee H, Penney D, Leamy J, *et al.* Three years on: a review of medical terminations performed in a sexual health service. *Sex Health* 2010;7:212–15.

21. Grimes DA, Creinin MD. Induced abortion: an overview for internists. *Ann Intern Med* 2004;140:620–6.

22. Diniz D, Madeiro A. Cytotec and abortion: the police, the vendors and women. *Cien Saude Colet* 2012;17:1795–804.

23. Asa I, de Costa C, Mola G. A prospective survey of cases of complications of induced abortion presenting to Goroka Hospital, Papua New Guinea, 2011. *Aust NZ J Obstet Gynaecol* 2012;52:491–3.

24. Petersen K. Abortion laws and medical developments: a medico-legal anomaly in Queensland. *J Law Med* 2011;18:594–600.

25. Faucher P, Hassoun D. *Interruption Volontaire de la Grossesse médicamenteuse,* 2nd edn. de Boeck/Estem, 2011.

Chapter

8

Vacuum aspiration

Pascale Roblin

Definition and indications

Vacuum aspiration (VA) is a surgical method of abortion. It is a transcervical procedure which consists of evacuating the contents of the uterus through a plastic cannula connected to a vacuum source. The pump may be electric (EVA) or manual (MVA) based on the same principle of gentle suction. VA, also referred to as suction evacuation or suction curettage, is one of the simplest and most common gynaecological procedures that can be safely carried out in an ambulatory day care setting. It is the recommended surgical technique for abortion for pregnancies of less than 14 weeks' gestation. Other indications include management of early pregnancy loss, incomplete abortion and as a back-up method for failed medical abortion [1].

VA is a procedure distinct from dilatation and evacuation (see Chapter 10) or sharp curettage; the latter uses a sharp metal curette for scraping the uterine wall and is considered obsolete in modern practice.

Until the early 1990s, VA was the established method of abortion but in recent years there has been a decreasing proportion of surgical abortions in Europe and the United States due to the popularity of the medical method (see Chapter 7). In Western Europe, surgical abortion still remains in widespread use in Germany, Belgium, Holland and Italy, but only for a minority in France and Britain and only marginally in Scotland, Sweden and Finland for instance.

Efficacy, safety and acceptability

VA is the most effective method for interrupting pregnancies, with success rates attaining 96–98% of complete abortions, marginally higher than for medical abortion (95–98%). Failure rates requiring repeat procedures are low and occur more often at gestations below seven weeks due to the small size of the gestation sac, which can be easily missed [2].

Numerous studies over past decades have documented the safety of the procedure in settings where abortion is legal and performed by appropriately trained personnel. The rate of complications is very low compared to unsafe abortions. In France, for example, the mortality rate for induced abortion before 14 weeks has been estimated at around 0.25 per million maternities [3]. The morbidity and mortality of early surgical abortion increase with gestational age but remain significantly lower than pregnancies carried to term. Overall, the risk of serious complications requiring hospitalization has been estimated at less than 0.1%

Abortion Care, ed. Sam Rowlands. Published by Cambridge University Press. © Cambridge University Press 2014.

in modern settings [4]. Surgical aspiration is not associated with future poor reproductive outcomes such as ectopic pregnancy, placental abruption or infertility (see Chapter 18). Nor is there any associated risk with breast cancer or mental health problems [1,5].

The acceptability of abortion is high for both surgical and medical methods. Although both methods are considered safe and effective, there is no best method since each has its drawbacks and complex inter-individual factors influence women's preferences [6]. Women choosing the surgical method may, for instance, prefer a highly predictable procedure with a limited number of visits, short duration of bleeding and minimal abdominal pain. The choice of the method will also depend on the legal setting, gestational age, availability of providers, operating room schedule constraints and cost but also the clinicians' preferences in terms of limits in operative skill and experience. See Chapter 7 for a fuller discussion of the choice between medical and surgical abortion.

Initial assessment and consent

Initial assessment includes relevant medical history and physical examination. Maternal age, last menstrual period (LMP), gestation, parity, previous caesarean section, conization of the cervix, uterine malformation, eligibility criteria for contraception, venous thrombo-embolism risk and allergies are determined. Body mass index, blood pressure and pulse are measured. A gynaecological examination may be an opportunity for updating cervical cytology or screening for sexually transmitted infections (STIs) according to local protocols. Bimanual pelvic examination combined with LMP may help determine gestational age. In high-resource settings, pregnancy is usually confirmed by hCG (urine or serum) or ultrasound, the latter being the most accurate method for determining gestational age. Although ultrasound is not a requirement, it is widely used in developed countries for confirming gestational age and localization, fetal number, cardiac activity, uterine scar, placental localization and adnexal structures (see Chapter 6). Laboratory pre-procedure investigations should, as a minimum, include determination of blood group and rhesus status. Haemoglobin is performed in many services. Cross-matching is not routinely done unless medically indicated.

During this initial consultation women should be informed that surgical abortion is a very safe procedure for which major complications are rare. Surgical aspiration and the alternative medical method with their respective benefits and risks should be explained [7]. The role of the clinician is to help the woman choose the method that is most suitable for her according to her preferences and gestational age. Women with significant medical conditions should be rapidly referred to relevant specialists [8] (see Chapter 15). Type of anaesthesia, cervical preparation, prevention of infective complications, available surgical time slots and common complications should also be discussed. Ideally, all pain control methods from paracervical block with or without sedation to general anaesthesia should be offered [9,10]. According to local protocols, a consultation with an anaesthetist may be required a few days before the operation. Advice on postabortion contraception to prevent further unwanted pregnancies is considered good practice since implants and intrauterine devices may be safely inserted intraoperatively (see Chapter 13).

Finally, providers should assess the certainty of the woman's decision to terminate the pregnancy, obtain consent and assure confidentiality. For women who need more time and support for the decision-making process, specific counselling should be provided by appropriately trained supportive staff (see Chapter 5). At the end of this initial consultation, women who choose the surgical method should be provided with an appointment for the procedure. They should be given the opportunity to have any questions answered before the procedure and should feel free to cancel the procedure if they change their mind.

Environment and pre-procedure medication

VA is an outpatient or ambulatory day care surgical procedure. There are various settings in which VA may be performed, mainly based on local resources, type of anaesthesia, provider preference and local legislation. In France, for example, an operating room within a hospital is usually the standard environment for surgical aspirations because general anaesthesia is still widely practised [11]. An operating theatre offers aseptic conditions, improved lighting, flexibility in patient positioning and continuous monitoring appropriate for all anaesthetic options. In other Western European countries, however, such as Germany or the Netherlands, VA is safely performed in dedicated procedure rooms within free-standing clinics. In the USA, MVA is performed in an office setting with lower costs [12]. In the UK, a mixture of all these is employed. No matter what the setting aseptic hand washing, protective barriers, adequate staffing and availability of an anaesthetist in case of emergencies are integral components of quality of care.

Concerning pain management, general anaesthesia is not recommended routinely for VA [1]. No evidence-based recommendations for optimal timing and type of analgesia during surgical abortion exist [13]. There is a continuum between local anaesthesia (paracervical block), minimal sedation (anxiolysis), moderate sedation and analgesia (conscious sedation), deep sedation and analgesia and general anaesthesia. Preoperative pain medication such as ibuprofen (400–800 mg) may be routinely combined with paracervical block or given before general anaesthesia. Paracetamol, however, is ineffective at reducing pain associated with surgical aspiration. Further details on pain control are in Chapter 11.

Cervical preparation (ripening the cervix) facilitates the procedure by reducing the mechanical force required to dilate the cervix, thereby reducing the incidence of uterine perforation, cervical injury, haemorrhage and incomplete abortion. Until recently cervical preparation was recommended only after 12–14 weeks or for young nulliparous women, in the presence of cervical abnormalities or for inexperienced providers. However, it is nowadays increasingly recommended routinely for all women in the first trimester [5,6,14]. Pharmacological agents such as misoprostol are popular in Europe; an effective and acceptable regimen consists of 400 µg vaginal misoprostol, three hours before the procedure. In the USA osmotic dilators are widely used but require women to undergo an extra visit for overnight insertion (see Chapter 10). Misoprostol used in combination with overnight osmotic dilators does not have an additional benefit in cervical dilation before 19 weeks [15].

All women having a surgical abortion should receive preoperative or perioperative antibiotic prophylaxis regardless of their risk of pelvic infection [1,5,7]. The ideal antibiotic, dosage and timing has not yet been established. Single doses of tetracyclines (doxycycline), nitro-imidazoles (metronidazole) or penicillins are commonly used because of clinical efficacy, oral availability, low cost and low risk of allergic reactions. For example, in the author's day care surgery unit, women fast for 6 h before the procedure (no smoking or fluids) and receive 3 h before surgery: 400 µg vaginal misoprostol, 400 mg oral doxycycline, 400 mg ibuprofen and have intravenous (IV) access placed regardless of the type of anaesthesia.

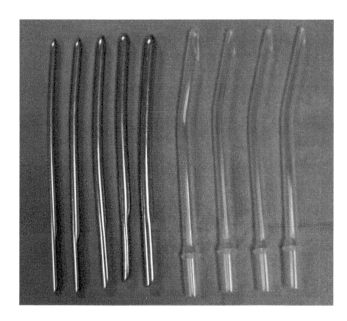

Figure 8.1 Hegar dilators (left) and rigid Karman cannulae (right). Courtesy of Dr Pascale Roblin.

Procedure

EVA in an operating theatre with appropriate staff and the presence of an anaesthetist is currently standard practice in France and the UK and will be described in this section [11,16]. There are some variations in the technique due to provider preference and experience. Typically, the entire procedure takes 15 to 20 minutes.

The woman is placed in the lithotomy position with her perineum just beyond the edge of the table. The table should be able to be tilted head-down in case of vasovagal episode, major blood loss or anaesthetic emergencies. The surgeon should wear adequate theatre equipment including sterile gloves and mask for prevention of infections such as *Streptococcus* A. When general anaesthesia is being used, induction may begin at this point. For procedures under local anaesthesia, it is useful to talk to the woman, warning her of various sensations, keeping her reassured and comfortable to reduce the chances of unexpected sudden movements. A complete description of paracervical block is provided in Chapter 11.

The pubis, vagina and cervix are cleaned with an iodine or chlorhexidine type of antiseptic solution followed by draping with a sterile sheet. Some clinicians find it useful to evacuate the bladder with a catheter. All instruments are sterile and a 'no touch' technique is used as a general rule; no parts of instruments that will enter the uterus are touched. A list of necessary equipment includes [17]: different sizes of speculum, a sharp-toothed tenaculum, a sponge forcep, a graduated sound, a series of cervical mechanical dilators, lubricating gel, a series of rigid or flexible cannulae, a uterine curette, gauze, bowl and antiseptic solution (Figure 8.1). If cervical block is being used, a syringe, needle and local anaesthetic agent such as lidocaine are necessary.

A gentle bimanual examination to confirm estimated gestational age, position of the cervix and uterus and to note extreme ante- or retroversion is performed. A speculum is then placed in the vagina. When using local anaesthesia, the paracervical 4 block technique may then begin and the cervix can be superficially infiltrated at the tenaculum clamp site. The anterior lip of the cervix is usually grasped horizontally with the single tooth tenaculum at 12 o'clock to stabilize and apply gentle traction to the uterus. Traction on the tenaculum straightens the angle between the cervical canal and the uterine cavity, preventing false tracks during dilatation or aspiration. Some providers prefer placing the tenaculum vertically at 12 o'clock with one tooth grasping inside the cervical canal. For a retroverted uterus, anterior lip traction can close the cervical canal and the tenaculum is better placed on the posterior lip. Transverse placement may result in cervical tears and repositioning and tightening of grip may be necessary during dilatation. It is important not to exert excessive traction force which risks cervical laceration and not to accidentally clamp the bladder at 12 o'clock or the rectum at 6 o'clock in cases of prolapse.

Following bimanual examination and cervical traction, some providers insert a sound through the cervical os until the fundus of the uterus is reached before mechanical dilatation. The advantage of uterine sounding is to ascertain the direction of the cervical canal and the overall depth of the uterine cavity by noting the level of mucus or blood on the graduated sound before mechanical dilatation. However, this procedure should be performed cautiously and should not be considered as routine since it may increase the risk of uterine perforation, especially during general anaesthesia. Mechanical dilatation of the cervical canal may be required to accommodate the aspiration cannula. This step is not mandatory if the cervix is already dilated following pre-procedure cervical preparation by misoprostol. Various types of rigid and tapered dilators such as Hegar, Pratt or Denniston can be used. Hegar dilators (Figure 8.1) are commonly used in Europe and correspond in diameter to the size of aspiration cannulae used. A majority of providers use a dilator and aspiration cannula equivalent to the gestational age. For example, an 8-week pregnancy is dilated with an 8 mm Hegar and aspirated with an 8 mm cannula. Each dilator is larger than the previous one and is gently passed in sequence to achieve the appropriate diameter required for the cannula. The dilator is inserted through the external os and passed to a depth just great enough to overcome the resistance of the internal os. In the event of resistance the dilator should not be excessively forced. Applying lubricating gel or antiseptic and tenaculum traction of the cervix may help. Usually the previous dilator is left for a minute in the cervical canal then immediately switched to the subsequent larger one. In difficult cases real-time ultrasound monitoring may guide the optimal dilatation route within the cervix. It is better to use a smaller sized dilator and cannula to reduce risk of cervical injury although it increases the duration of procedure.

Once cervical dilatation is considered optimal, a Karman cannula (Figure 8.1) in the form of a thin hollow tube attached to a vacuum source is inserted through the cervical os and positioned in the mid to upper uterine fundus. The Karman cannula is currently made of transparent plastic; it can be rigid or flexible, straight or curved and ranges in diameter from 6 to 16 mm. Choice of cannula varies according to gestational age, cervical opening and operator preference. For a majority of providers the diameter of the cannula corresponds to the gestational age. Both rigid and flexible cannulae have similar efficacy and are appropriate for EVA and MVA. For later gestations some providers prefer using a small cannula at the end of the procedure to complete evacuation of products.

Not until the cannula is correctly positioned in the uterus and attached by tubing to a bottle and pump, is the suction turned on. EVA provides rapid, gentle continuous suction of 60–80 mmHg negative pressure, aspirating the tissue out of the uterus. Gentle circular, back and forth movements within the uterine cavity are continued until the uterus is empty. This stage usually takes between 3 and 10 minutes according to gestational age. It is important to visualize the flow of amniotic fluid and passage of fetal tissue through the transparent cannula. Products of conception may occasionally obstruct the flow and the cannula should be withdrawn for cleaning. Before withdrawing the cannula outside the uterus, the aspiration is stopped. Occasionally, a sponge forcep may be needed to withdraw tissue in the cervix. The procedure is complete when a gritty sensation is felt as the cannula moves against the retracted uterine walls and no further products are aspirated.

At the end of the procedure products of conception in line with the gestational age should immediately be checked for before removing the tenaculum and speculum. The use of a sharp curette to ascertain complete abortion is not recommended and should be avoided [1]. An intrauterine device (IUD) or an implant can be inserted while the woman is still under anaesthesia. Continuous ultrasound monitoring during the procedure is not routinely required for uncomplicated procedures [5]. However, it may be a useful adjunct at advanced gestations or in cases where cervical dilatation is difficult. At the end of the procedure, ultrasound may ascertain uterine emptiness, integrity or ascertain correct IUD position. After removing the tenaculum the cervix is checked for absence of tearing. Compression with a gauze swab for a few minutes or a suture may be necessary to obtain haemostasis. Routine prophylactic oxytocics for prevention of excessive bleeding are not indicated [1,5].

Differences between EVA and MVA

MVA uses a hand-held 60 mL plastic syringe to which either a flexible or rigid Karman cannula of various sizes can be attached [17] (Figure 8.2). Vacuum is created by pulling back on the syringe plunger then releasing a valve to initiate suction. The same principle of circular, back and forth movements applies and it is critical to formally inspect aspiration products at the end of the procedure. The procedure takes between 5 and 15 minutes but can be longer and more difficult after 9 weeks. The syringe may be emptied one to three times before completion. A choice of available products is shown on the GLOWM website [18] and a chart explaining the procedure can be downloaded from Ipas [10].

Both EVA and MVA appear to be equally safe, effective and acceptable [19,20]. MVA has the advantage of being quiet and environmentally friendly since no electricity is required. Some models can be easily disassembled and sterilized in an autoclave therefore limiting the use of plastic compared to EVA. Although MVA is widely used in low-resource areas, it has gained renewed interest in the USA since the 1990s and is now widely used. Half of US abortion providers prefer MVA, particularly in the earliest weeks of pregnancy, and it is being successfully incorporated into family practice and in-office procedures with local anaesthesia at low costs. Modern protocols for very early procedures before 7 weeks rely on hCG assays, pre- and post-procedure ultrasound and careful immediate tissue inspection [2]. Currently, choice of MVA in developed countries depends primarily on provider training and experience.

Complications and prevention of common pitfalls

VA is a very safe procedure; the rate of serious complications is higher with less operator experience and greater gestational age. The main complications include: continuing pregnancy, incomplete evacuation, pelvic infection, excessive haemorrhage, cervical injury and uterine perforation. The management of these complications is detailed in Chapter 14.

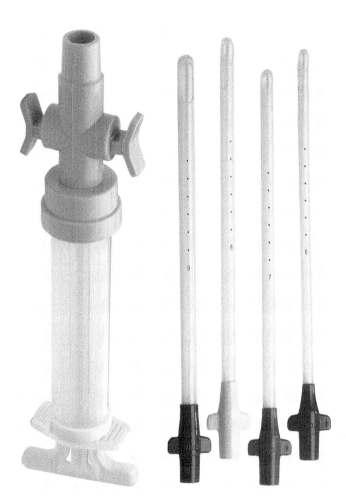

Figure 8.2 Ipas MVA syringe and cannulae. Courtesy of WomanCare Global.

One common pitfall in surgical aspiration is incomplete evacuation by using a cannula that is too small or stopping the aspiration too soon, resulting in retained tissue, haemorrhage and/or infection. It is therefore of paramount importance to verify intraoperatively that the quantity of aspirated tissue is compatible with gestational age. In the author's experience, in the event of doubt, intraoperative ultrasound is a simple non-invasive way to ascertain uterine emptiness and prevents the use of sharp curettage.

In the same vein, many clinicians are reluctant to perform surgical abortion before 7 weeks because of risk of failure and prefer deferring the procedure. A recent evidence-based guideline concluded that there was inadequate data to determine if rigid or flexible cannulae, routine ultrasound monitoring or light metallic curettage were beneficial in such cases [2]. Inspection of aspirated tissue, pre- and postoperative ultrasound or hCG assays may be potential safeguards.

In the case of false cervical track dilatation and suspicion of uterine perforation the surgical procedure should be immediately abandoned to prevent further serious complications. Although there are no evidence-based guidelines for the management of such scenarios, medical abortion or extensive cervical preparation with mifepristone followed by misoprostol may be a feasible option a few days later.

Finally, due to the rising rates of caesarean sections, special attention should be paid to anterior and low-lying placental implantations in women with uterine scars due to the increased risk of placenta accreta and subsequent bleeding. In such cases, preoperative ultrasound should select women for referral to tertiary centres.

Post-procedure management and follow-up

Once complete evacuation is confirmed with no excessive bleeding and the woman is awake, transfer to a nearby recovery room is possible. Length of stay for monitoring depends on type of anaesthesia used and gestational age but is usually short. A 30-minute stay in the recovery room following local anaesthesia is usually long enough. Common side-effects are abdominal cramping, slight bleeding and nausea or vomiting. Staff should pay special attention to excessive bleeding and/or acute pain, which may be indicative of complications including incomplete abortion, cervical laceration or uterine perforation. Analgesics and non-steroidal anti-inflammatory drugs are provided according to local guidance. All non-sensitized RhD-negative women should receive anti-D immunoglobulin. Hormonal contraception can be started at the same time as surgical abortion.

The woman can be discharged preferably accompanied by a friend or relative, as soon as she feels well enough, provided there is no excessive bleeding and she has normal vital signs [1,5]. Most women can return to their usual activities within hours or days. Women should be advised to expect some irregular bleeding or spotting for the first few days and pelvic pain similar to dysmenorrhoea may last for a few hours to few days. Tampon use, baths and sexual intercourse are usually not advised for at least a week. Written and oral instructions on how to recognize potential complications, regressing or continuing pregnancy-associated symptoms, gradual cessation of bleeding should be given, as well as analgesics. In case of warning signs such as fever, chills, fainting, increased pain, excessive or prolonged bleeding, the woman should have access to a 24-hour telephone advice helpline and be promptly informed of pathways to a gynaecology emergency unit.

Routine follow-up after an uncomplicated procedure is not mandatory if successful abortion has been confirmed at the time of the procedure. However, it can be an opportunity for additional services including: psychological support, advice on contraception, cervical smear and prevention of STIs (see Chapter 12).

Conclusions

Vacuum aspiration is a common, quick and simple outpatient surgical procedure with few office visits. It is highly effective, safe and acceptable for women who choose the method. However, VA is an invasive procedure, requiring anaesthesia and therefore a certain loss of autonomy for the woman. EVA and MVA appear to be equally safe, effective and acceptable. Local anaesthesia is considered to be the safest method of pain control. Both EVA and MVA require a skilled provider; choice of technique depends on provider experience, available equipment and legal setting.

References

1. WHO Department of Reproductive Health and Research. *Safe Abortion: Technical and Policy Guidance for Health Systems*, 2nd edn, 2012. www.who.int/reproductivehealth/unsafe_abortion/9789241548434/en/ (accessed 29 September 2013).

2. Lichtenberg ES, Paul M. Surgical abortion prior to 7 weeks of gestation. Society of Family Planning. *Contraception* 2013;88:7–17.

3. Report of the National Expert Committee on Maternal Mortality (CNEMM) 2001–2006. Institut de Veille Sanitaire, Saint Maurice, France. January 2010 (in French). www.invs.sante.fr/publications/2010/mortalite_maternelle/rapport_mortalite_maternelle.pdf (accessed 29 September 2013).

4. Hakim-Elahi E, Tovell HM, Burnhill MS. Complications of first trimester abortion: a report of 170,000 cases. *Obstet Gynecol* 1990;76:129–35.

5. Royal College of Obstetricians and Gynaecologists. *The Care of Women Requesting Induced Abortion. Evidence-based Clinical Guideline Number 7*. November 2011. www.rcog.org.uk/files/rcog-corp/Abortion%20guideline_web_1.pdf (accessed 29 September 2013).

6. Templeton A, Grimes DA. A request for abortion. *NEJM* 2011;365:2198–204.

7. Kapp N, White P, Tang J, Jackson E, Brahimi D. A review of evidence for safe abortion care. *Contraception* 2013;88:350–63.

8. Guiahi M, Davis A. First trimester abortion in women with medical conditions. Society of Family Planning Guideline. *Contraception* 2012;86:622–30.

9. National Abortion Federation. Clinical Policy Guidelines. 2013. www.guidelines.gov (accessed 3 March 2014).

10. Ipas. Clinical Updates in Reproductive Health, 2013. www.ipas.org/en/Resources/Ipas%20Publications/Clinical-updates-in-reproductive-health.aspx (accessed 29 September 2013).

11. Hamoda H, Templeton A. Medical and surgical options for induced abortion in first trimester. *Best Pract Res Clin Obstet Gynaecol* 2010;24:503–16.

12. Lyus RJ, Gianutsos P, Gold M. First trimester procedural abortion in Family Medicine. *J Am Board Fam Med* 2009;22:169–74.

13. Renner RM, Jensen JT, Nichols MD, Edelman AB. Pain control in first-trimester surgical abortion: a systematic review of randomized controlled trials. *Contraception* 2010;81:372–88.

14. Meirik O, My Huong NT, Piaggio G, Bergel E, von Hertzen H; WHO Research Group on Postovulatory Methods of Fertility Regulation. Complications of first-trimester abortion by vacuum aspiration after cervical preparation with and without misoprostol: a multicentre randomised trial. *Lancet* 2012;379:1817–24.

15. Newmann SJ, Dalve-Endres A, Diedrich JT, Steinauer JE, Meckstroth K, Drey EA. Cervical preparation for second trimester dilation and evacuation. *Cochrane Database Syst Rev* 2010;4:CD007310.

16. Flett G, Templeton A. Surgical abortion. *Best Pract Res Clin Obstet Gynaecol* 2002;16:247–61.

17. ARHP. *Manual Vacuum Aspiration (MVA). Quick Reference Guide for Clinicians*. Association of Reproductive Health Professionals, 2004.

18. Borgatta L, Kattan D, Stubblefield PG. Surgical techniques for first trimester abortion. Global Library of Women's Medicine. 2012. DOI 10.3843/GLOWM.10440 www.glowm.com/section_view/heading/Surgical%20Techniques%20for%20First-Trimester%20Abortion/item/439#t1 (accessed 29 September 2013).

19. IPPF. *First Trimester Abortion Guidelines and Protocols*. International Planned Parenthood Federation, September 2008. www.ippf.org.

20. Kulier R, Kapp N, Gülmezoglu AM, Hofmeyr GJ, Cheng L, Campana A. Medical methods for first trimester abortion. *Cochrane Database Syst Rev* 2011;9:CD002855.

Chapter 9

Medical abortion after nine weeks

Joyce Chai and Pak Chung Ho

Introduction

The ideal time to perform abortion is in the first trimester as abortion-related mortality and morbidity increase significantly as gestation advances. As described in Chapter 22, bio-psychosocial factors including failure to recognize an unplanned pregnancy in the first trimester, difficulties in accessing abortion services, late diagnosis of fetal anomalies (Chapter 17) and indecision in some women all contribute to the need for higher gestation abortions. In the literature higher gestation abortions usually means late first trimester and second/mid-trimester abortions. Late first trimester correlates to 9–12 weeks' gestation whereas second/mid-trimester is defined as a period ranging from 13 to 28 weeks' gestation.

The worldwide abortion rate is 28 per 1,000 women of childbearing age (Chapter 3) and abortion after nine weeks constitutes 10–15% of all induced abortions [1]. Although abortion after nine weeks represents a relatively small proportion of all abortions, it is associated with disproportionately high morbidity, accounting for two-thirds of major abortion-related complications [1]. Second trimester abortion by surgical means is one of the oldest and most commonly practised techniques in countries such as the USA and UK, but this procedure should only be performed by skilled gynaecologists with adequate knowledge and experience (see Chapter 10). When this surgical expertise is not available, the development of safe and effective medical techniques for higher gestation abortion is paramount. Ideally any method of medical abortion should have an overall efficacy comparable to that of surgical means, that is a rate of complete abortion of more than 95% and a continuing pregnancy rate of less than 1%. Over the decades effective medical abortion methods have been emerging with better safety profiles. Table 9.1 compares medical with surgical abortion at higher gestations.

Before the 1970s methods commonly employed in medical abortion were intra-amniotic injection of hypertonic saline or hyperosmolar urea and extra-amniotic administration of ethacridine lactate. Hypertonic saline was the mainstay of second trimester medical abortion prior to the development of prostaglandins (PG) despite its risks of hypernatraemia, coagulopathy and massive haemorrhage. Ethacridine lactate is primarily an antiseptic solution with abortifacient effect, when instilled extra-amniotically, and was found to be safer and better tolerated than hypertonic saline. Unfortunately these techniques achieved abortion with a relatively long induction–abortion interval, and they were invariably invasive requiring puncture of the intra-amniotic space or introduction of a Foley catheter into

Abortion Care, ed. Sam Rowlands. Published by Cambridge University Press. © Cambridge University Press 2014.

Table 9.1 Summary of methods for higher gestation abortion

	Surgical	**Medical**
Recommended method(s)	Dilatation and evacuation	Misoprostol with mifepristone (if available)
Cervical preparation	Osmotic dilators or misoprostol	Mifepristone or osmotic dilators if mifepristone not available
Efficacy	Complete abortion rate >95%	Complete abortion rate >95%
Pain relief	Paracervical block; conscious sedation; general anaesthesia	Non-steroidal anti-inflammatory; patient-controlled analgesic
Prerequisite	Experienced surgeon with adequate caseload; appropriate facilities	Mid-level medical staff/healthcare providers
Serious complications	Cervical injury, uterine perforation	Uterine rupture, haemorrhage requiring blood transfusion
Adverse effects	Vaginal bleeding	Higher incidence of pain, prolonged bleeding, nausea/vomiting, fever, incomplete abortion
Need for (repeat) evacuation	Less likely	More likely
Acceptability	High	High

the extra-amniotic space. Intravenous oxytocin, the most commonly-used induction agent at later gestational age, was another alternative but it fails to induce labour effectively as a single-agent therapy at mid-trimester as the number of myometrial oxytocin receptors increases with advancing gestation. Medical expertise was also required in the use of oxytocin because of the potential serious side-effect of water intoxication [2].

Prostaglandins

The introduction of prostaglandins and their analogues is a breakthrough in the field of medical abortion and their use has improved the efficacy of abortion and reduced side-effects. Prostaglandins are a group of lipid compounds that have the ability to stimulate myometrial contraction and interrupt pregnancy at all stages of gestation. In 1970, pioneering prostaglandin investigators Karim and Filshie first reported that intravenous infusion of either naturally occurring PGE_1 or $PGF_2\alpha$ could effectively induce abortion in the mid-trimester of pregnancy, despite a high incidence of gastrointestinal (GI) side-effects including diarrhoea, nausea and vomiting [3]. Subsequently intravenous administration was replaced by the intra-amniotic or extra-amniotic route in an attempt to reduce the GI side-effects and local irritation at the infusion site. When compared with intra-amniotic hypertonic saline, PGs had a shorter instillation–abortion interval and a higher success rate. In 1971 Karim and Sharma reported successful induction of abortion at gestations from 7 to 23 weeks with intravaginal administration of $PGF_2\alpha$ and PGE_2 suppositories [4]. The success rate was more than 95%, with a mean abortion time of 12 hours, but GI side-effects and fever were commonly reported.

Prostaglandin analogues

Prostaglandin analogues, synthetically made to resist enzymatic degradation, have a longer half-life and a more selective action on the myometrium than naturally occurring PGs, hence they are preferable for induction of abortion after nine weeks. Among all PGE analogues, sulprostone, gemeprost and misoprostol are most extensively studied.

Sulprostone, a 16-phenoxy-w-17,18,19,20-tetranor PGE_2 methyl sulphonylamide, was studied in the 1980s for second trimester medical abortion. It can be given intravenously or intramuscularly and is effective in inducing abortion. However, intramuscular sulprostone is no longer available due to its association with cardiovascular complications such as myocardial infarction and hypotension [5].

Gemeprost, a 16,16-dimethyl-trans-Δ^2 PGE_1 methyl ester, is formulated as a vaginal suppository that requires refrigeration. It is one of the most common PG analogues used for induction of abortion. Studies using a vaginal gemeprost-only regimen give a complete abortion rate of 88–96.5% in 48 hours and a mean induction–abortion interval of 14–18 hours [2]. However, its use is limited by its expense, instability at room temperature and single route of administration.

Misoprostol (15-deoxy-16-hydroxy-16-methyl PGE_1) is a PGE_1 analogue marketed for use in the prevention and treatment of peptic ulcer. Its abortifacient effect and its low cost and stability at room temperature has led to its 'off-label' use in medical abortion in many countries. When compared to gemeprost, misoprostol is equivalent in effect or more efficacious [6]. Misoprostol use is associated with less surgical intervention for delivery of the placenta than induction with other agents. All these favourable properties of misoprostol have led to its increasing use in medical abortion and it is now the PG analogue of choice for abortion care recommended by the World Health Organization (WHO) and the UK Royal College of Obstetricians and Gynaecologists (RCOG) [7,8].

Unlike gemeprost, misoprostol is rapidly absorbed by vaginal, sublingual, buccal and oral routes. For misoprostol vaginal administration appears to be the most efficient and is better tolerated when compared to both oral and sublingual regimens. Buccal misoprostol has been shown to be as effective as vaginal misoprostol in a small randomized controlled trial and further studies are required [9]. Vaginal misoprostol is therefore the recommended route of administration, although it may be less acceptable for some women. At onset of bleeding a non-vaginal route is usually preferred as the presence of blood may decrease misoprostol absorption when the drug is given vaginally [10].

Progesterone receptor modulators and prostaglandins

Mifepristone is a 19-norsteroid that blocks the receptors for progesterone and glucocorticoid. The history of the development of mifepristone was detailed in Chapter 7. Progesterone maintains the uterus in a quiescent state and is needed to sustain a pregnancy. By antagonizing this effect, mifepristone is approved for use clinically for induction of abortion. To date, mifepristone is licensed for medical abortion up to 9 weeks' gestation and over 13 weeks' gestation but not for 9–13 weeks' gestation although reports have demonstrated its efficacy in this gestational group [11]. Mifepristone not only inhibits the action of progesterone, it also increases the sensitivity of the uterus to prostaglandins. Indeed, mifepristone administration gradually elicits a five-fold increase in sensitivity to PG 24–48 hours after its administration. It can also produce uterine contractions and induce cervical ripening. The synergy between mifepristone and PG permits greater efficacy of PG at lower doses and achieves a shorter induction–abortion interval when compared to regimens in which either agent is used alone [12]. Unfortunately mifepristone is not available in all countries; it has only been licensed for use in 57 countries (www.gynuity.org).

Abortion at 9 to 13 weeks' gestation

Mifepristone with misoprostol has proven to be highly effective, safe and acceptable for abortions at up to 9 weeks' gestation (see Chapter 7). Data on pregnancies between 9 and 13 weeks' gestation are more limited and mainly come from case series. The recommended method for medical abortion by WHO and RCOG is 200 mg mifepristone administered orally followed 36–48 hours later by 800 μg misoprostol administered vaginally. Subsequent misoprostol doses should be 400 μg, administered either vaginally or sublingually, every three hours up to four further doses until expulsion of the products of conception occurs. Using this regimen the complete abortion rate is 95–96% [8]. When compared to the surgical method using vacuum aspiration in a randomized trial involving 368 women, the difference in complete abortion rates (95% in the medical group versus 98% in the surgical group) was not significant. Although women who undergo medical abortion experience more side-effects, 70% of them would opt for the medical method in the future reflecting its high acceptability [13].

When mifepristone is not available, misoprostol alone can be used but the effectiveness is expected to be lower. The time to complete abortion is longer and the requirement for misoprostol is higher. The recommended regimens are 800 μg administered vaginally or sublingually repeated at intervals of no less than 3 hours but no more than 12 hours for up to three doses. This regimen is 75–90% effective in completing abortion [7].

Abortion at 13 to 24 weeks' gestation

For medical abortion between 13 and 24 weeks both the WHO and the RCOG recommend 200 mg oral mifepristone followed 36–48 hours later by misoprostol 800 μg vaginally, then misoprostol 400 μg, vaginally or sublingually, every three hours up to a maximum of four further doses. This combined regimen offers the safest and most expeditious method with an abortion rate at 24 hours as high as 96% and a median induction–abortion interval as low as six hours [12]. A meta-analysis shows 200 mg of mifepristone is as effective as 600 mg for early pregnancy termination [14] and a randomized trial gives a similar recommendation in abortions after nine weeks [15]. The 36–48 h dosing interval poses several problems in the clinical setting including an increased duration of treatment, the requirement of repeat attendance at the hospital for drug administration and the fact that 0.2–0.4% of women may abort after the administration of mifepristone but before the administration of misoprostol [16]. Shortening this mifepristone–misoprostol interval to 24 hours [17] or giving both medications simultaneously [18] compromised efficacy with a longer induction–abortion interval and a higher requirement for misoprostol; hence it is not the method of choice.

Where mifepristone is not available the recommended method of medical abortion is 400 μg of misoprostol, administered vaginally or sublingually, repeated every three hours for up to five doses. The abortion rate at 24 hours is 80–90% with a median induction–abortion interval of 10–15 hours. Various studies have used doses ranging from 200 to 800 μg at intervals ranging from 3 to 12 hours [16]. A randomized trial comparing 400 μg of vaginal misoprostol given at 3-hour intervals or at 6-hour intervals showed that the regimen using 3-hour intervals was more effective without a significant increase in side-effects except for fever [19]. In general higher doses of misoprostol are associated with higher rates of fever, diarrhoea, nausea and vomiting. Medical abortion with misoprostol alone requires higher doses of misoprostol when compared to combined treatment with mifepristone, which invariably increases the frequency of side-effects.

Placement of osmotic dilators can be considered as an alternative to cervical preparation before the administration of PG in second trimester medical abortion when mifepristone is not available. Commonly-used dilators are laminaria (Lamicel®) derived from seaweed and Dilapan-S®, a synthetic osmotic dilator. A dry tent is inserted into the cervical canal the evening before PG administration and the tent will swell slowly in the presence of moisture, increasing to three to five times the original diameter, enhancing the softening of the cervix. Its use as a cervical ripening agent in surgical abortion is well-established but not so clear in medical abortion. It was shown to reduce the induction–abortion interval when used before sulprostone administration but not with vaginal misoprostol, although the laminaria tent was inserted with the first dose of misoprostol instead of 12 hours before. Mifepristone, if available, remains the drug of choice for cervical priming before misoprostol administration as it shortens the induction–abortion interval and is associated with less pain when compared to the laminaria tent [20].

Preabortion assessment and preparation

The principles of choice between medical and surgical abortion are the same as those outlined in Chapter 7 for early abortion. Studies have found that women are more likely to find a method of abortion acceptable if they have chosen it themselves [7]; therefore it is important to provide detailed information regarding all treatment options (including surgical methods if available) to women so that they can make an informed choice. Women who have opted for medical abortion should be informed of the details of the procedure and its risks and what to expect during and after the procedure.

A detailed medical history and physical examination should be performed to exclude possible absolute contraindications to medical abortion and to estimate gestational age. Absolute contraindications include allergies to mifepristone/misoprostol, inherited porphyria, chronic adrenal failure and known or suspected ectopic pregnancy. Caution is required in women who are on long-term corticosteroid therapy, or those with severe anaemia or pre-existing heart disease or cardiovascular risk factors. If there is doubt in the gestational age or the location of pregnancy, ultrasound scanning should be offered. Rhesus status should be determined and Rh negative women should receive anti-D prophylaxis.

Side-effects and complications

When abortion is performed by appropriately trained medical staff, in modern medical settings, complications are rare and the risk of death is negligible. Most of the side-effects in late medical abortion are related to the use of prostaglandins and frequently reported side-effects include vomiting, nausea, diarrhoea and fever which are usually self-limiting. There is a 2.5–10% chance of surgical intervention for retained placenta or incomplete abortion. Prolonged bleeding is an expected effect of medical abortion. On average, vaginal bleeding gradually diminishes over about two weeks after medical abortion but, in individual cases, bleeding and spotting may persist for up to 45 days. More serious complications such as haemorrhage requiring blood transfusion, uterine rupture and cervical tear are rare. Average blood loss in medical abortion in general is higher than that in surgical abortion and major bleeding is usually associated with prolonged retention of the placenta. Heavy bleeding requiring transfusion has been reported in less than 1% of women. Cases of uterine rupture occur with misoprostol with or without mifepristone. Risk factors for uterine rupture include previous uterine scar, grand multiparity, advanced gestation, prolonged PG therapy and use of oxytocin in addition to prostaglandins. However, uterine rupture has also been reported in women without these risk factors. Complications of medical abortion are considered further in Chapter 14.

Women in general can be reassured that the vast majority of them will not suffer any long-term effects to their general or reproductive health if the abortion is properly and safely induced. However, when the procedure is carried out by persons lacking the necessary skills or in an environment that does not conform to minimal medical standards, the risks increase substantially. In 2008, 21.6 million unsafe abortions were estimated to have occurred, causing the deaths of 47,000 women [21]. Deaths due to unsafe abortion are mainly caused by severe infections or bleeding resulting from the unsafe abortion procedure.

Pain management

Effective pain management is an important part of abortion care. Women undergoing medical abortion after nine weeks will inevitably experience some degree of abdominal pain related to the uterine contractions and the larger fetus passing through the cervical canal. The perception of pain varies in different individuals but in general the analgesia requirement is significantly higher in women of younger age, higher gestation, longer induction–abortion interval and with increased number of misoprostol doses while women with a previous live birth are less likely to use analgesia [22]. Women should be offered pain relief at the time of need. There are no evidence-based recommendations for optimal analgesia regimens in medical abortion after nine weeks.

Non-steroidal anti-inflammatory drugs (NSAIDs) inhibit the production of endogenous PGs, which are important messengers responsible for uterine contractions, cramps and pain sensation. NSAIDs such as ibuprofen have been shown to be more effective in mitigating pain when compared with paracetamol or placebo, and despite its effect on PGs it does not adversely affect the outcome of medical abortion. Paracetamol is found to be ineffective at reducing pain during medical abortion in randomized controlled trials and therefore its use is not recommended. Parenteral or patient-controlled analgesia using opioids is another option but it may not be readily available in some hospital settings [23]. See Chapter 11 for further details on pain control.

Feticide before abortion

The possibility of the fetus being born alive is significant for medical abortion after 20 weeks' gestation and feticide prior to the procedure should be considered. Feticide should be routinely offered to women undergoing medical abortion after 21 weeks and 6 days of gestation to avoid signs of life at abortion according to the RCOG recommendation [8]. Neither mifepristone nor misoprostol is directly feticidal and inducing fetal death before medical abortion may have beneficial emotional and ethical consequences. For some providers feticide is used in the belief that it shortens the induction–abortion interval in medical abortion but the evidence is lacking.

The RCOG recommends the use of intracardiac potassium chloride to ensure fetal asystole, which typically happens within minutes of injection. However, this technique requires a skilled operator for accurate needle positioning and continuous ultrasound monitoring to observe cardiac cessation. Other methods using intra-amniotic digoxin or hyperosmolar solutions such as urea require less expertise in ultrasound but they are not as effective as potassium chloride and usually take longer time for fetal death to occur. See Chapter 16 for more on feticide.

Medical abortion after nine weeks in women with a uterine scar

The incidence of caesarean section has increased gradually over the past few decades and it is now not uncommon to encounter women with a uterine scar requesting abortion. Uterine scar rupture is a potential complication of medical abortion using misoprostol and is associated with maternal morbidity and mortality in severe cases. A systematic review of 461 women with one prior low transverse caesarean scar undergoing second trimester pregnancy induction with misoprostol showed that the incidence of uterine rupture was 0.43% and none of the cases resulted in hysterectomy [24]. This risk is similar to the scar rupture rate during vaginal birth after caesarean section where there is spontaneous onset of labour, and it is considered to be acceptable by women and healthcare providers. Nonetheless it is important to be aware of the increased risk of scar rupture with the use of additional agents such as oxytocin and administration of both drugs should be avoided. Data on misoprostol use in women with more than one prior caesarean or with a prior classical caesarean delivery undergoing second trimester medical abortion are limited. The lack of clinical randomized trials precludes specific dosing recommendations and usage of misoprostol in these situations should be carried out with extra caution. It is wise to start with a lower dose or a less frequent dosing regimen. The dose can be increased gradually if the uterine contractions are not adequate. Whether surgical abortion by dilatation and evacuation (D&E) will be a safer option in these settings remains debatable as D&E in the second trimester is safe only when performed by experienced operators. Women should be appropriately informed of the risks before the procedure and access to experienced surgeons and an operating theatre should be available at the time of medical abortion.

The rising caesarean section rate also implies that healthcare providers may encounter placenta accreta more often than expected. The incidence of placenta accreta during the second trimester is reported to be comparable to that for third trimester deliveries. Routine ultrasound is not required for the provision of abortion; however, its use should be considered in women with a uterine scar who are resistant to medical abortion, to look for potential placenta accreta due to its inherent risk of massive haemorrhage.

Conclusion

With the high rate of unintended pregnancy and the increasing use of antenatal diagnosis to detect anomalies in mid-trimester, the need for abortion at higher gestations is likely to remain. The combined use of mifepristone and misoprostol in medical abortion after nine weeks has demonstrated high efficacy and safety, and such a regimen should be standard care, especially in institutions lacking skilled practitioners to carry out surgical abortion.

References

1. World Health Organization. Medical Methods for Termination of Pregnancy. *WHO Technical Report Series 871*. Geneva: World Health Organization, 1997.

2. Tang OS, Ho PC. Medical abortion in the second trimester. *Best Pract Res Clin Obstet Gynaecol* 2002;16:237–46.

3. Karim SMM, Filshie GM. Therapeutic abortion using prostaglandin F2α. *Lancet* 1970;1:157–9.

4. Karim SMM, Sharma SD. Therapeutic abortion and induction of labour by intravaginal administration of prostaglandin E_2 and $F_2α$. *J Obstet Gynaecol Br Commonw* 1971;78:294–9.

5. Ulmann A, Silvestre L, Chemama L, *et al.*
   Medical termination of early pregnancy
   with mifepristone (RU 486) followed
   by a prostaglandin analogue. Study in
   16,369 women. *Acta Obstet Gynecol Scand*
   1992;71:278–83.

6. Ho PC, Chan YF, Lau W. Misoprostol is
   as effective as gemeprost in termination
   of second trimester pregnancy when
   combined with mifepristone: a randomised
   comparative trial. *Contraception*
   1996;53:281–83.

7. WHO. *Safe Abortion: Technical and Policy
   Guidance for Health Systems*, 2nd edn.
   Geneva: World Health Organization, 2012.

8. Royal College of Obstetricians and
   Gynaecologists. *The Care of Women
   Requesting Induced Abortion: Evidence-
   based Clinical Guideline Number 7*.
   London: RCOG, 23 November 2011.

9. Ellis SC, Kapp N, Vragpvoc O, *et al.*
   Randomized trial of buccal versus
   vaginal misoprostol for induction of
   second trimester abortion. *Contraception*
   2010;81:441–5.

10. Tang OS, Schweer H, Lee SW, *et al.*
    Pharmacokinetics of repeated doses of
    misoprostol. *Hum Reprod* 2009;24:1862–9.

11. Hamoda H, Ashok PW, Flett GMM, *et al.*
    Medical abortion at 9–13 weeks' gestation:
    a review of 1076 consecutive cases.
    Contraception 2005;71:327–32.

12. Wildschut H, Both MI, Medema S, *et al.*
    Medical methods for mid-trimester
    termination of pregnancy. *Cochrane
    Database Syst Rev* 2011;(1):CD005216.

13. Ashok PW, Kidd A, Flett GM, *et al.* A
    randomized comparison of medical
    abortion and surgical vacuum aspiration
    at 10–13 weeks gestation. *Hum Reprod*
    2002;17:92–8.

14. Lievre M, Sitruk-Ware R. Meta-analysis of
    200 or 600 mg mifepristone in association
    with two prostaglandins for termination
    of early pregnancy. *Contraception*
    2009;80:95–100.

15. Webster D, Penney GC, Templeton
    A. A comparison of 600 and 200 mg
    mifepristone prior to second trimester

abortion with the prostaglandin
misoprostol. *BJOG* 1996;103:706–9.

16. Lalitkumar S, Bygdeman M, Gemzell-
    Danielsson K. Mid-trimester induced
    abortion: a review. *Hum Reprod Update*
    2007;13:37–52.

17. Nilas L, Glavind-Kristensen M, Vejborg
    T, *et al.* One or two day mifepristone-
    misoprostol interval for second trimester
    abortion. *Acta Obstet Gynecol Scand*
    2007;86:1117–21.

18. Chai J, Tang OS, Hong QQ, *et al.* A
    randomized trial to compare two dosing
    intervals of misoprostol following
    mifepristone administration in second
    trimester medical abortion. *Hum Reprod*
    2009;24:320–4.

19. Wong KS, Ngai CS, Yeo EL, *et al.*
    A comparison of two regimens of
    intravaginal misoprostol for termination of
    second trimester pregnancy: a randomized
    comparative trial. *Hum Reprod*
    2000;15:709–12.

20. Prairie BA, Lauria MR, Kapp N, *et al.*
    Mifepristone versus laminaria: a
    randomized controlled trial of cervical
    ripening in midtrimester termination.
    Contraception 2007;76:383–8.

21. WHO. *Unsafe Abortion: Global and
    Regional Estimates of Incidence of Unsafe
    Abortion and Associated Mortality in
    2008*, 6th edn. Geneva: World Health
    Organization, 2011.

22. Hamoda H, Ashok PW, Flett GMM,
    Templeton A. Analgesia requirements
    and predictors of analgesia use for
    women undergoing medical abortion
    up to 22 weeks of gestation. *BJOG*
    2004;111:996–1000.

23. Jackson E, Kapp N. Pain control in first-
    trimester and second-trimester medical
    termination of pregnancy: a systematic
    review. *Contraception* 2011;83:116–26.

24. Berghella V, Airoldi J, O'Neill AM,
    et al. Misoprostol for second trimester
    pregnancy termination in women with
    prior caesarean: a systematic review. *BJOG*
    2009;116:1151–7.

Chapter 10

Dilatation and evacuation

Patricia A. Lohr and Richard Lyus

Background

The widespread liberalization of abortion law in the latter part of the twentieth century led to steep reductions in abortion-related morbidity and mortality not only by increasing access to safe services but also through technological advances in abortion care [1]. At the time, surgical options for second trimester abortion were very limited. Hysterotomy and hysterectomy were performed but most women underwent induction of labour with intra-amniotic instillation of hypertonic solutions or prostaglandin. With the development of larger diameter cannulae, vacuum aspiration was demonstrated to be feasible in the early second trimester. However, advancement beyond 16 weeks' gestation required substantially greater cervical dilatation and the development of elongated, reinforced forceps to safely and efficiently extract the larger fetus and placenta. The procedure, now known as dilatation and evacuation (D&E), was demonstrated to be safer than instillation abortion and quickly supplanted it as the method of choice where available. In the USA, for example, the proportion of second trimester abortions conducted by D&E increased from 31% in 1974 to 96% in 2005 while instillation abortions decreased from 57% to 0.4% [2].

Vacuum aspiration, hysterotomy, hysterectomy, D&E and a variant of D&E called intact dilatation and extraction (D&X) are all procedures used for second trimester surgical abortion today. Vacuum aspiration is effective up to 16 weeks' gestation with 14–16 mm diameter cannulae, but forceps are often required to remove larger fetal parts such as the calvarium or spine (see Chapter 8). Hysterotomy and hysterectomy are reserved for cases where neither a medical induction nor a transcervical surgical approach is feasible, such as the presence of a large cervical tumour. Dilatation and evacuation remains the most commonly performed method of surgical abortion in the second trimester, with D&X utilized when preservation of fetal anatomy is desired.

In addition to its safety and effectiveness, advantages of D&E for both the woman and provider are that the procedure can be scheduled as a day case and operating times are short (about 10–15 minutes), as opposed to the unpredictable duration of a medical abortion, which requires hospitalization. The efficiency and predictability of D&E is also beneficial where women require an abortion for maternal medical conditions or complications of pregnancy, such as preterm premature rupture of membranes, which could deteriorate during the course of a lengthy labour induction. Lastly, D&E is an important back-up for failed second trimester medical abortion.

Abortion Care, ed. Sam Rowlands. Published by Cambridge University Press. © Cambridge University Press 2014.

This chapter will review the safety and prevalence of D&E and then focus on clinical aspects such as preoperative assessment, cervical preparation, surgical technique, postoperative care and complications. This chapter is a revised, expanded and updated version of a review article on D&E published in 2008 by the first author [3].

Safety and effectiveness

The comparative safety of D&E was established by large cohort studies and case series conducted in the USA. Instillation of saline, urea or prostaglandin $F_2\alpha$ was demonstrated to carry a significantly higher risk of serious complications than D&E, including death [4]. An analysis of abortion-related mortality from 1972 to 1981 revealed a rate of 4.9 per 100,000 with D&E and 9.6 per 100,000 with instillation methods [5]. Hysterectomy and hysterotomy were even higher at 60 deaths per 100,000 procedures.

In addition to being safer than the existing medical alternatives, D&E was associated with shorter hospital stays, less delay to treatment and better compliance [6]. While more complex than vacuum aspiration, D&E was shown to be a procedure that could be learned by experienced pelvic surgeons as well as those in training and safely undertaken as a day case procedure, thus reducing costs [3].

Modern methods of second trimester medical abortion use either a combination of the antiprogestogen mifepristone and the prostaglandin analogue misoprostol, or misoprostol alone (see Chapter 9). These regimens are faster and less morbid than instillation abortion but still have a higher overall risk of complications, greater pain and bleeding and more overnight hospital stays than D&E [7]. Second trimester surgical abortion is also associated with better short-term psychological outcomes than induction with mifepristone and misoprostol and is more acceptable to women. In a head-to-head trial significantly fewer women found surgical abortion to be worse than expected (0% versus 53%, p = 0.001), and more would opt for a surgical procedure again if needed (100% versus 53%, p ≤0.001) [8].

Prevalence

The proportion of second trimester abortions performed by D&E varies. It is the most common method of second trimester abortion in many parts of the world, such as the USA and England and Wales, but in others, like Scotland or Scandinavia, it is virtually never performed. Lack of training and motivation are important barriers to D&E availability. Surgical abortion in the second trimester is generally not taught in postgraduate training programmes. By contrast, the knowledge required to manage a second trimester medical abortion is similar to that required for induction of labour at term, which is within the scope of obstetrics and gynaecology. Some doctors find performing D&E distressing or unpleasant and are unwilling to accept the perceived additional burden of performing the operation [9]. Other obstacles are a lack of necessary equipment, local policies and staff acceptability.

The indication for abortion may also influence whether a medical or surgical procedure is offered or chosen. In the case of termination for fetal anomaly (see Chapter 17), induction abortion has been advocated because it allows for bonding with the fetus after delivery, which may help with the grieving process. Amongst women self-selecting medical or surgical abortion, however, no difference in grief resolution is apparent [10] and some evidence suggests that it may be psychologically beneficial for a woman to be able to obtain the procedure she feels would best suit her emotional coping style [11]. In addition, specimens obtained from D&E can be examined to confirm many pathological and cytological diagnoses [12]. Intact

D&X, where the fetus is extracted intact with the exception of the brain tissue, may also be used to effect a more thorough pathological examination.

Pre-procedure assessment

There are few contraindications to D&E, thus clinical assessment is focused on determining whether the procedure can safely take place in an outpatient setting and what anaesthesia can be offered. This should include a review of general health, observations, height and weight and targeted medical, obstetric and gynaecological histories. Indications for treatment in hospital include conditions that necessitate prolonged or intensive monitoring, such as severe cardiopulmonary disease, and those which place the woman at high risk of haemorrhage, such as placenta accreta or inherent or iatrogenic coagulopathy (see Chapter 15). Some conditions, such as obesity or uterine anomalies including large fibroids, can make D&E more challenging so prior knowledge is useful for procedure planning.

Options for pain management include conscious sedation, general anaesthesia, or a paracervical block with the addition of oral non-steroidal anti-inflammatory drugs (NSAIDs), narcotics or anxiolytics (see Chapter 11). In modern practice, general anaesthesia consists of deep intravenous sedation with propofol usually performed without intubation. This regimen has a very low complication rate; that of pulmonary aspiration was estimated in one large case series that included over 11,000 D&Es to be 0.03% [13]. Wherever possible, choice of pain management should be driven by the woman's preference. In those with complex medical histories a consultation with an anaesthetist is beneficial to determine which is most appropriate (see also Chapter 15).

While not a requirement gestational age is often determined by ultrasound. Accurate estimation of gestational age is important as it helps determine the cervical preparation regimen and underestimation is a risk factor for uterine perforation. Ultrasound is also used to determine placental location, which is of importance in women with prior caesarean delivery. If the placenta is anterior and either low-lying or a praevia, the risk for accreta can be substantial, resulting in torrential bleeding at the time of inadvertent evacuation. Further ultrasound examinations or magnetic resonance imaging can be used to exclude placental abnormalities or the decision can be taken to perform the operation in a fully functional operating theatre, with the ability to perform an emergency uterine artery embolization or hysterectomy if needed.

Determination of rhesus status is standard and guidelines recommend administration of anti-D immunoglobulin for all Rh-negative women, regardless of gestation [14]. While haemorrhage is rare after D&E haemoglobin is often obtained. Consideration should also be given to screening for chlamydia and gonorrhoea, which are strong risk factors for postabortion pelvic inflammatory disease [14].

As with all procedures, formal consent is essential and the woman should understand that the procedure begins with cervical preparation. If a woman decides to continue the pregnancy after this point she should be referred for obstetric care and observation as these agents may precipitate preterm labour and pregnancy loss.

Cervical preparation

Preparation of the cervix before D&E can be achieved using medication, such as misoprostol or mifepristone, or absorptive natural or synthetic cervical tents (osmotic dilators) [15]. Osmotic dilators swell after insertion and exert outward pressure on the endocervical canal and stimulate the release of endogenous prostaglandins to promote cervical ripening.

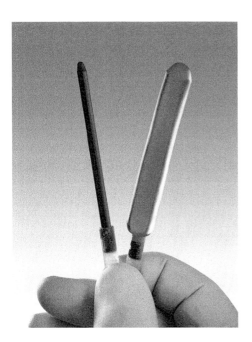

Figure 10.1 Dilapan-S® osmotic dilators in dry and swollen states. Copyright Medicem. Used with permission.

Laminaria is a natural osmotic dilator made of compressed stalks of seaweed (*Laminaria japonica* or *Laminaria digitata*). Sizes range from 2 to 10 mm in diameter and from 60 to 85 mm in length. After insertion, laminaria expand to three or four times their dry diameter without changing length. Although some dilatation is measurable three hours after insertion, 12–24 h are required for maximal expansion. Dilapan-S® is a synthetic osmotic dilator made of polyacrylate-based hydrogel (Figure 10.1). It is available in three sizes (3 × 55 mm, 4 × 55 mm and 4 × 65 mm). Dilapan-S® expansion occurs more rapidly, more consistently and to a greater degree than laminaria. Practically this means that fewer Dilapan-S® need to be inserted and for shorter periods of time. Dilapan-S® continue to expand for 24 h, but most dilatation is achieved in 4–6 h.

Dilapan-S® and laminaria are both safe and effective, therefore preferences are provider-dependent [15]. There is also no standard protocol for their use. In general, the number inserted and length of time the dilators are left in place increases with gestational age. Some providers use a combination of Dilapan-S® and laminaria or perform serial insertions over two days.

The placement of osmotic dilators requires insertion of a vaginal speculum, followed by optional cleansing of the cervix and administration of cervical anaesthetic. A tenaculum or vulsellum is used to stabilize the cervix. A dilator is grasped with a ring forcep at its proximal end and inserted until the distal tip extends beyond the internal os. This process is repeated until the desired number of dilators is achieved or until they fit snugly. Caution must be taken not to insert too many rods too tightly; if the os is resistant osmotic dilators can dilate at the ends but not the middle ('hourglass') and laminaria can congeal. Some providers insert a gauze sponge into the vagina to help hold the dilators in place if they are to be left overnight.

Discomfort or vasovagal reactions can occur during insertion and many women experience cramping and light bleeding as the dilators expand. NSAIDs are usually sufficient to control pain. Uncommonly, the dilators may fall out with progressive cervical expansion or

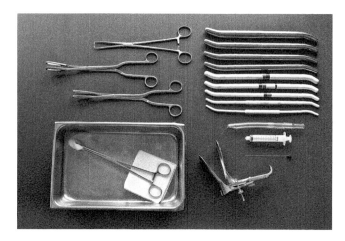

Figure 10.2 Typical instrument tray for D&E. Contents (clockwise from top left): tenaculum, Pratt and Denniston dilators, 14 mm rigid Karman cannula, 10 mL syringe, spinal needle, Graves speculum, tray, ring/sponge forcep, 4 × 4 gauze sponges, Sopher and Bierer forceps. Copyright Ipas. Used with permission.

if the membranes rupture. These are generally not emergencies but women do need to be guided as to signs suggestive of the onset of labour. Women may be discharged if the dilators are to remain in place overnight but should be provided with information on pain management and instructions on when and how to contact a healthcare professional.

Although osmotic dilators achieve greater cervical dilatation than medication [15], pharmacological methods of preparation may be more acceptable to some women. In addition, osmotic dilators are not available worldwide and overnight use may present a barrier for those travelling long distances to access care. Misoprostol is a cheap, widely available option which can be administered by the oral, vaginal, sublingual or buccal routes. The ideal regimen and upper gestational age limit have not been determined but observational studies have shown that buccal or vaginal misoprostol, in doses ranging from 400 to 800 μg, is effective [15]. Repeated doses and additional mechanical dilatation are frequently required. A single dose of misoprostol in combination with Dilapan-S® has been shown in two small case series to be an effective method of same-day cervical preparation up to 22 weeks' gestation [16].

Mifepristone causes cervical softening and dilatation when taken orally and its use as a ripening agent before D&E is an active area of research. When combined with misoprostol and osmotic dilators the risk of passage of the pregnancy before reaching theatre for surgical evacuation increases [15]. Used alone, the day prior to D&E at 14–16 weeks' gestation, 200 mg mifepristone results in procedure times equivalent to overnight laminaria or Dilapan-S®, albeit usually requiring additional mechanical dilatation [17].

Operative techniques

The standard method of D&E involves the removal of the fetus and placenta through the prepared cervix in multiple passes using strong, elongated extraction forceps. A typical tray of instruments for D&E is shown in Figure 10.2.

The woman is positioned in lithotomy, after induction if a general anaesthetic is used, and a bimanual examination is performed to assess uterine size and position. A bivalve or Sims speculum is placed and any osmotic dilators in situ are removed and counted. The cervix and vagina are cleansed with an antiseptic and, if being used, a paracervical block is administered. A tenaculum is applied to the cervix which is used to straighten the endocervical canal and draw the cervix closer to the introitus. Passive or active drainage of amniotic fluid by vacuum aspiration is then performed in order to bring the fetal parts

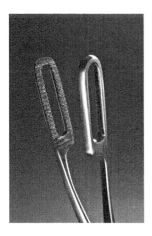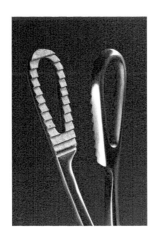

Figure 10.3 Left: close-up Sopher forcep jaw. Right: close-up Bierer forcep jaw. Copyright Ipas. Used with permission.

into the lower part of the uterus to facilitate extraction and reduce the risk of amniotic fluid embolism.

Specialized forceps are then used to remove the fetus and placenta. The choice of forcep depends on the amount of dilatation achieved, gestational age and surgeon preference. McClintock or ring forceps require minimal cervical dilatation (10–12 mm) but because of their small, relatively smooth grasping area are not sufficient beyond 17 or 18 weeks' gestation. At this point, a heavier forcep with a longer shank and wider, serrated surface (e.g. Sopher, Bierer) is more efficient but requires between 14 and 19 mm dilatation (Figure 10.3). As a minimum, the amount of dilatation must permit easy passage of the extraction forceps into the uterus. If this has not been achieved, mechanical dilatation can be performed with tapered dilators (e.g. Pratt, Denniston or Hawkin Ambler).

The jaw of the forcep is passed through the internal os, ideally under ultrasound guidance, and opened as widely as possible to encircle the presenting fetal parts in the lower uterine cavity. These are reduced in size by closing the forcep and brought out through the cervix with gentle rotation. The non-dominant hand can be used to palpate the size of parts as they are pulled against the internal os, or to palpate the uterus abdominally; these manoeuvres help the operator to avoid extracting large parts which could cause a cervical laceration or rupture and maintain an awareness of the forcep relative to the uterine fundus.

The fetal parts and the placenta should be noted as they are removed. Once completely extracted, a final vacuum aspiration is performed with a 10–14 mm rigid cannula to remove any remaining blood or tissue; care must be taken as the uterus will have contracted. The amount of bleeding is assessed and, with a sterile glove, a finger may be passed into the cervix and lower uterus to palpate for remaining fetal parts or injury. A bimanual examination can ensure the uterine tone is firm. Once all of the products of conception have been removed, and accounted for, and bleeding is determined to be minimal the woman is moved to the recovery area. Observation for 60–90 minutes is usual, dependent on the type of anaesthesia administered. A sanitary pad should be placed to aid in assessment of bleeding in the immediate postoperative period; bleeding should be light.

With D&X, wide cervical dilatation is achieved with two or more days of laminaria. This is followed by an assisted breech delivery of the trunk of the fetus, decompression of the calvarium, and delivery of the fetus otherwise intact. The degree of dilatation (reported as a median of 5 cm, range 2–10) and mode of evacuation means that fewer instrument passes are made with D&X than with D&E.

Feticide

Procedures to cause fetal demise before D&E are used in an effort to make the procedure safer but lack an evidence base. Their posited benefits are cervical ripening and the softening of fetal tissues to facilitate removal. The true incidence of use is not known and the gestational age at which feticide is administered differs among practitioners; however, it is typically reserved for procedures at 18 weeks' gestation or greater. The most common agents for inducing fetal demise are potassium chloride and digoxin. Potassium chloride is administered to the fetus by an intracardiac or intrathoracic route. Digoxin may also be injected into or near the fetal heart, but is usually administered into the amniotic fluid or other fetal tissues.

The only randomized controlled trial [18] available found that intra-amniotic digoxin administered 24 h prior to D&E did not reduce the duration of the procedure, complications or subjective difficulty compared to placebo. Women receiving feticide with digoxin do experience more side-effects, more spontaneous expulsions and more infections than when it is not administered, however [19]. Similarly, benefits have not been demonstrated with potassium chloride when used for feticide before D&E [20] but complications can be serious including cardiac arrest with inadvertent injection into the maternal circulation [21]. Further details of feticide are to be found in Chapter 16.

Complications

Overall, serious complications occur in about 1% of D&E cases [7]. Mortality is rare but is gestational age-dependent. US data from 1988 to 1997 indicate that the rate with abortions performed at 8 weeks or earlier was 0.1 deaths per 100,000 procedures, which increased to 1.7 at 13–15 weeks, 3.4 at 16–20 weeks, and 8.9 deaths per 100,000 abortions at 21 weeks or later [22]. Complications are further considered in Chapter 14.

Cervical laceration

The risk of cervical laceration is variably reported between 0.1 and 1%. The risk is increased with advancing gestational age, operator inexperience, nulliparity and young age; it is reduced by cervical preparation with osmotic dilators. Lacerations or tears of the external os, if large or bleeding, can be sutured immediately. High cervical tears can be associated with concealed bleeding into the broad ligament from the uterine vessels and require further investigations and inpatient monitoring, and may need laparotomy for repair.

Uterine perforation

Perforation of the uterus occurs in 0.2–0.5% of procedures. A perforation may be recognized at the time of the procedure or postoperatively if the woman complains of an unusual amount of pain or bleeding or becomes haemodynamically unstable. Although small perforations during first trimester abortions may be managed conservatively with observation, those occurring with the larger instruments used for D&E typically require exploratory laparotomy and are often associated with bowel injury, haemorrhage and, in some cases, hysterectomy. One retrospective study of an historical cohort, done in a training setting, found that use of intraoperative ultrasound to monitor the position of instruments reduced the rate of perforation from 1.4 to 0.2% [23]. Osmotic dilators also reduce the risk of uterine perforation.

Bleeding

The average blood loss with D&E is between 100 and 400 mL. Haemorrhage is defined as blood loss greater than 500 mL and is encountered in 0.9% of cases. The requirement for transfusion ranges from 0.09 to 0.6%. Excessive blood loss may occur as a result of injury to the uterus or cervix, an incomplete procedure, failure of the uterus to contract adequately, removal of an abnormally implanted placenta or coagulopathy. Atony is the most common cause and massage or uterotonics such as oxytocin, ergot alkaloids and misoprostol are effective treatments. Some operators routinely give prophylactic uterotonics at D&E but this has not been well investigated. One randomized controlled trial demonstrated a statistically significant reduction in blood loss when dilute vasopressin was injected into the cervix with local anaesthetic as part of a paracervical block [24]. Insertion and inflation of a 30 mL Foley catheter in the lower uterine segment can also stem bleeding.

Incomplete abortion

Retained tissue requiring re-aspiration occurs in 0.05 to 1% of D&Es. Women typically present in the days or weeks following their abortion with persistent or heavy bleeding and abdominal pain. Ultrasound is often used to diagnose retained tissue but is not reliable because of the variable appearance of the normal postabortion uterine cavity and can therefore lead to unnecessary intervention. Where it is clinically confirmed, retained tissue can be treated with uterine re-aspiration or with misoprostol.

Infection

Prior to the introduction of routine antibiotic prophylaxis, 0.8% of D&Es in one large case series were associated with febrile complications. Upper genital tract infection following first trimester surgical abortion is reduced by approximately 40% with antibiotic prophylaxis [25]; this benefit is likely to be similar with second trimester surgical abortion but this has not been studied. The optimal regimen has not been determined but both nitro-imidazoles (e.g. metronidazole) and tetracyclines (e.g. doxycycline) are effective [26]. Single- or multiple-dose regimens that cover chlamydia and commensurate vaginal flora are generally chosen. A 'no-touch' technique, which ensures that the tips of instruments never contact non-sterile surfaces before entering the uterus, is also used to reduce the risk of infectious complications.

Long-term sequelae

Some clinicians may be concerned that the amount of artificial dilatation needed to perform D&E may affect the integrity of the internal cervical os resulting in an increased risk of cervical incompetence, miscarriage and preterm birth. Neither retrospective case series nor a case-control study found an association between D&E preceded by cervical preparation with overnight osmotic dilators and future pregnancy complications [27]. However, see Chapter 18 for a general account of surgical abortion and longer-term outcomes.

Postabortion care

Professional guidance generally does not recommend routine follow-up after surgical abortion [14,28] but all patients should be able to arrange a follow-up appointment if desired, and should be given advice to contact the provider of their abortion if they have any concerning symptoms, such as excessive pain, bleeding or fever. See Chapter 12 for a detailed account of follow-up.

Resumption of ovulation occurs within 10–14 days of a surgical abortion. Therefore, initiation of contraception should be facilitated as soon as possible if required. All methods of contraception can be started immediately after D&E, including insertion of progestogen-only subdermal implants and intrauterine devices [14]. Older trials demonstrated significantly higher expulsion rates with IUD insertions immediately after D&E. However, more recent retrospective and prospective studies have shown expulsion rates similar to interval insertion, possibly due to the use of ultrasound guidance. Those studies comparing immediate to delayed insertion have also consistently shown that requiring a woman to return at a later time significantly reduces the likelihood that the intrauterine contraception will ever be inserted [29]. Chapter 13 provides further detail on contraception after abortion.

Conclusion

Dilatation and evacuation is safe, effective and highly acceptable in elective abortion as well as abortion for maternal or fetal indications. In many parts of the world multiple barriers prevent access to D&E. Professional organizations recognize that women requesting abortion should be able to choose between medical and surgical abortion methods [14,28]. Given the evidence that surgical abortion in the second trimester is superior, and preferred by a majority of women, it is incumbent upon providers of women's healthcare to strive to make D&E accessible to all.

References

1. Joffe C. Abortion and medicine: a sociopolitical history. In M Paul, ES Lichtenberg, L Borgatta, et al. (eds.) Management of Unintended and Abnormal Pregnancy: Comprehensive Abortion Care. Oxford: Blackwell Publishing, 2009.

2. Gamble SB, Strauss LT, Parker WY, Cook DA, Zane SB, Hamdan S; Centers for Disease Control and Prevention (CDC). Abortion surveillance – United States, 2005. MMWR Surveill Summ 2008;57:1–32.

3. Lohr PA. Surgical abortion in the second trimester. Reprod Health Matters 2008;16:151–61.

4. Cates W, Schulz KF, Grimes DA, et al. Dilatation and evacuation procedures and second-trimester abortions. The role of physician skill and hospital setting. JAMA 1982;248:559–63.

5. Grimes DA, Schulz KF, Cates W, et al. Mid-trimester abortion by dilatation and evacuation: a safe and practical alternative. NEJM 1977;296:1141–5.

6. Grimes DA, Hulka JF, McCutchen ME. Midtrimester abortion by dilatation and evacuation versus intra-amniotic instillation of prostaglandin F2 alpha: a randomised clinical trial. AJOG 1980;137:785–90.

7. Grossman D, Blanchard K, Blumenthal P. Complications after second trimester surgical and medical abortion. Reprod Health Matters 2008;16:173–82.

8. Kelly T, Suddes J, Howel D, Hewison J, Robson S. Comparing medical versus surgical termination of pregnancy at 13–20 weeks of gestation: a randomized controlled trial. BJOG 2010;117:1512–20.

9. Kaltreider NB, Goldsmith S, Margolis AJ. The impact of midtrimester abortion techniques on patients and staff. AJOG 1979;135:235–8.

10. Burgoine GA, Van Kirk SD, Romm J, et al. Comparison of perinatal grief after dilation and evacuation or labor induction in second trimester terminations for fetal anomalies. AJOG;192:1928–32.

11. Kerns J, Vanjani R, Freedman L, Meckstroth K, Drey EA, Steinauer J.

Women's decision making regarding choice of second trimester termination method for pregnancy complications. *Int J Gynecol Obstet* 2012;116:244–8.

12. Ernst LM, Gawron L, Fritsch MK. Pathologic examination of fetal and placental tissue obtained by dilation and evacuation. *Arch Pathol Lab Med* 2013;137:326–37.

13. Dean G, Jacobs AR, Goldstein RC, Gevirtz CM, Paul ME. The safety of deep sedation without intubation for abortion in the outpatient setting. *J Clin Anesth* 2011;23:437–42.

14. Royal College of Obstetricians and Gynaecologists. *The Care of Women Requesting Induced Abortion*. London: RCOG, 2011.

15. Newmann SJ, Dalve-Endres A, Diedrich JT, Steinauer JE, Meckstroth K, Drey EA. Cervical preparation for second trimester dilation and evacuation. *Cochrane Database Syst Rev* 2010;(8):CD007310.

16. Lyus R, Lohr PA, Taylor J, Morroni C. Outcomes with same-day cervical preparation with Dilapan-S osmotic dilators and vaginal misoprostol before dilatation and evacuation at 18 to 21+6 weeks' gestation. *Contraception* 2013;87:71–5.

17. Borgatta L, Roncari D, Sonalkar S, *et al.* Mifepristone vs. osmotic dilator insertion for cervical preparation prior to surgical abortion at 14–16 weeks: a randomized trial. *Contraception* 2012;86:567–71.

18. Jackson RA, Teplin VL, Drey EA, *et al.* Digoxin to facilitate late second-trimester abortion: a randomized, masked, placebo-controlled trial. *Obstet Gynecol* 2001;97:471–6.

19. Dean G, Colarossi L, Lunde B, Jacobs AR, Porsch LM, Paul ME. Safety of digoxin for fetal demise before second-trimester abortion by dilation and evacuation. *Contraception* 2012;85:144–9.

20. Singh S, Seligman NS, Jackson B, Berghella V. Fetal intracardiac potassium chloride injection to expedite second-trimester dilation and evacuation. *Fetal Diagn Ther* 2012;31:63–8.

21. Coke GA, Baschat AA, Mighty HE, Malinow AM. Maternal cardiac arrest associated with attempted fetal injection of potassium chloride. *Int J Obstet Anesth* 2004;13:287–90.

22. Bartlett LA, Berg CJ, Shulman HB, *et al.* Risk factors for legal induced abortion-related mortality in the United States. *Obstet Gynecol* 2004;103:729–37.

23. Darney PD, Sweet RL. Routine intraoperative ultrasonography for second trimester abortion reduces incidence of uterine perforation. *J Ultrasound Med* 1989;8:71–5.

24. Schulz KF, Grimes DA, Christensen DD. Vasopressin reduces blood loss from second-trimester dilatation and evacuation abortion. *Lancet* 1985;2: 353–6.

25. Sawaya GF, Grady D, Kerlikowske K, Grimes DA. Antibiotics at the time of induced abortion: the case for universal prophylaxis based on a meta-analysis. *Obstet Gynecol* 1996;87:884–90.

26. Achilles SL, Reeves MF; Society of Family Planning. Prevention of infection after induced abortion: release date October 2010: SFP guideline 20102. *Contraception* 2011;83:295–309.

27. Jackson JE, Grobman WA, Haney E, *et al.* Mid-trimester dilation and evacuation with laminaria does not increase the risk for severe subsequent pregnancy complications. *Int J Obstet Gynecol* 2007;96:12–15.

28. World Health Organization. *Safe Abortion: Technical and Policy Guidance for Health Systems*. Geneva: WHO, 2012.

29. Hohmann HL, Reeves MF, Chen BA, Perriera LK, Hayes JL, Creinin MD. Immediate versus delayed insertion of the levonorgestrel-releasing intrauterine device following dilation and evacuation: a randomized controlled trial. *Contraception* 2012;85:240–5.

Pain control

Ellen Wiebe and Regina-Maria Renner

Introduction

Pain management is essential in abortion care. In a random sample of clinics in North America, women undergoing surgical abortion reported a mean pain score of 5.2 with local anaesthesia and 4.7 with procedural sedation, using an 11-point numeric pain scale (0–10) [1]. Providers choose a pain management technique based on efficacy, cost, availability and patient preference. In a survey of 289 North American abortion clinics in 2009 (providing about one-third of all abortions in the USA and Canada), 46% reported using local anaesthesia with oral medications only, 33% used intravenous (IV) sedation and 21% used deep sedation or general anaesthesia [2]. An informal survey of International Federation of Professional Abortion and Contraception Associates (FIAPAC) in 2013 revealed that general anaesthesia and deep sedation are more commonly used in Europe, but it varies from 85% in the UK and Italy to 15% in Spain. The depth of sedation varies with the drugs, doses, route of administration and patient factors such as weight. In this chapter, we will concentrate on the types of pain control used by the abortion provider rather than general anaesthesia provided by an anaesthetist or nurse anaesthetist.

Pain is a complex and individual experience. Recognized components of pain include physical (sensory), psychological (affective, motivational, interpretive), and social (context, support) features and, importantly, their constant interplay. Physical pain is thought to be transmitted via parasympathetic fibres (S2–4), the Frankenhauser plexus that innervates the cervix and the lower uterine segment, and is anaesthetized with local anaesthesia. In addition, the fundus and lower uterine segment are innervated by sympathetic fibres from T10 to L1 via the inferior hypogastric nerve, and the ovarian plexus. The innervations of the endometrium are only poorly understood, and opioid receptors are thought to be few [3]. See Figure 11.1 for an example of local anaesthesia.

Factors associated with increased pain include fewer prior pregnancies, history of dysmenorrhoea, retroverted uterus and pre-procedure anxiety/depression. Less pain has been reported by women with a prior vaginal delivery, shorter operative time and increased provider experience. The impact of gestational age is controversial with some studies reporting more pain in very early and later gestations [4].

For surgical abortion care, all levels of pain management are used, including local anaesthesia with or without oral medications, minimal, moderate or deep procedural sedation, general anaesthesia and non-medication methods. We are using the definitions of

Abortion Care, ed. Sam Rowlands. Published by Cambridge University Press. © Cambridge University Press 2014.

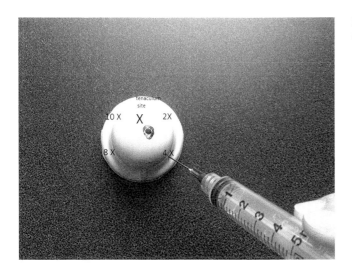

Figure 11.1 Sites for paracervical injection.

depth of sedation in the American Society of Anesthesiologists continuum of sedation (see Table 11.1).

Surgical abortion

Local anaesthesia is a frequently chosen method to decrease procedural pain. In theory, paracervical injection, especially when deep, infiltrates the Frankenhauser plexus and thereby decreases procedural pain. As the anaesthetic does not reach the uterine fundus, analgesia is incomplete.

Amides (e.g. lidocaine, bupivacaine and mepivacaine) are predominantly used, as they have less risk of allergic reaction than esters (e.g. procaine) [5]. According to the manufacturer's guidelines, the lidocaine dose for a healthy person should not exceed 4.5 mg/kg or a total of 300 mg [4]. The most common local anaesthetic used by North American providers is 10–20 mL 1% lidocaine [2]. Its half-life is 1.5–2 hours.

Allergic reactions usually start with erythema and may progress to urticaria, bronchospasm, anaphylaxis and death [3]. Side-effects include lightheadedness, tinnitus, circumoral tingling and metallic taste in the mouth. At a higher serum level muscular twitching, unconsciousness and seizures can occur. Signs of an increasing blood level include hypotension, bradycardia, cardiac arrest and death. Morbidity and mortality from lidocaine toxicity have been reported only infrequently and most were related to doses exceeding 300 mg [4]. Hypersensitivity is rare but can present with the same symptoms. Blood levels can help differentiate between toxicity and hypersensitivity.

Multiple studies have compared different local anaesthetics, techniques of para- or intracervical block or intrauterine administration and additives such as bicarbonate. The following section summarizes the best available data of randomized controlled trials (RCTs). More details can be found in the 2009 Cochrane Review on 'Pain control in first trimester surgical abortion' [4], which included 13 studies (1,961 women) on use of local anaesthesia. A meta-analysis is impossible due to the heterogeneity of the data. Several new studies have been published since then.

Table 11.1 American Society of Anesthesiologists continuum of depth of sedation: definition of general anesthesia and levels of sedation/analgesia*

Committee of origin: Quality Management and Departmental Administration (approved by the ASA House of Delegates on 13 October 1999 and amended on 21 October 2009).

	Minimal sedation/ anxiolysis	Moderate sedation/ analgesia (conscious sedation)	Deep sedation/ analgesia	General anaesthesia
Responsiveness	Normal response to verbal stimulation	Purposeful** response to verbal or tactile stimulation	Purposeful** response following repeated or painful stimulation	Unrousable even with painful stimulus
Airway	Unaffected	No intervention required	Intervention may be required	Intervention often required
Spontaneous ventilation	Unaffected	Adequate	May be inadequate	Frequently inadequate
Cardiovascular function	Unaffected	Usually maintained	Usually maintained	May be impaired

Minimal sedation (anxiolysis) is a drug-induced state during which patients respond normally to verbal commands. Although cognitive function and physical coordination may be impaired, airway reflexes, and ventilatory and cardiovascular functions are unaffected.

Moderate sedation/analgesia (conscious sedation) is a drug-induced depression of consciousness during which patients respond purposefully** to verbal commands, either alone or accompanied by light tactile stimulation. No interventions are required to maintain a patent airway and spontaneous ventilation is adequate. Cardiovascular function is usually maintained.

*Monitored anaesthesia care does not describe the continuum of depth of sedation, rather it describes 'a specific anesthesia service in which an anesthesiologist has been requested to participate in the care of a patient undergoing a diagnostic or therapeutic procedure'.

**Reflex withdrawal from a painful stimulus is NOT considered a purposeful response.

Source: www.asahq.org/For-Members/Standards-Guidelines-and-Statements.aspx.

Local anaesthesia compared to placebo or no intervention

A paracervical block (PCB) with 20 mL 1% buffered lidocaine deeply (2–3 cm) injected at five sites (12 o'clock intracervical, and 2, 4, 8, 10 o'clock paracervical, see Figure 11.1) significantly decreased cervical dilatation pain and uterine aspiration pain compared to a sham-PCB in non-sedated patients [6]. In sedated patients the effect of a PCB or cervical block compared to no intervention was non-significant. Chloroprocaine has been found superior to normal saline, while in a lower quality study, 1% buffered lidocaine did not differ from normal saline. Distension was thought to have an analgesic effect, but there was no non-intervention arm to verify an effect of either study arm [4].

Local anaesthetics and additives for PCB

Buffered lidocaine was superior to plain lidocaine, while no difference was shown between 0.5% lidocaine and 1% lidocaine as well as 1% lidocaine and 0.25% bupivacaine [4]. Ropivacaine is a new analgesic product with possibly fewer side-effects. It decreased aspiration pain compared to 1% lidocaine [7]. Adding ketorolac, a potent non-steroidal anti-inflammatory drug (NSAID), to 1% lidocaine decreased dilatation pain, but not aspiration pain [8]. Vasopressin is added by many providers to achieve vasoconstriction and decrease procedural blood loss; especially in the second trimester [2,9].

Injection technique
Deep injection (3 cm) has been shown to more effectively decrease dilatation and aspiration pain than superficial injection. Two- versus four-site injection as well as a wait time between injection and cervical dilatation have not been clearly shown to be beneficial. However, slow injection (60 seconds) decreased pain with PCB administration compared to fast injection [4].

Injection site
Cervical versus paracervical injection has not been shown to make a difference [10]; however, data are limited and a possible difference might be masked by IV sedation in one of the studies. Four per cent intrauterine lidocaine decreased dilatation and aspiration pain compared to intrauterine normal saline [4].

Adjunct medications
Pre-procedure medications used in surgical abortion care include anti-anxiety medications, analgesics and cervical ripening agents. The NSAID ibuprofen is one of the most frequently used medications. Ibuprofen 600 mg and naproxen 550 mg one to two hours pre-procedure have been shown to improve pain scores [4]. Oral paracetamol (acetaminophen)/hydrocodone has been shown not to decrease pain [11]. Pre-procedure use of 1 mg lorazepam has not been shown to improve pain scores [4]. In first trimester abortions, misoprostol has been shown to shorten procedure time and difficulty of dilatation but not to improve pain scores [12].

Procedural sedation: safety, effectiveness
Moderate IV sedation, previously called conscious sedation, is a drug-induced depression of consciousness, during which the patient responds purposefully to verbal commands or tactile stimulation and adequately maintains ventilation and usually also cardiovascular function. As there is a continuum to deep sedation, which might require support of the airway, moderate IV sedation should only be offered by skilled providers and in a setting allowing airway management if needed.

Commonly used medications are narcotics, such as fentanyl, and benzodiazepines, such as midazolam; both have a rapid onset of action when given IV with half-lives of 3.7 and 2.5 hours respectively. North American abortion providers use minimal or moderate sedation with IV fentanyl (50–200 µg) and midazolam (1–3 mg) [2].

Adding IV fentanyl (50–100 µg) alone as well as in combination with diazepam to a PCB decreased pain compared to a PCB alone in several RCTs [4]. Women reported increased dizziness and drowsiness, but no difference in nausea. Another RCT compared adding only 25 µg fentanyl and 2 mg midazolam versus placebo to a PCB and found increased satisfaction but no difference in pain scores [4]. IV fentanyl 100 µg and midazolam 2 mg decreased pain compared to oral oxycodone 10 mg and sublingual lorazepam 1 mg in women who all received a PCB [13].

General anaesthesia

General anaesthesia (GA) is usually not provided by the abortion provider, but by staff trained in anaesthesia as it involves airway management. Therefore, we will not discuss associated medications in detail in this chapter.

Deep IV sedation, on the continuum to GA, is a drug-induced depression of consciousness (see Table 11.1 for details). Patients cannot be easily roused but respond purposefully following repeated or painful stimulation. The ability to maintain respirations may be impaired and patients may require assistance.

GA is a drug-induced depression of consciousness. Patients are not rousable even by painful stimulation and often require ventilatory assistance or positive pressure ventilation. Cardiovascular function may be impaired.

Regimens studied included combinations of inhalational agents and IV agents propofol, etomidate, midazolam, fentanyl, alfentanil, thiopental, ketamine and methohexital. The most common outpatient regimen is propofol and fentanyl with or without midazolam (total IV anaesthesia). Studies have shown that propofol is superior to ketamine, which has been associated with increased pain and more side-effects (dreams, hallucinations) [4]. The most common pain control used in Europe and Australia is deep sedation with IV propofol (100–200 mg) and fentanyl (50–100 μg) with or without midazolam (2.5–5 mg); nitrous oxide is used rarely (informal survey of FIAPAC members).

Postoperative pain can be decreased by adding IV narcotics such as fentanyl and nalbuphine. Oral or rectal paracetamol or narcotic have not been shown to be beneficial [9]. Studies have shown that adding a 10 mL PCB to GA does not decrease postoperative pain [4,14]. However, one study compared GA (alfentanil and propofol) versus moderate sedation (midazolam 0.1 mg/kg and alfentanil 0.01 mg/kg) with a PCB (mepivacaine 20 mL with adrenaline). Postoperative pain was lower in the sedation/PCB group [4]. Postoperative pain when adding various NSAIDs to GA has been studied: lornoxicam (8 mg by mouth 1 h preoperatively) was found to be superior to paracetamol (1 g by mouth 1 h preoperatively). While oral diclofenac 50 mg given 10–20 minutes pre-anaesthesia was not more effective than placebo, intramuscular (IM) diclofenac 75 mg as well as IM ketorolac 30 mg given 10–20 min pre-anaesthesia were more effective than placebo or oral diclofenac.

Non-pharmacological pain management

Although women who are more anxious experience more pain [4], it is not clear how best to reduce anxiety and how much reducing anxiety reduces pain. A randomized trial of hypnotic suggestion showed reduced IV sedation and nitrous oxide use during abortion and increased satisfaction. The amount of time and training required by staff in that study would not be feasible for most abortion clinics. The use of IV anxiolytics clearly reduces anxiety, but a randomized placebo trial of 1 mg of sublingual lorazepam showed no effect on anxiety or pain scores. The same study showed that if women knew they were taking the lorazepam, they did have a reduction in anxiety, showing the benefit of placebo [4]. Music has been associated with decreased pain in some studies and no difference in others [4,15]. Randomized trials are not always the best method to pinpoint exactly what works best to reduce anxiety, because all the confounders such as personality of clinicians and ambience of the clinic cannot be controlled for. Experienced providers understand that 'vocal anaesthesia' works well and use a combination or choice of various methods such as distraction (talking about her last vacation), guided imagery ('imagine yourself at the beach on a sunny day'), deep slow breathing, progressive relaxation, music, low lighting and humour.

Medical abortions

First trimester

The proportion of first trimester abortions induced with medication (versus surgical aspiration) varies around the world: about 30% in the UK, 20% in the USA, 70% in Portugal, 15% in Spain, 55% France, etc. (informal survey of FIAPAC members).

A majority of women require analgesia [9]. The most common medication used for pain is ibuprofen, which has been shown to decrease pain and further analgesic use without decreasing efficacy [16]. A systematic review of pain control in first and second trimester medical abortion showed that in the first trimester, prophylactic paracetamol (acetaminophen), paracetamol with codeine, or alverine (an antispasmodic) did not reduce pain [16].

The pain experienced during medical abortion varies with the dose and timing of the misoprostol; in two studies comparing different misoprostol doses and timing after mifepristone, 400 µg was less painful than 600 µg, 600 µg was less painful than 800 µg and three doses of 800 µg within 24 h were more painful than when used 24 h apart. More pain was experienced with higher gestational ages. The mean worst pain score women reported was about 6/10 with a range from 0 to 10. Narcotics, such as codeine and oxycodone, are also used. Information is important to help women cope with the pain using medications appropriately as well as non-pharmacological methods such as heat [16].

Second and third trimester induction

Pain associated with induction in the second trimester increases with gestational age. As noted above, pain tolerance varies substantially between women.

The same analgesics as used in first trimester medical abortion should be considered, including oral NSAIDs or narcotics. Additional analgesic options are IV medications, either as individual doses that can be repeated or as a patient-controlled analgesia (PCA). Commonly, morphine or hydromorphone are used, especially for a PCA. One study showed that a fentanyl (50 µg) PCA resulted in higher satisfaction and pain relief than a fentanyl (25 µg) or morphine PCA. Individual doses of NSAIDs such as ketorolac can be given. Diclofenac given with the first dose of misoprostol has been shown to decrease subsequent opioid analgesia requirements in women at 15 weeks' gestation or above without interfering with the misoprostol efficacy. This effect was not seen with paracetamol/codeine [16]. Data on the benefit of metoclopramide are conflicting. A PCB has been shown to decrease pain [16]. Depending on the resources available, some women might prefer an epidural or spinal analgesia. In a French survey of second and third trimester induction abortions, epidural or more rarely combined spinal-epidural analgesia was performed in more than 90% of cases [17]. Few studies have compared different analgesic regimens and an effective treatment of pain is not well established [3]. A wide range of oral and parenteral analgesics should be available [9].

Non-pharmacological support should be considered as well and has been described above.

Conclusions

In summary, pain management is a central aspect of providing abortion services, surgical and medical, and a range of options is available. As Figure 11.2 depicts, selection of

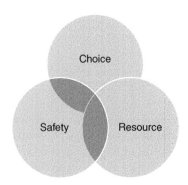

Figure 11.2 Choice of pain management.

pain management should be informed by individual choice, safety concerns and available resources and their interplay. Safety is affected by co-morbidities and free-standing clinic versus hospital setting. Resources are determined for example by equipment, personnel and cost. Pain management is included in documents and guidelines published by organizations such as the World Health Organization (www.who.int/reproductivehealth/publications), UK Royal College of Obstetricians and Gynaecologists [9], the National Abortion Federation (www.prochoice.org/about_abortion/index.html) and the Society for Family Planning (www.societyfp.org) for readers who wish to undertake further study.

References

1. Rawling MJ, Wiebe ER. Pain control in abortion clinics. *Int J Gynecol Obstet* 1998;60:293–5.

2. O'Connell K, Jones HE, Simon M, Saporta V, Paul M, Lichtenberg ES. First-trimester surgical abortion practices: a survey of National Abortion Federation members. *Contraception* 2009;79:385–92.

3. Paul M, Lichtenberg ES, Borgatta L, Grimes DA, Stubblefield PG (eds.) *Management of Unintended and Abnormal Pregnancy*. Chichester: Wiley-Blackwell, 2009.

4. Renner RM, Jensen JT, Nichols MD, Edelman A. Pain control in first trimester surgical abortion. *Cochrane Database Syst Rev* 2009:CD006712.

5. Nichols MD, Halvorson-Boyd G, Goldstein R, Gevirtz C, Healow D. Pain management. In M Paul, ES Lichtenberg, L Borgatta, DA Grimes, PG Stubblefield, (eds.) *Management of Unintended and Abnormal Pregnancy*. Chichester: Wiley-Blackwell, 2009: 90–110.

6. Renner RM, Nichols MD, Jensen JT, Li H, Edelman AB. Paracervical block for pain control in first-trimester surgical abortion:

   a randomized controlled trial. *Obstet Gynecol* 2012;119:1030–7.

7. Agostini A, Provansal M, Collette E, *et al.* Comparison of ropivacaine and lidocaine for paracervical block during surgical abortion. *Contraception* 2008;77:382–5.

8. Cansino C, Edelman A, Burke A, Jamshidi R. Paracervical block with combined ketorolac and lidocaine in first-trimester surgical abortion: a randomized controlled trial. *Obstet Gynecol* 2009;114:1220–6.

9. Royal College of Obstetricians and Gynaecologists. *The Care of Women Requesting Induced Abortion*. London: RCOG Press, 2011. www.rcog.org.uk/files/rcog-corp/Abortion%20guideline_web_1.pdf (accessed 1 March 2013).

10. Owolabi OT, Moodley J. A randomized trial of pain relief in termination of pregnancy in South Africa. *Trop Doct* 2005;35:136–9.

11. Micks EA, Edelman AB, Renner RM, *et al.* Hydrocodone-acetaminophen for pain control in first-trimester surgical abortion: a randomized controlled trial. *Obstet Gynecol* 2012;120:1060–9.

12. Kapp N, Lohr PA, Ngo TD, Hayes JL. Cervical preparation for first trimester surgical abortion. *Cochrane Database Syst Rev* 2010:CD007207.

13. Allen RH, Fitzmaurice G, Lifford KL, Lasic M, Goldberg AB. Oral compared with intravenous sedation for first-trimester surgical abortion: a randomized controlled trial. *Obstet Gynecol* 2009;113:276–83.

14. Lazenby GB, Fogelson NS, Aeby T. Impact of paracervical block on postabortion pain in patients undergoing abortion under general anesthesia. *Contraception* 2009;80:578–82.

15. Wu J, Chaplin W, Amico J, *et al.* Music for surgical abortion care study: a randomized controlled pilot study. *Contraception* 2012;85:496–502.

16. Jackson E, Kapp N. Pain control in first-trimester and second-trimester medical termination of pregnancy: a systematic review. *Contraception* 2011;83:116–26.

17. Dubar G, Benhamou D. Anesthesiologists' practices for late termination of pregnancy: a French national survey. *Int J Obstet Anesth* 2010;19:395–400.

Chapter

12

Follow-up

Sharon Cameron

Introduction

A routine follow-up visit with a healthcare provider at two to three weeks used to be considered an integral part of abortion care and an opportunity to confirm successful abortion, detect any complications of the procedure (e.g. infection, retained products of conception) and ensure that effective contraception had been commenced (and, if not, to discuss contraceptive methods and prescribe or administer the chosen method). It was also perceived as an important opportunity to discuss the woman's emotional wellbeing and arrange further psychological counselling or support, as required. However, with the high efficacy and safety of modern medical and surgical methods of inducing an abortion, the increasing emphasis on the importance of commencing effective contraception immediately after abortion, and the consistent evidence that abortion does not have adverse effects upon mental health, it is clear that a follow-up is no longer necessary for all women. What does need to be considered is under what circumstances is follow-up necessary after abortion. And what should that follow-up consist of?

Confirmation of successful abortion

The incidence of a continuing pregnancy following a surgical abortion is rare at approximately 2.3 per 1,000 cases [1]. At vacuum aspiration, the operator can visualize the products of conception and so further follow-up to exclude a continuing pregnancy (or an ectopic pregnancy, if this has not been excluded at the preabortion assessment) is only required in those cases where products have not been clearly observed. Likewise, if a woman is having a medical abortion in a clinic or hospital setting, passage of the pregnancy can be confirmed by the clinician, with follow-up reserved for those cases where products of conception have not be visualized. In most countries where early medical abortion with mifepristone and misoprostol is available, women can choose to receive the medication and pass the pregnancy at home. The incidence of continuing pregnancy is uncommon with regimens using mifepristone and misoprostol: in the region of 0.5–1% [1].

In view of this the UK Royal College of Obstetricians and Gynaecologists (RCOG) in their evidence-based guideline on abortion state that routine follow-up is no longer necessary after an uncomplicated surgical or medical abortion, where products of conception have been visualized [1]. This viewpoint has also been endorsed by the World Health Organization (WHO) in their guidance *Safe Abortion: Technical and Policy Guidance for Health Systems* [2].

Abortion Care, ed. Sam Rowlands. Published by Cambridge University Press. © Cambridge University Press 2014.

Confirmation of the success of the procedure is important, since the consequences of a continuing pregnancy could mean that the woman would need to have a further abortion procedure at a higher gestation (if within the legal limit) or that a continuing pregnancy would have been exposed to the uncertain effects of abortifacient drugs.

How to exclude a continuing pregnancy

Whilst a routine ultrasound at a follow-up clinic visit after abortion will reliably exclude a continuing pregnancy, ultrasound equipment is costly, requires the availability of skilled staff and so limits the settings in which this can be provided to women. A disadvantage of routine postabortion ultrasound is that the identification of ultrasonically visible, but clinically unimportant, blood clot/tissue within the uterus may lead inexperienced providers to institute unnecessary medical or surgical intervention [3].

Furthermore, observational studies have shown that as many as 50% of women do not attend this follow-up clinic visit, which is wasteful in terms of staffing resources [3]. There is also evidence that the need for this 'extra visit' may deter women from choosing a medical method in the first place, particularly those women who live at a distance from the clinic [4]. It is also possible that returning for a follow-up to the service where the woman had her abortion may be distressing for some.

Alternative modalities to ultrasound for detecting continuing pregnancy after early medical abortion that have been tested have included women's self-assessment, clinician assessment, serum human chorionic gonadotrophin (hCG) measurement both pre and post treatment, and urine pregnancy testing (Table 12.1). In a systematic review, a woman's self-assessment of continuing pregnancy following medical abortion was found to be fairly accurate compared to ultrasound examination or clinician assessment, but less accurate at gestations over 50 days when continuing pregnancy is unfortunately more likely [5].

With early medical abortion, serum hCG falls dramatically (70%) within 24 hours of misoprostol administration and then declines more gradually [6]. By two weeks after medical abortion hCG levels are reduced by 99%. In a study of women at less than seven weeks' gestation, a fall in hCG (by 6–18 days after mifepristone) of less than 20% of the pre-treatment value, strongly predicted a continuing pregnancy [7]. However, serum hCG requires a visit to a provider or laboratory, the discomfort of venepuncture and interpretation by a clinician. It is also time-consuming. In addition, the studies that have assessed the accuracy of serum hCG in detecting failed medical abortion have been limited by the inherent high success rate of medical abortion and the small numbers of continuing pregnancies [5].

In contrast, the use of simple, cheap 'qualitative' urinary pregnancy tests to screen women who may have a continuing pregnancy appears promising. Studies have been conducted using both low sensitivity urine pregnancy tests (LSUP) with typical detection thresholds of around 1,000 mIU/mL and high sensitivity urine pregnancy tests (HSUP) with typical detection thresholds around 25 mIU/mL. A large US study of more than 3,000 women attending a clinic after early medical abortion for an assessment at two weeks that included a routine ultrasound, questions on duration of bleeding and presence of pregnancy symptoms and an LSUP evaluated different algorithms that could best predict continuing pregnancy [8]. Although the study showed that use of an LSUP on its own would not have detected all the continuing pregnancies, a combination of self/clinician assessment and LSUP did identify all continuing pregnancies.

Table 12.1 Advantages and disadvantages of alternative methods of detecting continuing pregnancy after early abortion

	Advantages	Disadvantages
Ultrasound	• Reliably excludes continuing pregnancy • Can be performed any time after pregnancy expulsion	• Equipment costly • Trained staff needed to conduct • May lead to unnecessary intervention for ultrasonically visible but clinically unimportant retained tissue • Requires further clinic visit for woman
Serum hCG monitoring	• Validated for <7 weeks' gestation • May be used 1–2 weeks after treatment • Can be performed remotely at another clinic or laboratory	• Needs pre- and post-treatment samples • Invasive • Clinician to interpret • Time-consuming
Qualitative urine pregnancy test (and telephone call* to ask about bleeding, signs and symptoms of pregnancy*)	• HSUP test widely available and cheap • LSUP test can be performed at 2 weeks • Women can perform this themselves at home • Cheap	• HSUP test cannot performed before one month • LSUP not widely available • Needs to be performed correctly
Semi-quantitative urine hCG test	• May be used one week after treatment • Women could possibly perform this themselves at home	• Needs pre- and post-treatment samples • Not widely available • Needs to be performed correctly • Not yet fully evaluated for home use

*Ongoing research to determine if this may be replaced by text messaging, or asking the woman to call provider if a concern.

HSUP test = high sensitivity urinary pregnancy test; LSUP test = low sensitivity urinary pregnancy test.

A study from the UK determined women's views (n = 258) on alternative methods of follow-up [9]. Women stated a theoretical preference for performing a urinary pregnancy test themselves at home rather than attend a clinic for this or attend a clinic for an ultrasound. The main reasons women gave for this preference were that it would be more convenient for them, less stressful and would avoid another visit to the clinic. Following on from this, a simplified follow-up regimen for women who chose to go home to expel the pregnancy after receiving treatment for early medical abortion (mifepristone/misoprostol) was developed and evaluated in the UK. This consisted of women performing their own LSUP test at home two weeks after treatment with a telephone call from clinic staff to ask about the result of the LSUP test and questions about bleeding duration and quantity and any persisting pregnancy symptoms [9]. Women who screened 'positive' on the basis of a positive LSUP test, scant bleeding or persisting pregnancy symptoms then attended a clinic for an ultrasound scan to confirm/exclude continuing pregnancy. The investigators reported that a combination of telephone call and LSUP test at two weeks had a high negative predictive value (NPV 99.7%; 95% CI 98.4–99.9) for detecting continuing pregnancy. Only 10% of women in this study screened positive and were required to attend a clinic [9]. The authors concluded that this simplified follow-up regimen was feasible and likely to be a cost-effective alternative to providing a routine follow-up visit with ultrasound for all women [9]. The authors also highlighted how no test is perfect and that even if the LSUP is negative, women should still have a clinic review if they had scant bleeding, signs/symptoms of continuing pregnancy or absence of the next period after treatment. Data from the same centre of a larger series of almost 1,000 women having this method of follow-up has confirmed these findings [10]. In a smaller study of telephone follow-up from the USA that involved women (n = 139) performing an HSUP test themselves at home at one month after treatment (mifepristone/misoprostol regimen), one-third of women 'screened positive' with the telephone call/HSUP test and were required to attend a clinic to confirm complete abortion [11]. Whilst some providers might prefer to perform the telephone follow-up at one month, using the widely available and cheap HSUP test, rather than a two-week follow-up with an LSUP test, there is evidence that women would prefer a pregnancy test at two weeks rather than waiting until four weeks after the procedure to know the outcome of treatment [9].

Other areas of ongoing research include the use of self-performed urine pregnancy tests in combination with the use of mobile phone technology such as SMS/texting as an alternative to a clinic visit. Simplifying the follow-up even further to eliminate the routine telephone call to women, i.e. the woman takes responsibility for contacting the abortion service if there is concern, is another avenue of research. In the UK study of telephone follow-up, just over one-half of respondents felt they would have been likely to choose self-assessment (i.e. to perform the LSUP test without a telephone call from the service) and only contact the abortion service if there was a problem, if this had been an option [9]. Preliminary findings from an observational study from the UK of self-assessment using an LSUP test at home in combination with clear written and pictorial advice (Figure 12.1) about what signs/symptoms are suggestive of failed abortion are now available [12]. These show that this self-assessment option is chosen by the majority of women and that only a few women contact the service with concerns; those that make contact with a complication do so promptly and appropriately. This demonstrates that a significant proportion of women do feel capable and comfortable with taking more responsibility themselves for their treatment and verification of the success of this procedure.

Another promising alternative to the qualitative urine pregnancy tests (LSUP or HSUP) is a semi-quantitative urine pregnancy test that is performed at the time of medical abortion and one week later; it appears highly predictive in screening for continuing pregnancy [13]. A large study to determine the feasibility of women performing and interpreting these more complicated (and costly) tests themselves in a home setting is therefore required.

Detection of complications

Complications following safely performed medical and surgical methods of abortion are rare; less than 1% of women have serious abortion-related complications [1]. In a recent study from the UK that was a retrospective review of over 1,000 women having early medical abortion, only 4% of women had to make an unscheduled attendance to the abortion service for a complication related to the procedure [14]. This re-attendance rate did not differ between women who chose to go home to expel the pregnancy and those who remained on a hospital ward to pass the pregnancy. Most attendances were due to pain and/or bleeding and most were not serious and required oral antibiotic treatment only. There were three cases of haemorrhage (0.3% of women) that occurred at 0, 8 and 11 days after mifepristone respectively. This highlighted how the time-course of a 'traditional' routine follow-up consultation at two to three weeks would have been too late to detect or prevent these serious

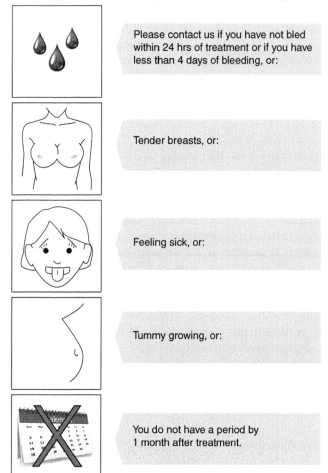

Even if your pregnancy test is negative, please remember you might still be pregnant if you have any of the following

Please contact us if you have not bled within 24 hrs of treatment or if you have less than 4 days of bleeding, or:

Tender breasts, or:

Feeling sick, or:

Tummy growing, or:

You do not have a period by 1 month after treatment.

Figure 12.1 Pictoral information to alert women to signs/symptoms that might be indicative of a continuing pregnancy after early medical abortion (courtesy of Dr Sharon Cameron, University of Edinburgh).

complications. Rather than arranging to review women (who may not have any problems and fail to attend), both the RCOG and WHO advise that women should be provided with information on signs/symptoms suggestive of a complication (heavy bleeding, fever) and where to go to seek medical care in such circumstances [1,2].

Contraception

Health professionals often underestimate a woman's need for contraception in the immediate postabortion period. There is good evidence that most women ovulate in the month following abortion and so are at risk of another pregnancy if they resume sexual intercourse [1]. There is evidence that 50% of women have resumed sexual activity by two weeks postabortion and that as many as 15% have resumed intercourse within one week of mifepristone [15]. Rather than waiting for a follow-up visit to commence contraception both the RCOG and WHO advise that hormonal methods can be started immediately [1,2]. This does, however, mean that contraception be discussed with women at presentation for abortion. This is also an important opportunity to provide accurate information to women and dispel any misconceptions about contraception that they may have, particularly about the most effective methods such as the intrauterine method and contraceptive implant [16]. Contrary to concerns that women may be too distressed or overloaded with information to consider contraception, it has been shown that women value the opportunity to have a discussion about future contraception at this time [17].

For women who choose to have a surgical method both the intrauterine system (IUS) and the intrauterine device (IUD) can safely be inserted intraoperatively [18]. This is convenient for the women and avoids another vaginal examination at a later date. There is also global evidence that women who choose to have immediate insertion of an IUD/IUS have a significantly reduced risk of having another abortion [18]. For women who choose to have a medical method of abortion, the IUD/IUS can be inserted when it is reasonably certain they are no longer pregnant [1,2]. There is good evidence that delaying the insertion after medical abortion constitutes a barrier to uptake of the IUD/IUS and that uptake rates are higher if this appointment for insertion is scheduled for as soon as possible after the medical procedure [15]. In view of this, it might be appropriate to offer women a temporary 'bridging' method of contraception until they can have the IUD/IUS inserted.

There is also evidence that women who choose to have immediate insertion of a contraceptive implant at the time of abortion (surgical or medical) have a significantly reduced risk of having another abortion within the next two years [18]. In a British study women who chose immediate insertion of an implant were 16 times less likely to have another abortion within two years than women choosing an oral contraceptive pill [19].

Health professionals may be concerned that hormonal methods will have an adverse effect upon postabortion bleeding patterns. However, it has been shown that the combined oral contraceptive pill does not affect the duration of bleeding after medical abortion [19]. Furthermore, it has also been shown that women who opt for an IUS at surgical abortion or soon after early medical abortion may benefit from the reduction in days of heavy bleeding at this time [15].

Further details on contraception after abortion can be found in Chapter 13.

Emotional wellbeing

Although support and reassurance may be appreciated by some women, studies show that most women who terminate a pregnancy are certain of their decision and do not experience serious regret [20]. Furthermore, several studies have reported that for most women measures of depression and anxiety are lower after abortion compared to just prior to the procedure [20]. This would suggest that it is the state of being pregnant with an unwanted pregnancy itself that is stressful for many women and that this is reduced once the decision to terminate has been agreed and the procedure has been completed [20].

Rather than arranging routine follow-up for all women to determine emotional wellbeing, information should be provided beforehand for women on pathways to further support or counselling if required after the procedure [1]. In addition, clinicians should try to identify those women with risk factors (such as pre-existing mental health problems) who may require more support after the abortion and ensure that they know how to access support and therapeutic counselling if required [1] (see also Chapter 5).

Conclusions

There is no medical need for routine follow-up after an uncomplicated medical or surgical abortion, assuming that successful abortion has been confirmed at the time of the procedure, that the woman has information on when and where to seek care for complications and has received an ongoing method of contraception. For those women for whom success of the procedure has not been confirmed (usually an early medical abortion) then exclusion of a continuing pregnancy is required. There is growing evidence that a simple urinary pregnancy test performed by the woman herself at home, coupled with simple instructions on signs/symptoms of continuing pregnancy and possibly combined with a telephone call, can replace an in-person visit to a clinic in most cases. Avoiding additional routine clinic visits is more convenient for women and reduces travel, time off work and child care costs. Fewer routine follow-up visits will also have benefits for the abortion service by reducing the disruptions to clinical activity that are incurred from high failure-to-attend rates.

All women should, however, be provided with high quality information on the signs/symptoms indicative of a complication (such as increasing pelvic pain, heavy bleeding and fever) that would warrant urgent medical attention.

In addition, abortion providers should offer the most effective methods of contraception to women on the day of the abortion procedure (where appropriate) and provide information for women who choose not to start a method immediately about the availability of local contraceptive services. Women should also be given information on where further emotional support/therapeutic counselling is available if required after the abortion.

References

1. Royal College of Obstetricians and Gynaecologists. *The Care of Women Requesting Induced Abortion. Guideline Number 7.* 2011. www.rcog.org.uk/files/rcog-corp/Abortion guideline_web_1.pdf (accessed 4 January 2013).

2. World Health Organization. *Safe Abortion: Technical and Policy Guidance for Health Systems,* 2nd edn. 2012. www.who.int/reproductivehealth/publications/unsafe_abortion/9789241548434/en/ (accessed 20 February 2013).

3. Grossman D, Ellertson C, Grimes DA, Walker D. Routine follow-up visits after first-trimester induced abortion. *Obstet Gynecol* 2004;103:738–45.

4. Cameron ST, Glasier AF, Logan J et al. Impact of the introduction of new medical methods on therapeutic abortions at the Royal Infirmary of Edinburgh. *Br J Obstet Gynaecol* 1996;103:1222–9.

5. Grossman D, Grindlay K. Alternatives to ultrasound for follow-up after medication abortion: a systematic review. *Contraception* 2011;83:504–10.

6. Honkanen H, Ranta S, Ylikorkala O, et al. The kinetics of serum hCG and progesterone in response to oral and vaginal administration of misoprostol during medical termination of early pregnancy. *Hum Reprod* 2002;17:2315–19.

7. Fiala C, Safar P, Bygdeman M, et al. Verifying the effectiveness of medical abortion; ultrasound versus hCG testing. *Eur J Obstet Gynecol Reprod Biol* 2003;109:190–5.

8. Clark W, Bracken H, Tanenhaus J, et al. Alternatives to a routine follow-up visit for early medical abortion. *Obstet Gynecol* 2010;115:264–72.

9. Cameron ST, Glasier A, Dewart H, et al. Telephone follow-up and self-performed urine pregnancy testing after early medical abortion: a service evaluation. *Contraception* 2012;86:67–73.

10. Michie L, Cameron ST. Simplified follow-up after early medical termination: 12-month experience of a telephone call and self-performed low-sensitivity urine pregnancy test. *Contraception* 2014;89:440–5.

11. Perriera LK, Reeves MF, Chen BA, *et al.* Feasibility of telephone follow-up after medical abortion. *Contraception* 2010;81:143–9.

12. Cameron S, Glasier A, Dewart H, *et al.* Self assessment of success of early medical termination of pregnancy: a service evaluation. *BJOG* 2012;119: Issue Supplement s2, P8.07.

13. Blum J, Shochet T, Lynd K, *et al.* Can at-home semi-quantitative pregnancy tests serve as a replacement for clinical follow-up of medical abortion? A US study. *Contraception* 2012;86:757–62.

14. Astle H, Cameron ST, Johnstone A. Comparison of unscheduled re-attendance and contraception at discharge, among women having the final stage of early medical abortion at home and those remaining in hospital. *J Fam Plann Reprod Health Care* 2012;38:35–40.

15. Sääv I, Stephansson O, Gemzell-Danielsson K. Early versus delayed insertion of intrauterine contraception after medical abortion – a randomized controlled trial. *PLoS One* 2012;7:e48948.

16. Michie L, Cameron ST, Glasier A, *et al.* Myths and misconceptions about intrauterine contraception among women seeking termination of pregnancy. *J Fam Plann Reprod Health Care* 2014;40:36–40.

17. Powell-Jackson R, Glasier A, Cameron ST. Benefits of using a digital video disk for providing information about abortion to women requesting termination of pregnancy *Contraception* 2010;81:537–41.

18. Steenland MW, Tepper NK, Curtis KM, *et al.* Intrauterine contraceptive insertion postabortion: a systematic review. *Contraception* 2011;84:447–64.

19. Cameron ST, Glasier A, Chen ZE, Johnstone A, Dunlop C, Heller R. Effect of contraception provided at termination of pregnancy and incidence of subsequent termination of pregnancy. *BJOG* 2012;119:1074–80.

20. Cameron S. Induced abortion and psychological sequelae. *Best Practice & Research Clinical Obstetrics & Gynaecology* 2010;24:657–65.

Chapter

13

Contraception after abortion

Oskari Heikinheimo, Satu Suhonen and
Pekka Lähteenmäki

Introduction

The highest rates of unplanned pregnancy and induced abortion in many European countries, as well as globally, are seen among 20- to 29-year-old women [1]. Besides high fecundity and sexual activity in this age group, the high rate of abortion may also reflect the fact that these women are in the process of gaining their own independence, are often in the middle of their studies and economically in an unstable situation.

When planning postabortion contraception it is important to appreciate that these women have demonstrated their fertility. In some cases there will have been problems with contraceptive adherence [2]. Thus an effective contraceptive method with minimal user-dependence is likely to be the most cost-effective.

In many developing countries, clandestine abortions still constitute a major cause of maternal morbidity and mortality, especially in those countries in which the abortion law is restrictive. Even though global abortion-related mortality is on the decline, an estimated 13% of all maternal mortality continues to be attributable to unsafe abortion. This makes unsafe abortion the second commonest single cause of maternal death (haemorrhage being the first) [3]. For women living in these parts of the world, prevention of further unwanted pregnancy and abortion is therefore of the utmost importance.

Optimizing postabortion contraception as regards both contraceptive methods offered as well as service provision has become a major issue in recent years. Also, the importance of postabortion contraception as a key component in family planning has recently been endorsed by several global advocates of female reproductive health including the International Federation of Gynecology and Obstetrics (FIGO), International Confederation of Midwives (ICM) and United States Agency for International Development (USAID) [4].

Usually only the effects of postabortion contraception on future reproductive health outcomes (such as risk of subsequent abortion) are highlighted. The overall effect of contraceptive options on various health, quality of life and cost-benefit outcomes in different healthcare settings has traditionally received little research attention.

This chapter reviews the return of pituitary-ovarian axis function after induced abortion, the safety and efficacy of reversible postabortion contraceptive options as well as their recommended time of initiation following both surgical and medical abortion. Special emphasis is given to the efficacy of long-acting reversible contraceptives (LARCs) as postabortion contraception.

Abortion Care, ed. Sam Rowlands. Published by Cambridge University Press. © Cambridge University Press 2014.

Return of ovulation after abortion

A continuing pregnancy suppresses the secretion of pituitary gonadotrophins and ovarian steroids. In early pregnancy the production of pituitary luteinizing hormone (LH) is replaced by the production of placental human chorionic gonadotrophin (hCG), and follicle stimulating hormone (FSH) secretion becomes completely suppressed. The developing placenta gradually starts to take over the production of estradiol and progesterone around the seventh week of pregnancy.

After surgical abortion, with rapid removal of the placenta, plasma levels of estradiol and progesterone fall rapidly within a few days followed by a more gradual elimination within a period of about a week [5]. The disappearance of circulating hCG occurs in several phases. The initial half-life of hCG is rapid, less than 20 h following both surgical and medical abortion. However, the total elimination of hCG takes an average of 37 days after termination of a first trimester pregnancy. This means that a sensitive pregnancy test remains positive after a successful abortion and can be positive even after a first postabortion menstrual period.

Recovery of pituitary gonadotrophin secretion after a first trimester abortion is fast. Plasma FSH starts to increase 4–9 days after abortion. Ovarian recovery shows a wider variation. Plasma estradiol concentrations start to follow the initial FSH rise. First ovulation, as indicated by a plasma LH/FSH peak and/or progesterone rise to the ovulatory level, takes place approximately 16 days after first trimester surgical abortion and 21 days after mifepristone administration in medical abortion [5,6]. However, it may occur as early as 8 days after early medical abortion [6]. About 80–90% of women undergoing a first trimester abortion have an ovulatory first postabortion cycle, indicating the absolute need for effective contraception without delay after the abortion procedure [5–7].

Risk factors for subsequent abortion

Sociodemographic factors

As detailed in Chapter 21, risk factors for subsequent abortion in women undergoing abortion have been well characterized in several countries. These include young age, proven fertility (history of an abortion or childbirth), socio-economic disadvantage (such as low level of education or unstable relationship status) or living in urban areas. In addition, in some studies a history of domestic violence and substance abuse have been associated with an increased risk of subsequent abortion. Figure 13.1 shows some sociodemographic risk factors for subsequent abortion according to a study utilizing the Finnish national abortion registry [8].

Also, an advanced gestation at index abortion increases the risk of subsequent abortion. In comparison with first trimester abortion, an abortion performed during the second trimester increases the risk of another abortion 1.5-fold, and nearly 4-fold for a subsequent second trimester abortion [9].

Postabortion contraception

When assessing the typical effectiveness of various contraceptive methods several factors are important. These include fecundity of the woman, her level of sexual activity, efficacy of the contraceptive method and adherence to the method used.

The importance of the efficacy of the postabortion contraceptive method used has been recognized in recent years. A safe and highly effective method with minimal user-dependence,

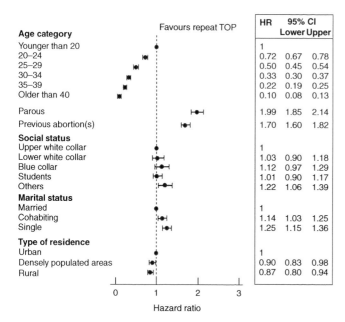

Figure 13.1 Sociodemographic risk factors for subsequent abortion according to Finnish national abortion registry data. TOP, termination of pregnancy. Modified from Niinimäki *et al.* [8].

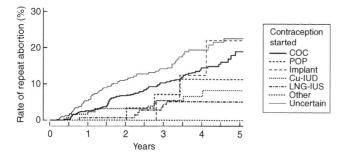

Figure 13.2 Rate of subsequent abortion according to the contraceptive method started at the time of a first trimester medical abortion. COC: combined oral contraception; POP: progestogen-only pill; Cu-IUD: copper-IUD; LNG-IUS: levonorgestrel intrauterine system. 'Other' refers mainly to female or male sterilization; 'uncertain' mainly to active postponement/non-start of postabortion contraception. Modified from Heikinheimo *et al.* [10].

i.e. a long-acting reversible contraceptive (LARC), is clearly of value. Figure 13.2 shows the cumulative percentage of women presenting for a subsequent abortion following first trimester medical abortion according to the method of contraception started at the time of index abortion [10]. Use of oral contraceptives or postponing initiation of contraception was associated with a significantly increased risk of subsequent abortion when compared to the use of LARCs and especially intrauterine contraception.

Postabortion contraception using intrauterine devices, either copper-IUD or levonorgestrel intrauterine system (LNG-IUS), has received increasing attention in recent years [10–16]. The results of some of these studies are summarized in Table 13.1. The studies show that postabortion use of intrauterine devices is associated with a significant decrease in the risk of a further abortion. In addition, in both a Canadian cohort study and a US

Table 13.1 Postabortion use of intrauterine contraception versus the risk of subsequent abortion

Reference	Country	Risk of subsequent abortion
Goodman *et al.*, 2008 [11]	USA	HR 0.38 (0.27–0.53) IUD vs non-IUD contraception
Heikinheimo *et al.*, 2008 [10]	Finland	HR 0.33 (0.16–0.7) copper-IUD and HR 0.39 (0.18–0.83) LNG-IUS vs COC
Roberts *et al.*, 2010 [12]	New Zealand	OR 0.3 (0.2–0.5) IUD vs COC
Rose and Lawton, 2012 [13]	New Zealand	HR 0.36 (0.17–0.77) IUD vs OC

Figures in parentheses are 95% confidence intervals. HR = hazard ratio; OR = odds ratio; LNG-IUS = levonorgestrel intrauterine system; COC = combined oral contraception.

cost analysis study, provision of postabortion intrauterine devices resulted in significantly reduced healthcare expenditure [15,16].

Initiation of contraception after abortion

In the vast majority of cases an abortion is performed other than for fetal anomaly. Therefore information about and provision of all methods of contraception should be offered to all women undergoing an abortion. Following appropriate information provision, women's right to choose the method according to their individual preferences and retain autonomy is most important.

Hormonal methods

Combined hormonal contraceptives including pills (COCs), vaginal rings and transdermal patches can all be started on the day of a surgical abortion or on the following day. If medical abortion is chosen, these methods can be started on the day of misoprostol administration or after passage of the products of conception (Table 13.2).

Although the first months after starting combined hormonal contraception are associated with an increased risk of venous thromboembolism, the preceding abortion does not seem to increase the risk of these adverse events. According to the World Health Organization (WHO) Medical Eligibility Criteria for contraceptive use [17], initiation of oestrogen-containing contraception is classified as category 1 (a condition for which there is no restriction in use) after either first or second trimester abortion.

Progestogen-only pills (POPs), implants or injectables can also be started according to the same timetable as combined methods of hormonal contraception [17,18]. However, the use of all user-dependent methods (pills, rings, patches) carries an increased risk of a further abortion as adherence and continuation rates are lower.

Intrauterine contraception

Surgical abortion

Placement of an intrauterine device (copper-IUD or LNG-IUS) immediately at the time of first trimester surgical abortion is routine practice and is also recommended in various international guidelines [14,17,18]. The only contraindication to immediate IUD/IUS insertion is septic abortion.

Table 13.2 Recommended timing of initiation of various reversible methods of contraception following medical and surgical abortion

	Medical	Surgical
Hormonal contraceptives		
Oral contraceptives	After administration of misoprostol/passage of pregnancy	Immediately after abortion
Contraceptive patch/vaginal ring	After administration of misoprostol/passage of pregnancy	Immediately after abortion
Contraceptive implant	After administration of misoprostol/passage of pregnancy At the time of mifepristone administration (Sonalkar *et al.* 2013 [25])	At the time of abortion
Contraceptive injection	After administration of misoprostol/passage of pregnancy	Immediately after abortion
Intrauterine contraception		
Copper-IUD	After verified abortion At 1–3 weeks after abortion (Sääv *et al.*, 2012 [21])	At the time of abortion
LNG-IUS	After verified abortion At 1–3 weeks after abortion (Sääv *et al.*, 2012 [21])	At the time of abortion

In comparison to delayed insertion the expulsion rate is somewhat higher (5 vs 3%) following immediate insertion. However, the number of IUD/IUS users during follow-up is increased when compared to delayed insertion (92 vs 77%) [19]. There is no evidence that IUD/IUS placement at the time of surgical abortion is associated with a risk of uterine perforation or infection higher than that with interval insertion.

Thus, an effective, immediately-started long-acting contraceptive should be the goal of management as long as another pregnancy is not planned. Attending for insertion at a later date can be problematic; failure to attend such an appointment is common. There are studies showing low attendance; fewer than one-third of women scheduled for a later IUD/IUS insertion subsequently attend [20]. These women have a higher risk of a further unintended pregnancy.

Medical abortion

After a medical abortion, the effective start of intrauterine contraception is more challenging. According to Faculty of Sexual and Reproductive Healthcare guidelines for contraceptive use, an IUD/IUS can be inserted after the second part of medical abortion [19]. In studies assessing intrauterine contraception following medical abortion, IUDs have been inserted from one week onwards following abortion (Table 13.2 and [21]).

However, more and more women choose medical abortion and administer the misoprostol at home. Scheduled follow-up visits are poorly attended, and the chance of not attending the additional visit needed for an IUD insertion is high (see Chapter 12). Even when tailored 'fast track' appointments have been scheduled for IUD insertion after medical abortion [22], the attendance has been shown to be similarly low to the situation after surgical abortions. Thus adequate provision of 'bridging' contraception such as oral contraceptives to be started immediately after the abortion and to be used up to IUD/IUS insertion is important.

Table 13.3 Comparison of early versus delayed initiation of LARC methods in postabortion contraception

	Early start	Delayed start
Adherence during follow-up	Optimal	Decreased adherence likely due to decreased uptake
Rate of subsequent abortion	Decreased	Possibly increased
Need for additional visits	Not needed	Needed
Cost-effectiveness	Optimal	Decreased

LARC

Long-acting reversible contraception (LARC) includes injectables, progestogen-only implants and intrauterine devices. There are several studies showing the efficacy of LARC methods in reducing the risk of subsequent abortion. Women who say that they do not need any contraception after an induced abortion carry the highest risk of a subsequent abortion (Figure 13.2). Also young age and a previous abortion are risk factors for a further abortion. When considering the age at sexual debut and the age at first delivery, especially in developed countries, there is a need for effective, long-term contraception which depending on the method could also relieve menstrual problems. In developing countries every pregnancy, whether terminated or continued, carries a risk of maternal morbidity. Therefore, it is of the utmost importance to offer every woman the option of a LARC method after abortion or delivery.

Early start of an effective method is cost-effective

As mentioned above, LARC methods, especially intrauterine devices [10–16] and subdermal implants [23], have been shown to reduce the risk of a further unintended pregnancy in several studies. LARC methods also have higher continuation rates compared to user-dependent contraceptive methods. This is highlighted in a report from New York where a policy change from delayed to immediate provision of LARC methods at the time of surgical abortion resulted in a significantly reduced rate of pregnancy (27 vs 15%) and abortion (17 vs 10%) during the first year after the abortion [24].

Thus every institution taking care of women seeking abortion should weigh the cost-effectiveness of providing LARC methods at the time of abortion against the costs of a possible further abortion. Providing an effective contraceptive method, preferably LARC, does save money, reduces the need for the services of healthcare providers and also helps the woman in question physically, psychologically, socially and economically. Comparison of some of the effects of an early versus delayed initiation of LARC methods in postabortion contraception is presented in Table 13.3.

Areas of current research

Evolving abortion care, with an increasing use of the medical method, poses challenges to effective provision of postabortion contraception. Immediate provision of a LARC method is difficult to organize in a setting where medical abortion with home administration of misoprostol is widespread. However, progestogen-only implants inserted immediately after mifepristone administration could offer one solution [25]. Post-placental insertion of a copper-IUD has become standard practice in many countries, and is classified as category 1 by

WHO [17]. Analogously, there are ongoing studies evaluating IUD/IUS insertion immediately after passage of the products of conception in medical abortion. The need for additional visits would be avoided and an effective, long-acting contraceptive, with all its added health benefits, offered.

References

1. Sedgh G, Bankole A, Singh S, Eilers M. Legal abortion levels and trends by woman's age at termination. *International Perspectives on Sexual and Reproductive Health* 2012;38:143–53.

2. Westhoff C. Contraceptive adherence and continuation rates. In A Glasier, K Wellings, H Critchley (eds.) *Contraception and Contraceptive Use*. RCOG Press, 2005: Chapter 10.

3. Åhman E, Shah I. New estimates and trends regarding unsafe abortion mortality. *Int J Gynecol Obstet* 2011;115:121–6.

4. Post abortion family planning: a key component of post abortion care. Consensus Statement: International Federation of Gynecology and Obstetrics (FIGO), International Confederation of Midwives (ICM), International Council of Nurses (ICN), United States Agency for International Development (UNAID), White Ribbon Alliance (WRA), Department for International Development (DFID), and Bill and Melinda Gates Foundation. Released on 1 November 2013.

5. Lähteenmäki P. Influence of oral contraceptives on immediate postabortal pituitary-ovarian function. *Acta Obstet Gynecol Scand Suppl.* 1978;76:1–43.

6. Schreiber C, Sober S, Ratcliffe S, Creinin M. Ovulation resumption after medical abortion with mifepristone and misoprostol. *Contraception* 2011;84:230–3.

7. Cameron IT, Baird D. The return of ovulation following early abortion: a comparison between vacuum aspiration and prostaglandin. *Acta Endocrinologica* 1988;118:161–7.

8. Niinimäki M, Pouta A, Bloigu A, *et al.* Frequency and risk factors for repeat abortions after surgical compared with medical termination of pregnancy. *Obstetrics & Gynecology* 2009;113:845–52.

9. Mentula M, Niinimäki M, Suhonen S, *et al.* Young age and termination of pregnancy during the second trimester are risk factors of repeat late abortion. *American Journal of Obstetrics & Gynecology* 2010;203:107. e1–7.

10. Heikinheimo O, Gissler M, Suhonen S. Age, parity, history of abortion and contraceptive choices affect the risk of repeated abortion. *Contraception* 2008;78:149–54.

11. Goodman S, Hendlish SK, Reeves MF, Foster-Rosales A. Impact of immediate postabortal insertion of intrauterine contraception on repeat abortion. *Contraception* 2008;78:143–8.

12. Roberts H, Silva M, Xu S. Post abortion contraception and its effect on repeat abortions in Auckland, New Zealand. *Contraception* 2010;82:260–5.

13. Rose A, Lawton B. Impact of long-acting reversible contraception on return for repeat abortion. *American Journal of Obstetrics & Gynecology* 2012;206:37.e1–6.

14. Grimes D, Lopez L, Schulz K, Stanwood N. Immediate postabortal insertion of intrauterine devices. *Cochrane Database of Systematic Reviews* 2010; Issue 6. Art. No.: CD001777. DOI. 10.1002/14651858. CD001777.pub3.

15. Ames C, Norman W. Preventing repeat abortion in Canada: is the immediate insertion of intrauterine devices postabortion a cost-effective option associated with fewer repeat abortions? *Contraception* 2012;85:51–5.

16. Salcedo J, Sorensen A, Rodriguez MI. Cost analysis of immediate postabortal IUD insertion compared to planned IUD insertion at the time of abortion follow-up. *Contraception* 2013;87:404–8.

17. World Health Organization. *Medical Eligibility Criteria for Contraceptive Use*, 4th edn. Geneva: WHO, 2009.

18. Faculty of Sexual and Reproductive Healthcare. *UK Medical Eligibility Criteria for Contraceptive Use*, 2nd edn. 2009.

19. Bednarek P, Creinin M, Reeves M, *et al.* Immediate versus delayed IUD insertion after uterine aspiration. *New England Journal of Medicine* 2011;364:2208–17.

20. Stanek A, Bednarek P, Nichols M, *et al.* Barriers associated with the failure to return for intrauterine device insertion following first-trimester abortion. *Contraception* 2009;79:216–20.

21. Sääv I, Stephansson O, Gemzell-Danielsson K. Early versus delayed insertion of intrauterine contraception after medical abortion – a randomized controlled trial. *Plos ONE* 2012;7: e48948.

22. Cameron ST, Berudoga N, Johnstone A, Glasier A. Assessment of a "fast-track" referral service for intrauterine contraception following early medical abortion. *J Fam Plann Reprod Health Care* 2012;38:175–8.

23. Cameron ST, Glasier A, Chen ZE, *et al.* Effect of contraception provided at termination of pregnancy and incidence of subsequent termination of pregnancy. *BJOG* 2012;119:1074–80.

24. Langston A, Joslin-Roher S, Westhoff C. Immediate post-abortion access to IUDs, implants and DMPA reduces repeat pregnancy within one year in a New York City practice. *Contraception* 2014;89:103–8.

25. Sonalkar S, Hou M, Borgatta L. Administration of the etonogestrel implant on the day of mifepristone for medical abortion: a pilot study. *Contraception* 2013;88:671–3.

Complications and safety

Rodica Comendant, Stelian Hodorogea and
Irina Sagaidac

Abortion-related morbidity and mortality

The frequency and severity of abortion complications depends mostly on whether abortion is safe or unsafe. Unsafe abortion, defined by the World Health Organization (WHO) as a procedure for terminating a pregnancy that is performed by an individual lacking the necessary skills or in an environment that does not conform to minimal medical standards, or both, continues to be a major cause of maternal mortality and morbidity worldwide [1].

Although the estimated annual number of deaths from unsafe abortion has decreased substantially from 69,000 in 1990 and 56,000 in 2003 to 47,000 in 2008, and the unsafe abortion mortality ratio has declined from 50 in 1990 to 30 in 2008, the proportion of maternal mortality due to unsafe abortion is stable and continues to represent 13% of all maternal deaths. Most of these cases occur in developing countries; Africa is the region with the highest number of maternal deaths attributable to unsafe abortion [2]. The epidemiology of abortion is covered fully in Chapter 3.

The main causes of unsafe abortion deaths are haemorrhage, sepsis, peritonitis and trauma of genital and abdominal organs, frequently as consequences of insertion of foreign bodies or poisoning during attempts to provoke abortion. Unsafe abortion is also an important cause of complications and long-term disabilities, including infertility, among women in the developing world. It is estimated that in 2005 more than 8.5 million women had complications from unsafe abortion requiring medical attention and that 3 million of these women did not receive the care they needed.

In contrast, abortion performed by trained healthcare providers with approved equipment, correct techniques and sanitary standards is considered by WHO to be one of the safest medical procedures. In countries and regions with good access to safe abortion services which use modern methods, the likelihood of dying as a result of an abortion is less than one per 100,000 procedures [1]. For example, in the USA legal abortion results in 0.6 deaths per 100,000 procedures; in the UK, between 1994 and 2005, abortion-related mortality was even lower, constituting approximately 0.45 deaths per 100,000 procedures. In France, in a recent 10-year period, abortion-related deaths (miscarriage or induced abortion) accounted for 4% of all maternal deaths or 0.7 cases per 100,000 procedures [3].

Currently, women's risk of death during safely performed first trimester abortion is lower than from an allergic reaction to a penicillin injection and ten times lower than the risk of death during pregnancy and childbirth [1]. At the same time, the risk of death following complications of unsafe abortion procedures in developing countries is hundreds of times

Abortion Care, ed. Sam Rowlands. Published by Cambridge University Press. © Cambridge University Press 2014.

higher than that of abortion performed professionally under safe conditions. According to WHO estimates, the global case-fatality rate (220 per 100,000 procedures) associated with unsafe abortion is almost 350 times higher than the rate associated with legal abortions in the USA; in sub-Saharan Africa, for instance, the rate is more than 800 times higher (460 per 100,000). Even in developed countries, the case-fatality rate for unsafe abortion is 40 times higher than that for safe abortion [2].

Venous thromboembolism, infection, severe bleeding and adverse reactions to anaesthesia are the main causes of the rare deaths occurring during legal abortion procedures. In France, out of 14 deaths caused by abortion complications between 1996 and 2006, 4 were the result of infection and 3 the result of haemorrhage, 2 were caused by anaphylactic shock during anaesthesia and 5 were due to thromboembolism [3].

Possible associations with longer-term adverse effects are considered in Chapter 18.

Factors influencing the incidence of complications of safe abortions

As mentioned above, the most relevant factor influencing the incidence and severity of abortion complications is whether abortions are safe or unsafe, their legal status and ease of access to services. Other important factors are the gestational age of the pregnancy; the method of abortion used; the skill of the abortion provider; and use of preventive measures during the procedure such as cervical ripening and routine administration of antibiotics [1,2].

Gestational age of pregnancy

Generally, the earlier the abortion is done, the safer it is. The case-fatality rate for surgical abortion is: 0.1 per 100,000 procedures at gestations of less than 9 weeks; 0.4 per 100,000 procedures at 11–12 weeks; 1.7 per 100,000 procedures at 13–15 weeks; 3.4 per 100,000 at 16–20 weeks; and almost 9.0 per 100,000 procedures done at after 20 weeks [1]. So, one of the ways to reduce the risk of complications is to have the abortion procedure as early as possible.

Skill of the abortion provider

A study of practices in hospitals in the USA immediately after liberalization of the abortion law found a high rate of cervical injury (10.3 per 1,000 procedures), much higher than in Denmark – a country with longer experience in provision of legal abortion (0.89 per 1,000) [4,5]. It is noteworthy that, in the 15 years following liberalization of abortion law in the USA, the mortality rate associated with legal abortion procedures declined substantially from 4.1 to 0.6 per 100,000 abortion procedures.

Antibiotic prophylaxis and cervical priming

Routine use of antibiotics at the time of surgical abortion, and cervical priming before surgical abortion, in specific circumstances, are recommended by WHO as technologies with proven efficacy in reducing the incidence of complications.

Method of abortion

Vacuum aspiration is associated with significantly fewer complications than dilatation and curettage (D&C), including the incidence of haemorrhage, pelvic infection and cervical and uterine injury. Early medical abortion has a similar safety profile to first trimester aspiration abortion. WHO and the International Federation of Gynecology and Obstetrics (FIGO) now recommend manual vacuum aspiration (MVA) or electric vacuum aspiration (EVA) as the preferred surgical methods of uterine evacuation. WHO suggests that sharp curettage, if still practised, should be replaced by vacuum aspiration or medical abortion [1].

Complications of surgical abortion

Complications of surgical abortion include, but are not limited to, the following.

Vasovagal reaction

Vasovagal reaction, also called vasovagal response or vasovagal syncope, can occur during administration of paracervical block, cervical dilatation or venepuncture. Clinically this reaction is characterized by a rapid onset of bradycardia, a drop in the blood pressure, pallor and faintness. Frequently no treatment is needed apart from leg elevation and oxygen support. In the event that the symptoms persist, injection of atropine (0.4–1.0 mg) intravenously or subcutaneously is recommended [6]. The procedure should be stopped if the clinician observes the onset of a vasovagal reaction. The abortion procedure can be completed when symptoms disappear, and the woman feels comfortable. Administration of atropine (0.4 mg or 0.5 mg) mixed with the local anaesthetic in a paracervical block has been shown to prevent vagal effects and syncope [7].

Cervical laceration

Cervical laceration is a complication caused by overdilatation of the cervix, injury to the cervix by fetal parts and, in certain cases (especially in nulliparous women), due to resistance of the internal os to forced dilatation. The incidence of this complication varies between 0.1 and 1% [8]. In the second trimester the incidence of cervical laceration is slightly higher at 3% [9]. The risk of complications is increased in cases in which the woman is a teenager, general anaesthesia is used and/or the procedure is performed by an inexperienced operator [8].

Clinically the onset is characterized by bright red bleeding that increases while withdrawing the cannula. The amount of bleeding depends on the size of the laceration. In small lacerations, applying direct pressure can stop the bleeding; additionally silver nitrate may be used.

Cervical priming makes the procedure quicker and easier to perform by reducing the need for mechanical cervical dilatation. Cervical priming is described in detail in Chapters 8, 9 and 10.

Uterine perforation

Uterine perforation occurs most frequently during dilatation of the cervix. The risk of a perforation is increased by: cervical stenosis, severe uterine anteflexion or retroflexion, uterine abnormalities, difficult and prolonged uterine evacuation and an inexperienced operator [10].

Perforation is suspected if the woman experiences generalized abdominal pain, fat or bowel is found in the tissue removed from the uterus and/or the instrument passes without resistance into the uterine cavity further than expected. If perforation is suspected the procedure should be stopped immediately.

If perforation occurs when the abortion procedure is complete and the woman has stable vital signs, uterotonics and antibiotics are recommended with close monitoring. If vital signs are not stable, intravenous fluids and oxygen are required in addition. When bleeding cannot be controlled with uterotonics, laparotomy may be required to repair the source of bleeding or to diagnose the type of injury to pelvic organs.

In some authors' opinions, if evacuation is not complete, the abortion should be completed as soon as feasible or delayed until the perforation heals. In the event of unhealed uterine perforation it is recommended that the procedure be completed under ultrasound or laparoscopic visualization; laparotomy is indicated when severe perforation is suspected [11]. There is an option to complete the abortion with a medical method, but there is no strong evidence to support this.

Lindell and Flam analysed 84,850 legal abortions performed in the Stockholm area during the period 1982 to 1992; uterine perforation occurred in 145 cases (0.17%). The authors advocate conservative management of uterine perforation (which occurs during vacuum aspiration) because the results of their review showed that, even though in half of the cases immediate exploration of the abdomen was decided upon, in only 18 cases was the decision justified by bleeding and lacerations to organs of the pelvis [12].

Haemorrhage

Haemorrhage after surgical abortion is rare; it occurs in less than 1% of cases [13]. The haemorrhage may be caused by retained products of conception, uterine atony, cervical laceration, abnormal placentation (e.g. placenta accreta), uterine perforation and coagulopathy. Advanced gestational age, use of general anaesthesia, lack of use of uterotonic drugs in dilatation and evacuation (D&E) and prolonged procedure time are all factors that increase the risk of haemorrhage [13].

Uterine atony and incomplete abortion are the most frequent causes of bleeding. Treatment should begin with complete uterine evacuation, uterine massage, uterotonics and blood volume replacement with fluids [1]. In the event that the bleeding continues after evacuation and administration of uterotonics, providers should suspect cervical laceration or uterine perforation. The causes and management of these complications have been described above.

If haemorrhage continues, ultrasound examination, monitoring of vital signs, evaluating blood loss and laboratory assessment are important (haemoglobin, coagulation parameters and a cross-match for possible blood transfusion). One of the options to treat atony is tamponade with a Foley catheter with a 30 mL balloon inflated up to 60 mL [13].

Disseminated intravascular coagulopathy (DIC) may be diagnosed in cases of extremely heavy or prolonged bleeding, associated with anaemia and protracted clotting time. Treatment of DIC is complex and may include transfusion of fresh frozen plasma, cryoprecipitate, platelets and red cells to correct the anaemia. In settings where uterine artery embolization is available, it is recommended to attempt this prior to invasive measures [13].

Surgery is a last resort. The woman may be examined by laparoscopy, if perforation is suspected. Hysterectomy is the definitive treatment for postabortion haemorrhage, but the decision should be taken only when all other methods of treatment have failed.

Incomplete abortion

The incidence of retained products of conception ranges from 0.5 to 2% [4]. This complication occurs more frequently in medical than in surgical abortions. Correct estimation of gestational age and operator experience are factors that may influence the frequency of this complication. Tissue examination after the aspiration procedure contributes substantially to a decrease in incidence of this complication and is recommended by WHO [1].

Incomplete abortion is suspected if the woman returns with symptoms of vaginal bleeding and abdominal pain. On bimanual examination the uterus is tender and possibly enlarged. Ultrasound examination will provide information about retained tissue in the uterine cavity; however, sometimes the information is ambiguous. In some cases fever is reported. In this case infection should also be suspected and antibiotics should be initiated.

Incomplete abortion may be treated using either vacuum aspiration or misoprostol [1]. The recommended misoprostol dose is 600 µg orally or 400 µg sublingually [1]. Complete abortion rates were analysed in cases of re-aspiration of the uterine cavity and administration of misoprostol for women with incomplete abortions (uterine size up to 13 weeks' gestation) and no differences were demonstrated [1]. Expectant management can also be considered, if women are comfortable with this, when vital signs are stable and there is no heavy bleeding.

Haematometra

Haematometra is a collection or retention of blood in the uterine cavity. Haematometra can manifest itself immediately after the procedure, or several days later. This complication is rare; the cause of retention of blood clots is atonia or hypotonia of the uterus after abortion [14].

In haematometra, the endometrium is distended by blood and blood clots, and the uterus is unable to contract effectively to expel the contents. Because of the existing lower abdominal pressure, one of the first symptoms the woman may experience is cramping. On pelvic examination, the uterus is enlarged and tender. The size of the uterus correlates with the volume of blood or blood clots in the cavity [11]. The treatment of haematometra includes re-aspiration of the uterine cavity, uterotonics and antibiotics.

Anaesthesia-related complications

The evidence shows that local anaesthesia is safer than general anaesthesia, both for vacuum aspiration in the first trimester and for D&E in the second trimester [1]. The risk of death from first trimester abortion under general anaesthesia is two to four times higher than with local anaesthesia [15].

One of the important advantages of local anaesthesia is that the woman is alert, able to communicate with the operator during the procedure and to describe the symptoms she is experiencing [11].

It is important to emphasize that the spectrum of complications with general and local anaesthesia is different. General anaesthesia is associated with higher rates of cervical injury, uterine perforation and haemorrhage [14]. Local anaesthesia may be associated with fever and convulsions, but the overall number of major complications is fewer.

Infection

The incidence of endometritis varies between 0.5 and 5% [14]. Infection is more likely to affect the genital tract after abortion because the cervix is still dilated. A history of pelvic inflammatory disease increases the risk of developing infection again after an abortion. In addition untreated chlamydia and gonorrhoea increase the rate of postabortion infection; treatment can be initiated before or at the time of the procedure.

According to the UK Royal College of Obstetricians and Gynaecologists, the following regimens are suitable for periabortion antibiotic prophylaxis:

1. azithromycin 1 g orally on the day of abortion plus metronidazole 1 g rectally or 800 mg orally prior to, or at the time of, abortion;

OR

2. doxycycline 100 mg orally twice daily for seven days, starting on the day of abortion, plus metronidazole 1 g rectally or 800 mg orally prior to, or at the time of, abortion;

OR

3. metronidazole 1 g rectally or 800 mg orally prior to, or at the time of, abortion for women who have tested negative for *C. trachomatis* infection [8].

First symptoms of endometritis may appear in the first or second days after the procedure, but usually the woman returns to the clinic in three to four days and reports cramping, fever, pelvic tenderness and prolonged vaginal bleeding. Bimanual examination reveals a tender, enlarged uterus and offensive cervical discharge. The white cell count may or may not be elevated.

There are few studies regarding treatment of postabortion endometritis. In mild infections the treatment can start with oral antibiotics. If other infections are suspected (bacterial vaginosis or chlamydia), use of broad spectrum antibiotics should be considered. Treatment of bacterial vaginosis at the time of abortion decreases the rate of infection by 75% [16].

Sometimes incomplete abortion is associated with endometritis; in this case re-aspiration of the uterine cavity is necessary. Antibiotics should be administered as soon as endometritis is suspected, before the re-aspiration. In severe, generalized infections or in cases of high risk of sepsis immediate aggressive treatment is required.

Continuing pregnancy

The incidence of this complication is less than 1% [17]. The causes of a continuing pregnancy, in relation to surgical abortion, may be: uterine perforation; aspiration of one horn of the uterus while the pregnancy is localized in the other one (uterine anomalies); or multiple pregnancy.

A potential continuing pregnancy may be suspected by the operator when the gestation sac or chorionic villi are not seen during the post-procedure tissue examination. The woman may still report symptoms related to pregnancy such as morning sickness, breast tenderness and urinary frequency. Continuing pregnancy can also be suspected at the two-week follow-up visit when, at bimanual examination, the uterus is found to be tender and enlarged.

When a continuing pregnancy is suspected an ultrasound scan is needed in order to confirm the presence of the pregnancy, its viability, localization (uterine or ectopic) and to

safety and effectiveness when used for the treatment of incomplete abortion [28]. Surgical evacuation (vacuum aspiration) or expectant management can be offered, as well, depending on women's preferences.

Providers' fear of incomplete abortion and bleeding, when they are starting to offer medical abortion, may lead to unnecessary surgical interventions and hence lower efficacy of the medical method. Over time, gaining experience and confidence in providing medical abortion, providers develop patience and do not intervene unnecessarily. Offering the necessary support and reassurance to women and obtaining their understanding and cooperation is also crucially important when a complication is suspected.

Continuing pregnancy

A continuing pregnancy should be suspected if women, after taking the medications, still experience pregnancy symptoms or have had bleeding for just one day or not at all after misoprostol administration. Clinical examination, which reveals an enlarged uterus, may be enough for the diagnosis but ultrasound examination may help to clarify if the pregnancy is viable. Also measurement of plasma hCG may be used. Women with a continuing pregnancy may be offered either vacuum aspiration or repeat administration of mifepristone/misoprostol to complete the abortion.

There are some concerns regarding a potential risk of a teratogenic effect of mifepristone or misoprostol. Available data regarding a potential risk of fetal abnormality after an unsuccessful medical abortion are limited and inconclusive; therefore, it is unnecessary to insist on termination of an exposed pregnancy if the woman wishes to continue it. Women should, nevertheless, be informed that due to the unquantified risk of abortifacient drugs to the fetus, follow-up is important, with special attention at the anomaly scan during antenatal care [1].

Haemorrhage, incomplete abortion and uterine rupture in medical abortion after 12 weeks

The rate of major complications from second trimester medical abortion using mifepristone and misoprostol is low although minor complications such as retained placenta or bleeding, needing a procedure, are more frequent than from D&E [29]. In a review of 1,002 cases of second trimester medical abortion with mifepristone and misoprostol, 8.1% of women needed surgical evacuation of the uterus, the majority of them for retained placenta. Only 2 out of the 1,002 women needed a surgical evacuation to terminate the pregnancy. Serious complications such as haemorrhage, blood transfusion or hysterectomy occurred in less than 1% of cases [27].

Uterine rupture is a rare complication in medical abortion after 12 weeks' gestation. It is associated with later gestational age and uterine scarring, but has also been reported in women without these risk factors [1]. The risk of uterine rupture among women with a prior caesarean delivery undergoing second trimester abortion using misoprostol is less than 0.3% in a meta-analysis and this may be acceptable to both patients and providers [30]. Nevertheless, caution is needed in the use of misoprostol alone for pregnancies in the second trimester and the dosages of misoprostol must be reduced as the duration of pregnancy increases because, beyond 16 weeks, the uterus becomes very sensitive to prostaglandins [31].

References

1. WHO. *Safe Abortion: Technical and Policy Guidance for Health Systems*. Geneva: World Health Organization, 2012.

2. WHO. *Unsafe Abortion: Global and Regional Estimates of the Incidence of Unsafe Abortion and Associated Mortality in 2008*, 6th edn. Geneva: World Health Organization, 2011.

3. Saucedo M, Deneux-Tharaux C, Bouvier-Colle M-H. Ten years of confidential inquiries into maternal deaths in France, 1998–2007. *Obstet Gynecol* 2013;122:752–60.

4. Schulz KF, Grimes DA, Cates W. Measures to prevent cervical injury during suction curettage abortion. *Lancet* 1983;1:1182–4.

5. Zhou W, Nielsen GL, Moller M, Olsen J. Short-term complications after surgically induced abortions: a register-based study of 56 117 abortions. *Acta Obstet Gynecol Scand* 2002;81:331–6.

6. Saxena R. *Tips and Tricks in Operative Obstetrics and Gynecology*. Jaypee Brothers Medical Pub., 2011: 243.

7. Fritz MA, Speroff L. *Clinical Gynecologic Endocrinology and Infertility*, 8th edn. Wolters Kluwer/Lippincott Williams & Wilkins, 2011.

8. Royal College of Obstetricians and Gynaecologists. *The Care of Women Requesting Induced Abortion. Evidence-based Clinical Guideline Number 7.* November 2011.

9. Ben-Ami I, Schneider D, Svirsky R, Smorgick N, Pansky M, Halperin R. Safety of late second-trimester pregnancy termination by laminaria dilatation and evacuation in patients with previous multiple cesarean sections. *Am J Obstet Gynecol* 2009;201:154 e151–5.

10. Cooper JM, Brady RM. Intraoperative and early postoperative complications of operative hysteroscopy. *Obstet Gynecol Clin North Am* 2000;27:347–66.

11. Hern WM. Surgical abortion: management, complications, and long term risks. In JJ Sciarra, PV Dilts (eds.)

Gynecology and Obstetrics. Philadelphia: J.B. Lippincott Company, 1994: Chapter 59.

12. Lindell G, Flam F. Management of uterine perforations in connection with legal abortions. *Acta Obstet Gynecol Scand* 1995;74:373–5.

13. Kerns J, Steinauer J. Management of postabortion hemorrhage: release date November 2012 SFP Guideline #20131. *Contraception* 2013;87:331–42.

14. Borgatta, L, Kattan, D, *et al.* Surgical techniques for first-trimester abortion. *Glob Libr Women's Med* 2012; DOI 10.3843/GLOWM.10440.

15. Peterson HB, Grimes DA, Cates W, Rubin GL. Comparative risk of death from induced abortion at less than or equal to 12 weeks' gestation performed with local versus general anesthesia. *Am J Obstet Gynecol* 1981;141:763–8.

16. Larrson PG, Platz-Christensen JJ, Theijls H, *et al.* Incidence of pelvic inflammatory disease after first-trimester legal abortion in women with bacterial vaginosis after treatment with metronidazole: a double-blind, randomized trial. *Am J Obstet Gynecol* 1992;166:100.

17. Faucher P, Hassoun D. *Interruption Volontaire de la Grossesse médicamenteuse*, 2nd edn. de Boeck/Estem, 2011.

18. Henshaw RC, Naji SA, Russell IT, Templeton AA. A comparison of medical abortion (using mifepristone and gemeprost) with surgical vacuum aspiration: efficacy and early medical sequelae. *Hum Reprod* 1994;9:2167–72.

19. Chan YF, Ho PC, Ma HK. Blood loss in termination of early pregnancy by vacuum aspiration and by combination of mifepristone and gemeprost. *Contraception* 1993;47:85–95.

20. Niinimäki M, Pouta A, Bloigu A, *et al.* Immediate complications after medical compared with surgical termination of pregnancy. *Obstet Gynecol* 2009;114:795–804.

21. Allen RH, Westhoff C, De Nonno L, Fielding SL, Schaff EA. Curettage after mifepristone-induced abortion. Frequency,

timing and indications. *Obstetr Gynecol* 2001;98:101–6.

22. ICMA. ICMA Information Package on Medical Abortion. www. medicalabortionconsortium.org/articles/ for-health-care-providers/health/?bl=en (accessed 31 October 2013).

23. Gynuity. *Providing Medical Abortion in Developing Countries: An Introductory Guidebook*. New York: Gynuity Health Projects, 2004.

24. Shannon C, Brothers LP, Philip NM, Winikoff B. Infection after medical abortion: a review of the literature. *Contraception* 2004;70:183–90.

25. Meites E, Zane S, Gould C. Fatal *Clostridium sordellii* infections after medical abortions. *New England Journal of Medicine* 2010;363:1382–3.

26. Fjerstad M, Trussell J, Sivin I, Lichtenberg ES, Cullins V. Rates of serious infection after changes in regimens for medical abortion. *New England Journal of Medicine* 2009;361:145–51.

27. Ashok PW, Templeton A, Wagaarachchi PT, Flett GM. Factors affecting the outcome of early medical abortion: a review of 4132 consecutive cases. *BJOG* 2002;109:1281–9.

28. Diop A, Raghavan S, Rakotovao J-P, Comendant R, Blumenthal PD, Winikoff B. Two routes of administration for misoprostol in the treatment of incomplete abortion: a randomized clinical trial. *Contraception* 2009;79:456–62.

29. Autry AM, Hayes C, Jacobson GF, Kirby RS. A comparison of medical induction and dilation and evacuation for second-trimester abortion. *American Journal of Obstet Gynecol* 2002;187:393–7.

30. Goyal V. Uterine rupture in second-trimester misoprostol-induced abortion after cesarean delivery: a systematic review. *Obstet Gynecol* 2009;113:1117–23.

31. Shannon CS, Winikoff B, eds. *Misoprostol: An Emerging Technology for Women's Health*. Report of a Seminar: May 7–8, 2001. New York: Population Council, 2004.

Chapter

15

Women with medical problems

Kate Paterson and Helgi Johannsson

Introduction

Within the terms of the 1967 Abortion Act, abortion in England, Scotland and Wales is now readily available providing two doctors state that it is being performed under one or more of the specified grounds. In 2012, of 185,122 abortions provided to residents of England and Wales 179,398 (97%) were funded by the National Health Service (NHS). In 2002 there were 175,932 abortions of which 78% were funded by the NHS [1].

Despite this improved availability there remains a group of women who still have difficulty accessing abortion. These are women who suffer from medical co-morbidity. In 2002, 53% of NHS-funded abortions were performed in NHS hospitals and the remainder by agencies in the specialist independent sector funded by the NHS. However, by 2012 the proportion performed in NHS hospitals had fallen to 36%. The abortion skills and standard of care is high in both provider groups but the ability to manage more complex medical problems is only available in hospitals and this is complicated by the fact that the skills to provide second trimester surgical abortion tend to be concentrated in the independent sector.

Medical problems include both medical illnesses and physical problems (such as uterine scars, malformations and congenital or acquired disabilities). There are no national data relating to co-morbidity in women requesting abortion but there is a general feeling within obstetrics and gynaecology that the number of these women is increasing. Most published material relates to perinatal outcome and there is little relating specifically to abortion. The authors have based their choice of topics for this chapter on the experience gained in a tertiary unit which, in addition to running a local abortion service, also accepts referrals from the independent sector and other NHS hospitals.

Performing an abortion is little different from any other minor surgical procedure. Managing women with medical problems requires teamwork, particularly with the anaesthetist but also with other specialist physicians. It is important to understand the reason a woman is requesting an abortion; if it is mainly due to concern about a medical problem, this should be further discussed with both an obstetrician and the physicians normally providing care for that condition so that the risks and benefits of the choice between abortion and continuing the pregnancy are fully explored and understood.

Abortion Care, ed. Sam Rowlands. Published by Cambridge University Press. © Cambridge University Press 2014.

General principles of management

Cervical preparation

All women should be considered for cervical preparation [2,3]. In the first trimester miso-prostol 400 μg can be given 2–3 h prior to surgery, either vaginally or buccally. At later gestations oral mifepristone 200 mg can be added 24–48 h prior to surgery or Dilapan-S® (a hygroscopic cervical dilator) can be placed in the cervix on the morning of surgery. For gestations greater than 20 weeks the Dilapan-S® can be placed the night before and the woman scheduled to return in the morning for surgery.

Ultrasound

Real-time ultrasound should be available in the operating theatre, especially for late gestations or where there is a uterine problem.

Anaesthesia

Traditionally, day surgery facilities have been limited to those who are American Society of Anesthesiology (ASA) 1 and 2, with a body mass index (BMI) of under 35. Practice is changing considerably: there is now little evidence that more obese patients or those with more serious co-morbidities do worse when treated as a day case. In fact, there is evidence that preoperative testing can be kept to a minimum for these patients [4].

The choice of anaesthetic is important. For some women medical abortion can remove the need for general anaesthesia (GA); there is evidence that local anaesthesia (LA) is safer than GA [5,6] and intuitively may seem the better option. However, modern anaesthesia expertly provided in an appropriately equipped environment is generally very safe. Abortion requires a short, relatively deep anaesthetic. The mainstay of this is the use of propofol and an opiate such as fentanyl or alfentanil. Anaesthetic gases such as sevoflurane may be used, but some operators find this relaxes the uterus and disrupts the 'feel' of the empty uterus.

Most anaesthetic agents vasodilate and depress respiratory drive and laryngeal reflexes. This is of particular significance in valvular heart disease, where blood pressure may drop precipitously, and in obesity where the airway may be compromised.

Abortion under GA gives a controlled environment, offers a better experience for anxious patients [7], reduces the operating time and is also easier for surgeons who may have limited experience operating under LA, particularly at higher gestations. For women with severe pulmonary dysfunction spinal anaesthesia is a useful option.

Even when the first choice is medical abortion or abortion under LA it is important to be aware of the possible need for surgical intervention under GA so theatre facilities need to be available. The woman's preference should always be considered, but ultimately it is best to use the safest option chosen by the team.

Women should be fasted for the minimum time prior to anaesthesia. They should not ingest solids or milky drinks later than six hours prior to anaesthesia but can take clear fluids up to two hours beforehand to maintain hydration [8] and almost all women should continue their standard medications as prescribed. Morning doses can be taken on rising with a sip of water.

Environment

A day care surgery unit, working with a familiar team, is safe and suitable for women with all but the most severe conditions. Although many women undergoing early medical abortion have the option to complete the procedure at home, women with co-morbidities should stay on hospital premises for observation and support until abortion occurs. Medical abortions after nine weeks can be managed on a gynaecology ward by suitably trained nursing staff but the best option for late medical abortion with serious medical conditions is a high dependency area such as the labour ward as it has 24-hour medical cover and the midwives are trained to manage high-risk pregnancies.

Specific medical conditions

Obesity

One of the most common secondary referrals is for obese women. The World Health Organization estimates that 23% of females in the UK have a BMI greater than 30 kg/m² [9]; those with a BMI greater than 40 present a particular challenge. Diagnosis of pregnancy may be delayed or these women may have difficulty finding a unit able, or willing, to perform an abortion. This leads to a disproportionate number presenting in the second trimester of pregnancy. It is worth considering medical abortion for these women while appreciating that there may be a need for surgical intervention. Both medical and surgical procedures require equipment able to support high weights and sufficient manpower to assist moving the woman.

Those with extreme obesity also present a challenge to the anaesthetist. The airway may be difficult to maintain and lipophilic drugs such as propofol are redistributed faster, leading to higher doses being needed which may result in a longer recovery time. The woman may have undiagnosed obstructive sleep apnoea or type 2 diabetes and intravenous access may be difficult. In addition positioning these women correctly is vital to prevent injuries; manual handling devices such as hoists and operating table extensions may be necessary.

Access to the cervix can be extremely difficult [10]. During the abortion it is often helpful to have assistants to help support and abduct the woman's legs and further assistance may be required to hold lateral wall retractors as the vaginal walls may fall across the cervix. Once the cervix has been stabilized the abortion will usually be straightforward. Preoperative cervical preparation is helpful and, if an assistant holds up the panniculus, it is usually possible to get a relatively good transabdominal ultrasound view of the uterus. During the abortion fundal pressure may also be required to bring the fundus of the uterus within reach of the cannula.

Thromboprophylaxis should be considered in obese women [11].

Diabetes

Type 1 diabetes can usually be managed providing that hypoglycaemia is avoided and treatment is not given while a woman is ketoacidotic. With good preoperative planning a sliding scale insulin regimen can usually be avoided [12], except for later medical abortions. For early medical abortion food and insulin should be taken as normal. At later gestations surgical abortion is usually easier. A woman can fast and take no insulin providing the abortion is done early on a list. When she has recovered she can administer her usual morning dose of insulin and be given breakfast. Most people with type 1 diabetes are very good at managing their own diabetes; they should always be consulted about how best to alter their insulin regimen during perioperative fasting. If good cervical preparation is required the woman can either take mifepristone 200 mg 36–48 h prior to surgery, followed by 400 µg vaginal misoprostol on the morning of surgery, or have Dilapan-S® inserted the evening prior to surgery.

After ending the pregnancy, insulin requirements fall and the woman should be advised to monitor her glucose values carefully.

Thyroid disease

This is rarely a problem when well controlled. However, if the woman is thyrotoxic or clinically hypothyroid this needs to be treated prior to the abortion, either by her endocrinologist or general practitioner.

Asthma and other respiratory diseases

Asthma is the most common chronic disease, affecting 11% of women in the UK. Women with asthma can often be managed by medical abortion; however, most women with asthma have very mild symptoms that usually have no impact on anaesthesia. They should be advised to bring, and use, their own prescribed medication and pre-treatment with salbutamol should be considered, especially in severe asthma.

Most people with mild asthma are able to tolerate non-steroidal anti-inflammatory drugs. Women recently treated with systemic steroids should be given an additional dose of intravenous steroid to cover the procedure. Spinal anaesthesia should be considered in women with severe lung disease (e.g. cystic fibrosis).

Those with asthma can deteriorate quickly under anaesthesia; resuscitation facilities and drugs to treat severe bronchoconstriction should be available.

Renal disorders

There is no evidence linking pyelonephritis with abortion. If a woman is on dialysis the procedure should be discussed with her renal physician but problems are rare. The woman should have dialysis either earlier the same day or the previous day, with post-dialysis blood results available.

Women who have had renal transplants also do well but the immunosuppressant drugs and their interactions should be discussed with a nephrologist.

Hepatic impairment

Coagulation can be deranged in those with liver disease and may have to be corrected prior to the procedure. Ascites and generalized oedema may pose technical difficulties and hepatic encephalopathy may get worse perioperatively.

Anaemia

Unexpectedly low haemoglobin in a clinically well woman is often well compensated. It is usually best to do a surgical procedure to minimize the blood loss and be in a position to manage any unexpected bleeding efficiently. Blood transfusion should not be considered unless the haemoglobin is less than 7 g/dL. Advice from a haematologist should be sought as the anaemia can usually be fully investigated and treated conservatively after the abortion.

Platelet disorders

These are surprisingly common in a tertiary referral centre. Most women are already under the care of a haematologist and have a diagnosis. It is essential to have haematological input as, if the platelet count is low, the woman may need preoperative treatment with steroids and possibly a platelet transfusion. The platelet level should be at least 50×10^9/L and preferably 70×10^9/L before any surgery is undertaken. Some women have normal platelet counts but dysfunctional platelets and require cross-matched platelets to be available and some, such as those with von Willebrand's disease or mild haemophilia A, need to be treated with desmopressin acetate. Providing the preparation is meticulous, the procedure itself should be straightforward. Tranexamic acid has been used in orthopaedic surgery but has not been shown to be effective in abortion care.

Thrombophilias and women at risk of venous thromboembolism

The most common thrombophilia is factor V Leiden deficiency; antithrombin III and protein C and S deficiency may also be seen. These women are all at risk of venous thromboembolism (VTE). In addition, women who have had a previous VTE, those with synthetic heart valves, atrial fibrillation and antiphospholipid syndrome are also at risk.

Management of women at risk of VTE is as follows. If a woman is on warfarin this should be changed to low molecular weight heparin. The last dose should be taken the day before surgery, and the heparin can be commenced later in the day following surgery. Aspirin should be stopped five days before surgery but a shorter time rarely causes a problem if this is not possible. For high-risk women it may be safer to continue aspirin in the perioperative period. A careful assessment of risk and benefit will need to be conducted. Longer-term anticoagulation after the abortion will depend on the underlying pathology and it is best to refer the woman back to a haematologist to manage this. Abortion is a short procedure compared to other forms of surgery and the woman should be mobilized as quickly as possible. Women at risk of VTE who are not normally on anticoagulation can be managed using graduated compression stockings, but care must be taken to avoid the 'tourniquet' effect especially in obese women. A single dose of low molecular weight heparin may be preferable. The woman should be encouraged to continue to mobilize in the weeks after the abortion.

Sickle cell disease

Sickle cell trait is not associated with any problems. Women with homozygous sickle cell disease often have a low haemoglobin but are well compensated; the woman can be asked what level she normally runs at. Any recent exacerbations or blood transfusions should be carefully noted. It is important that she remains warm and well oxygenated both during and after the procedure. The fasting period should be minimized to ensure the woman is well hydrated. The abortion can usually be performed as a day case and early medical abortion works well at earlier gestations.

Acute intermittent porphyria

This may be exacerbated in pregnancy and contributing to the decision to end the pregnancy. Abortion can be safely performed under regional anaesthesia [13]; a review of all types of anaesthetic for those with porphyria has been published by James and Hift [14].

Cardiovascular disease

In women who have no cyanosis and non-dilated ventricles together with a good functional status, such as the ability to climb stairs, a short abortion procedure under general anaesthesia is unlikely to cause problems. Mitral and aortic stenosis, corrected Fallot's tetralogy, moderate mitral and aortic regurgitation and porcine valve replacements can be similarly managed. Women on anticoagulation should be discussed with the anaesthetist in advance. In some cases (e.g. lone atrial fibrillation) the warfarin can simply be stopped four days in advance, but more generally the warfarin cessation should be covered with low molecular weight heparin, which can be given as an outpatient.

Women with significant cardiomyopathy, valvular heart disease or coronary artery disease are at high risk of further cardiac compromise or even death whether they undergo abortion or continue the pregnancy. They need to have their abortion in a fully equipped theatre with an anaesthetist with experience of anaesthetizing those with cardiac disease. Valvular heart disease with a fixed cardiac output such as in mitral and aortic stenosis poses a particular risk and women with these conditions should be carefully assessed by the anaesthetist in advance.

Cardiac medication (such as β-blockers) should not be omitted simply because the patient is 'nil-by-mouth'. These drugs can safely be given with a little water preoperatively.

It is no longer recommended to give routine prophylactic cardiac antibiotics [15].

Epilepsy

Those with epilepsy are probably easier to manage surgically as most anaesthetic drugs have antiepileptic properties. It is important that the woman takes her antiepileptic medication as prescribed. She will require careful postoperative observation as there is a risk of seizure in the recovery period. The purported link between propofol and epilepsy has now been disproven; it is safe to use propofol in those with epilepsy [16].

Human immunodeficiency virus (HIV) infection

There is no evidence of an adverse effect from abortion. The woman should continue taking her prescribed antiretroviral drugs and, if she is healthy and well established on medication with a suppressed viral load and adequate CD4 count, there are few implications for anaesthesia. However, if she has severe immunosuppression or a high viral load it is important to liaise with an HIV physician.

Psychiatric conditions and substance use

Women with psychiatric problems need careful consideration given to assessing the impact of abortion versus continuing the pregnancy and may need formal psychiatric and social assessment before making the decision to have an abortion, considering the impact both for themselves and for any child born.

Substance users have additional clinical problems: venous access is important and can be difficult to achieve; heroin and methadone users may require a change of dose of fentanyl/alfentanil given on induction of anaesthesia; cocaine and amphetamines are very unpredictable and can be associated with major cardiac arrhythmias, coronary vasospasm and cardiac arrest. In addition, the history from substance users is often unreliable and it is important to expect the unexpected.

Anticipated surgical problems

Uterine conditions

Women may be referred with uterine anomalies which may be developmental or acquired. Probably the most common acquired anomalies are uterine fibroids. Careful ultrasound scanning, both abdominal and vaginal, can help to assess whether these will impede an abortion. Fundal fibroids are rarely a problem although the woman may suffer from post-operative pain when large fibroids involute after the pregnancy has ended. However, low fibroids may distort the cervix and in some cases completely fill the pelvis preventing access to the gestation sac. Cervical preparation and the use of real-time ultrasound scanning are essential. If the sac is very high in the uterus, medical abortion with mifepristone and miso-prostol may succeed when surgical abortion is not possible or has been incomplete [17]. As a last resort, particularly at later gestations, a hysterotomy may be required. The fibroids should be reassessed after involution of the uterus and long-term management discussed.

Women with known pelvic venous anomalies should be operated on in a centre with access to the skills and equipment for interventional radiology and where severe bleeding can be managed by selective artery embolization [18].

Another increasingly common problem is women who have had several deliveries by caesarean section (CS). Most women in the UK have been delivered by lower segment CS, which minimizes the risk of scar dehiscence; however, women with an upper uterine scar, either for caesarean section or following a myomectomy, are at particular risk. In the first trimester there are rarely any problems when the abortion is performed after cervical prep-aration and under ultrasound surveillance. However, at advanced gestations of pregnancy, especially during medical induction, there is a real risk of scar dehiscence and haemorrhage. Surgical abortion by dilatation and evacuation (D&E) after cervical preparation is the most controlled way to terminate these pregnancies and allows the uterine scar to be assessed digitally at the end of the procedure or if there are any concerns about the integrity of the uterus intraoperatively. However, the woman needs to be aware that there is a risk of haem-orrhage which could lead to hysterectomy. If surgical intervention at laparotomy fails to control the bleeding, or there is generalized bleeding, an interventional radiologist may be able to assist with transfemoral selective artery embolization. In women of high parity with multiple CS scars the risk of a further pregnancy should be discussed and it may be safer to perform a planned hysterotomy and tubal ligation.

Developmental anomalies affecting abortion range from a vaginal or uterine septum to a full duplication of the reproductive organs; monitoring the procedure using ultrasound scanning usually allows a successful abortion. Medical abortion will also usually be straight-forward and effective.

When there is difficulty finding or dilating a cervix, medical preoperative cervical prepa-ration, using mifepristone and misoprostol usually makes it easier to locate the external os and then the cervical canal can be navigated with a fine dilator while monitoring by ultrasound scan. Where there is a suspicion that a false passage has been made, flexible hys-teroscopy, with tension on the cervix to straighten the cervical canal, is a useful tool to find the correct direction [19]. Using ultrasound guidance the dilator can then follow the path taken by the hysteroscope. Once the correct path has been found it is usually relatively easy to introduce larger dilators.

Failure to dilate the cervix, especially by inexperienced operators, may simply be due to failure to recognize a retroverted uterus, or an extreme ante- or retroflexed uterus.

Twin pregnancy

Abortion of a twin pregnancy should be uneventful as any difficulty with an abortion is usually related to the size of the fetus. However, the uterus is more extended and there is a small risk of uterine atony and haemorrhage which can usually be managed with intravenous fluids and oxytocics or prostaglandins.

Physical disabilities

These can cause a problem, particularly when there is difficulty abducting the hips. It is often more comfortable and easier to access the cervix if the legs are supported manually and, if possible, the hips are well flexed. In achondroplasia the uterus may be above the pelvis and access is improved if the operator is seated on a low stool. The option of medical abortion should also be considered but this can also be fraught with difficulties when there is severe pelvic distortion.

Trophoblastic disease

If this is suspected either before or during the abortion, the products of conception need to be sent for histopathological examination and, if the diagnosis is confirmed, reported to a national trophoblastic disease centre for follow-up and management. Vacuum aspiration of the uterus should be straightforward but there is an increased risk of bleeding, particularly at higher gestations.

Contraception

For all these women good contraceptive advice is essential (see Chapter 13). Care must be taken to avoid drug interactions. Surgical abortion offers a good opportunity to consider a levonorgestrel intrauterine system or copper intrauterine device, which are both very effective and have few contraindications. Women planning pregnancy in the future should consult with an obstetrician for pre-pregnancy planning to minimize complications. In women with a badly damaged uterus (some of whom have been advised by their obstetrician never to have another pregnancy) it is appropriate to discuss sterilization.

Conclusion

Generally speaking abortion is a short and straightforward procedure and, even in women with medical problems, the risk of abortion is less than that of a pregnancy carried to term [20]. Where there is the potential for complications requiring specialist multidisciplinary input the abortion should always be performed in a hospital where these skills are available. In practice, with good assessment, liaison with medical specialists, adequate cervical preparation, the availability of real-time ultrasound monitoring and an experienced surgeon and anaesthetist there are rarely problems.

References

1. Department of Health. *Abortion Statistics, England and Wales: 2012.* www.gov.uk/government/uploads/system/uploads/attachment_data/file/213386/ Commentary1.pdf (accessed 2 November 2013).

2. Royal College of Obstetricians and Gynaecologists. *The Care of Women Requesting Induced Abortion. Evidence-based Clinical Guideline Number 7.*

London: RCOG, 2011. www.rcog.org. uk/womens-health/clinical-guidance/ care-women-requesting-induced-abortion (accessed 2 November 2013).

3. Kapp N, Whyte P, Tong J, Jackson E, Brahmi D. A review of evidence for safe abortion care. *Contraception* 2013;88:350–63.

4. Chung F, Yuan H, Yin L, Vairavanathan S, Wong DT. Elimination of preoperative testing in ambulatory surgery. *Anesth Analg* 2009;108:467–75.

5. Grimes DA, Schultz KF, Cates W, Tyler CW. Local versus general anaesthesia: which is safer for performing suction curettage abortions? *Am J Obstet Gynecol* 1979;135:1030–5.

6. MacKay HT, Schulz KF, Grimes DA. Safety of local versus general anaesthesia for second-trimester dilatation and evacuation abortion. *Obstet Gynecol* 1985;66;661–5.

7. Keder LM. Best practices in surgical abortion. *Am J Obstet Gynecol* 2003;189:418–22.

8. Preoperative fasting for adults to prevent perioperative complications (Cochrane review). *The Cochrane Library*, Issue 4. Chichester: Wiley, 2003.

9. World Health Organization. Global database on Body Mass Index. http://apps. who.int/bmi/index.jsp?introPage=intro_3. html (accessed 3 March 2014).

10. Borgatta L, Stubblefield PG. The challenging abortion. In *Management of Unintended and Abnormal Pregnancy*. Chichester: Wiley-Blackwell, 2009: 193–207.

11. Kimball AM, Hallum AV, Cates W. Deaths caused by pulmonary thromboembolism after legally induced abortion. *Am J Obstet Gynecol* 1978;132:169–74.

12. Davis A, Easterling T. Medical evaluation and management. In *Management of Unintended and Abnormal Pregnancy*. Chichester: Wiley-Blackwell, 2009: 78–89.

13. Sahu MT, Rajaram S, Saxena AK, Goel N, Ghumman S. Medical termination of pregnancy in acute intermittent porphyria. *Gynecol Obstet Invest* 2008;62:38–40.

14. James MFM, Hift RJ. Porphyrias. *Br J Anaesth* 2000;85:143–53.

15. National Institute for Health and Care Excellence. *Prophylaxis against Infective Endocarditis (NICE Clinical Guideline 64)*. London: NICE, 2008.

16. Prabhakar H, Bindra A, Singh GP, Kalaivani M. Propofol versus thiopental sodium for the treatment of refractory status epilepticus. *Cochrane Database Syst Rev* 2012;8:CD009202.

17. Creinin MD. Medically induced abortion in a woman with a large myomatous uterus. *Am J Obstet Gynecol* 1996;175:1379–80.

18. Alanis M, Hurst BS, Marshburn PB, Matthews ML. Conservative management of placenta increta with selective arterial embolization preserves future fertility and results in a favorable outcome in subsequent pregnancies. *Fertility and Sterility* 2006;86:1514. e3–e7.

19. Setchell T, Paterson C, Higham J. Flexible hysteroscopic exploration in surgical termination of pregnancy in a patient with uterine abnormality. *J Gynaecol Surg* 2007;4:215–16.

20. Raymond EG, Grimes DA. The comparative safety of legal induced abortion and childbirth in the United States. *Obstet Gynecol* 2012;119:215–19.

- Where the fetal abnormality is not lethal and abortion is being undertaken after 22 weeks' gestation, failure to perform feticide could result in a live birth and survival, an outcome that contradicts the intention of the abortion. In such situations, the baby should receive the neonatal support and intensive care that is in the infant's best interest and its condition managed within published guidance for neonatal practice.

These recommendations are also supported by the clinical guideline from the US Society of Family Planning (SFP) which (based primarily on consensus and expert opinion) recommends that inducing fetal demise before induction abortion avoids signs of life at delivery; this may have beneficial emotional, ethical and legal consequences [1]. Based on limited or inconsistent scientific evidence the SFP recommended that feticide may decrease the induction–delivery time when completing a medical abortion in the second trimester.

There are limited data to support the role of feticide prior to surgical abortion. There has only been one randomized, placebo-controlled trial that studied the use of preoperative intra-amniotic digoxin, which did not reveal a surgical benefit of feticide [6]. The authors found no difference in procedure duration, difficulty, estimated blood loss, pain scores or complications between the groups but concluded that preference of the woman may justify its use. A retrospective analysis of women who underwent second trimester D&E between 13 and 23 weeks also did not find any benefit for preoperative feticide with intracardiac potassium chloride (KCl) [13]. The authors concluded that presurgical feticide with KCl was not associated with shorter anaesthesia time and that the decision to perform feticide should be based on other considerations, such as preference of the woman.

Methods for feticide and their effectiveness

Mechanical and pharmacological methods have been used for induction of fetal demise over the past three to four decades. The mechanical methods described in the literature are as follows:

- cord occlusion or transection
- air embolization
- cardiac puncture and exsanguination
- hysterotomy
- umbilical cord (intrafunic) steel coil placement
- gestation sac aspiration.

The pharmacological methods described in the literature include:

- sclerotic agents (intrafunic and intrahepatic injections of ethanol or enbucrilate)
- normal saline injection
- hypertonic saline injection
- hyperosmolar urea injection
- calcium gluconate injection
- lidocaine injection
- potassium chloride (KCl) injection
- digoxin injection.

Most of the above methods have now been consigned to history. They have been reported mostly as case-series of single agents and no randomized trials have compared their modalities of inducing fetal demise. It is therefore difficult from published information to make a valid comparison regarding safety and efficacy between these methods. Data also remain scarce about the effect of these techniques upon the safety of the abortion itself.

Pharmacological agents are the most commonly used methods for inducing fetal demise nowadays. The majority of information and experience centres on two agents: KCl and digoxin. In the USA, KCl is used generally by specialists in infertility and maternal-fetal medicine, whereas digoxin is used more commonly by abortion providers [1].

Potassium chloride (KCl)

Potassium chloride injected into the fetal circulation is the most frequently used procedure for inducing fetal demise. The most common route of KCl administration is via transabdominal intracardiac injection performed with ultrasound guidance. Intrathoracic and intrafunic injections through the transabdominal route have been reported. Transcervical procedures have also been reported but there have been no randomized controlled trials comparing routes of administration of concentrated KCl. In the UK the RCOG recommends intracardiac KCl 2–3 mL strong (15%) injection into a cardiac ventricle [12]. A further injection may be required if asystole has not occurred after 30–60 seconds. Asystole should be observed for at least two minutes and fetal demise should be confirmed by ultrasound scan after 30–60 minutes. Potassium chloride achieves its effect by disrupting the balance of intra- and extracellular potassium ions, decreasing the conduction of action potentials in cardiac myocytes thus leading to bradycardia and, eventually, asystole [1]. The reported first injection failure rate for KCl ranges from 0% [14] to 9% [15]. The potential advantages of KCl use are that it causes immediate cessation of the fetal heart, there are no drug contraindications and, at doses under 10 mEq, it is virtually free of maternal side-effects or complications as long as accurate needle placement is assured [14].

Digoxin

Digoxin, on the other hand, has been used for inducing fetal demise via intra-amniotic, intrafetal or intrathoracic injection. Digoxin functions by inhibiting the sodium-potassium ATPase – which regulates sodium and calcium concentrations indirectly – increasing cardiac contractility, eventually leading to atrioventricular block [1]. The effectiveness of digoxin in achieving fetal demise is dependent on the dose and the route of administration. Intrafetal digoxin has shown better efficacy in achieving fetal demise than intra-amniotic digoxin. The reported first injection failure rate ranges from 0% with intrafetal injection of 1.0 mg digoxin to 70% with intra-amniotic injection of 0.25 mg digoxin [16]. In a large retrospective review, Molaei et al. concluded that the overall failure rate with digoxin was 7%, although there were no failures with an intrafetal dose of 1.0 mg. A failure rate of 8% was reported in the only RCT that used 1.0 mg intra-amniotic digoxin before surgical abortion at 20–23 weeks' gestation [6].

Intracardiac injection of KCl or intrathoracic injection of digoxin requires considerably more skill than intra-amniotic injection of digoxin. While the latter may be slightly less effective in inducing fetal demise, its use may be an option for services that lack personnel with sufficient skill in administering intracardiac injections [11].

Risks, side-effects and safety of feticidal agents

The medicines or compounds used for feticide have some potential for maternal toxicity or side-effects. The safety of administration of digoxin or KCl for feticide depends on injection of the agent into the desired location and avoiding maternal intravascular injection. Based on limited data, injection of KCl and digoxin to cause fetal demise appears to be a safe procedure with low complication rates. The reported side-effects and complications of inducing fetal demise with these agents include vomiting, early labour or deliveries before reaching theatre for surgical evacuation, infection, cardiac events, coagulopathy, pain from injection and emotional distress [1].

Feticide in non-tertiary settings

In the UK, abortion can only be carried out in a National Health Service (NHS) hospital or in a place approved for the purpose by the Secretary of State for Health (non-NHS setting otherwise called specialist independent sector), and after 24 weeks, only in an NHS hospital [17]. It has been suggested that feticide is under-reported nationally [14]. Pasquini and colleagues [14] also suggested that although the vast majority of feticide procedures are performed within NHS units, it is well known that some procedures are carried out within the private sector (non-tertiary settings). An 11-year review of the abortion statistics for England and Wales residents (Table 16.1) shows that:

- 61% of abortions at all gestations were performed in non-NHS settings while the remaining 39% were performed in NHS hospitals
- there is an increasing trend in the number of abortions being performed in non-NHS settings while the trend is decreasing in NHS settings
- 1.5% of total abortions were carried out at 20 weeks and over
- in 2012, 65% (1858/2860) of the procedures at 20 weeks and over were carried out in non-NHS settings
- only about 1% of all abortions, and 41% of abortions at 20 weeks and over, were reported as involving feticide
- the distribution of the feticide procedures between the two settings was not obvious from the published data.

Historically, feticide was mostly carried out within the NHS in specialist feto-maternal medicine units. However, given that most abortions at 20 weeks and above (65%) are carried out in non-NHS settings, the requirement for feticide in such settings cannot be over-emphasized. One of the specialist independent abortion service providers in the UK, in its quest for clinical excellence and to address the gap in skill, decided in 2004 to train some doctors to provide feticide by intracardiac KCl and in 2007 by intra-amniotic digoxin. The decision to address this skill gap was also necessitated by the need to discontinue a 'two-stage procedure' for late surgical abortion involving cord transection because of the associated complications and to discontinue the use of urea for feticide prior to late medical abortion because it had become obsolete and because of a failed case in which the fetus survived.

The provision of feticide training outside the tertiary centres is in full compliance with the RCOG recommendation that feticide should always be performed by an appropriately trained practitioner (under specialist supervision) using aseptic conditions and with continuous ultrasound monitoring [12]. However, there are a limited number of doctors willing or able to carry out the procedures and a limited number of nurses and other support staff willing to participate in the procedure or to witness them. Individuals involved in abortion care have different levels of tolerance to different procedures and it is important for service providers to recognize this and support them appropriately. An analytical review of

Table 16.1 The proportion of abortions performed in NHS and non-NHS settings and the percentages of abortions carried out at 20 or more weeks and involving feticide (England and Wales residents – 2002 to 2012) [17]

Year	Total no. abortions	% NHS	% non-NHS	>20 weeks		Feticide		% >20 weeks
				Number	% total abortions	Number	% total abortions	
2002	175 932	42	58	2874	2	1056	1	37
2003	181 582	42	58	2927	2	2043	1	64
2004	185 713	40	60	2914	2	1833	1	58
2005	186 416	40	60	2637	1	815	0.4	31
2006	193 737	39	61	2948	2	1002	0.5	34
2007	198 499	38	62	2927	1	1024	0.5	35
2008	195 296	38	62	2889	1	1040	0.5	36
2009	189 100	38	62	2786	1	1086	0.6	39
2010	189 574	37	63	2744	1	988	0.5	38
2011	189 931	35	65	2729	1	1119	0.6	41
2012	185 122	35	65	2860	2	1115	0.6	39
Average	**188 264**	**39**	**61**	**2840**	**1.5**	**1193**	**0.65**	**41**

Table 16.2 Equipment for intracardiac potassium chloride injection

- Dressing pack to include receiver and gallipot
- Sterile gloves
- Cook 17-gauge 16 cm Chiba needle (Ref J-SN-171660)
- 25-gauge needle (× 1)
- 21-gauge needle (× 1)
- 10 mL syringe (× 1; for local anaesthetic)
- 5 mL syringe (× 1; for potassium chloride)
- 1 sterile 'feticide' label for syringe to contain potassium chloride
- Antiseptic solution for skin preparation
- 1% lidocaine (10 mL, if under LA)
- Potassium chloride concentrate: 15% (2 mmol/mL) in 10 mL ampoules
- High resolution ultrasound scanner with curvilinear array transducer and sterile ultrasound gel
- Sterile transducer cover
- Adhesive dressing

the understanding of feticide by Graham *et al.* [18] points out that there is little knowledge about how participation in feticide is conceptualized or experienced by those most closely involved – the women, their partners and the health professionals. The authors argue that the procedure of feticide is a complex and personal experience for those involved and suggest that there is a need to take seriously the views of health professionals at the level of professional opinion, but also at the level of personal ethics, experiences and feelings. In a qualitative study of health professionals' and parents' views about the role of feticide in the context of higher gestation abortion, Graham *et al.* [19] concluded that both the health professionals who provide and facilitate feticide and the women making decisions about abortion and feticide see the procedure as a necessary rather than as a chosen activity. Nevertheless, a survey of providers (physicians, nurses and midwives) on the use of feticide prior to abortion [20] showed that professionals have positive thoughts about the practice of feticide, stating that it avoids fetal or neonatal 'agony or pain'.

Procedure for KCl administration

This procedure is carried out either under local anaesthetic (LA) or general anaesthetic (GA) according to the woman's preference. Using a sterile technique, the equipment (Table 16.2) is prepared. Strong KCl (15%, 2 mmol/mL) is drawn into a labelled 5 mL syringe while 1% lidocaine is drawn into a 10 mL syringe if the procedure is being done under LA.

Women should be advised to empty their bladder immediately before the procedure. With the woman in a supine position on the surgical table, the abdomen is cleansed with non-spirit based antiseptic solution and draped to create a sterile window. A sterile cover containing ultrasound gel is placed over an abdominal transducer and an ultrasound examination performed to check fetal lie, presentation, cardiac motion and location of the placenta. If the procedure is not done under GA, the site for LA is chosen and 5–10 mL 1% lidocaine infused using a 25-gauge needle.

The fetal heart chambers are identified (Figure 16.1) and, under ultrasound guidance, a Chiba needle (Cook 17-gauge 16 cm Chiba needle) is inserted into the uterus and ultimately into the left ventricle of the fetal heart (Figure 16.2). Correct placement of the Chiba needle is confirmed by aspiration of fetal blood. An assistant may be required to steady the needle in order to avoid displacement of a correctly placed needle when the syringe is applied. The

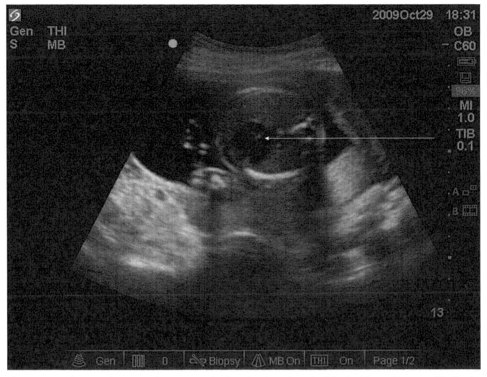

Figure 16.1 Ultrasound image to demonstrate the four chambers (arrow) of the fetal heart. Courtesy of Dr Emeka Oloto.

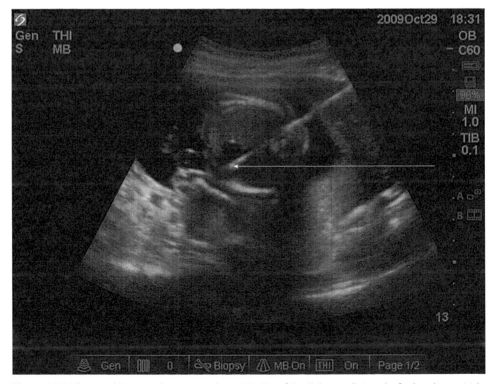

Figure 16.2 Ultrasound image to demonstrate the positioning of the Chiba needle into the fetal cardiac ventricle (arrow) before injection of potassium chloride. Courtesy of Dr Emeka Oloto.

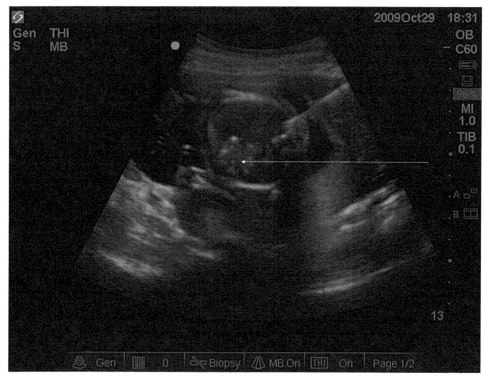

Figure 16.3 Ultrasound image to demonstrate the fetal heart with Chiba needle in situ immediately after injection of 5 mL of potassium chloride (arrow). Courtesy of Dr Emeka Oloto.

drawn KCl is injected into the fetal cardiac ventricle, 1 mL at a time (Figure 16.3), until fetal cardiac asystole is induced. The maximum total volume of KCl to be given is 20 mL. The fetal heart is observed for at least two minutes to confirm asystole. In the case of multiple gestations, the procedure is repeated and KCl administered into each fetal heart. The Chiba needle is then removed, ensuring haemostasis, and a dressing applied to the puncture site. Use of digoxin should be considered in the event of failure of the intracardiac KCl injection.

Procedure for digoxin administration

The equipment is the same as for KCl administration except for the following:
- 22-gauge spinal needle
- sterile 'feticide' label for syringe to contain digoxin
- digoxin: 3 × (2 mL) ampoules (250 µg/mL; total dose 1.5 mg).

The procedure is also similar to that of KCl except for ultrasound identification of an appropriate pocket of amniotic fluid and insertion of the spinal needle into it through the uterus under ultrasound guidance. Intrafetal or intracardiac administration of digoxin is also acceptable for those practitioners with the necessary additional skill.

Correct needle placement is confirmed by aspiration of a few millilitres of clear amniotic fluid into a 5 mL syringe. If bloody fluid is aspirated, the needle is repositioned until clear amniotic fluid is obtained before injecting the digoxin. In the case of multiple gestations, digoxin must be administered into each amniotic sac. The needle is removed, ensuring haemostasis, and a dressing applied to the puncture site.

Failed feticide with digoxin

If the woman is planning a medical abortion and the injection cannot be performed for technical reasons she may be referred to another non-tertiary unit or to a tertiary unit for intracardiac KCl injection. If a surgical abortion is planned, the need for a further injection or procedure without feticide should be considered.

Conclusions

Feticide by ultrasound-guided intracardiac KCl injection or intra-amniotic or intrafetal injection of digoxin is an acceptable, safe and effective method prior to abortion especially at higher gestations. Intracardiac KCl injection requires more technical skill than intra-amniotic or intrafetal digoxin injection. Inducing fetal demise prior to medical abortion at or near viable gestational ages to avoid signs of life at delivery is widely practised and supported by professional guidelines both in the UK and in the USA. The role of feticide in surgical abortion, especially dilatation and evacuation, remains unclear but may be justified by preference of the pregnant woman.

In the USA, KCl is used generally for inducing fetal demise by tertiary centres whereas digoxin is used more commonly by abortion providers outside tertiary settings. In the UK, most abortions at 20 weeks and above (65%) are carried out outside tertiary centres. The need for feticide in non-tertiary centres in the UK, especially prior to medical abortion at or above 22 weeks, cannot be overemphasized.

References

1. Diedrich J, Drey E. Induction of fetal demise before abortion. SFP guideline 21101. Release January 2010. *Contraception* 2010;81:462–73.

2. Royal College of Obstetricians and Gynaecologists. *Further Issues Relating to Late Abortion, Fetal Viability and Registration of Births and Deaths.* RCOG Statement. London: RCOG Press, 2001.

3. Clark P, Smith J, Kelly T, Robinson MJ. An infant who survived abortion and neonatal intensive care. *Journal of Obstetrics and Gynaecology* 2005;5:73–4.

4. Elimian A, Verma U, Tejani N. Effect of causing fatal cardiac asystole on second trimester abortion. *Obstet Gynecol* 1999;94:139–41.

5. Hammond C, Chasen S. Dilation and evacuation. In M Paul *et al.* (eds.) *Management of Unintended and Abnormal Pregnancy.* Chichester: Wiley-Blackwell, 2009: Chapter 11.

6. Jackson RA, Teplin VL, Drey EA, Thomas LJ, Darney PD. Digoxin to facilitate late second-trimester abortion: a randomized, masked, placebo-controlled trial. *Obstet Gynecol* 2001;97:471–6.

7. Evans MI, Goldberg JD, Horenstein J, *et al.* Selective termination for structural, chromosomal, and mendelian anomalies: international experience. *Am J Obstet Gynecol* 1999;181:893–7.

8. Ruano R, Dumez Y, Cabrol D, Dommergues M. Second- and third-trimester therapeutic terminations of pregnancy in cases with complete placenta previa – does feticide decrease post-delivery maternal haemorrhage? *Fetal Diagn Ther* 2004;19:475–8.

9. Bush MC, Eddleman KA. Multifetal pregnancy reduction and selective termination. *Clin Perinatol* 2003;30:623–41.

10. Morris RK, Kilby MD. Fetal reduction. *Obstetrics, Gynaecology and Reproductive Medicine* 2010;20:341–3.

11. Royal College of Obstetricians and Gynaecologists. *The Care of Women Requesting Induced Abortion*. London: RCOG, 2011.

12. Royal College of Obstetricians and Gynaecologists. *Termination of Pregnancy for Fetal Abnormality in England, Scotland and Wales. Report of a Working Party*. London: RCOG, 2010.

13. Singh S, Seligman NS, Jackson B, Berghella V. Fetal intracardiac potassium chloride injection to expedite second-trimester dilatation and evacuation. *Fetal Diagn Ther* 2012:31:63–8.

14. Pasquini L, Pontello V, Kumar S. Intracardiac injection of potassium chloride as method for feticide: experience from a single UK tertiary centre. *BJOG* 2008;115:528–31.

15. Bhide A, Sairam S, Hollis B, *et al.* Comparison of feticide carried out by cordocentesis versus cardiac puncture. *Ultrasound Obstet Gynecol* 2002;20:230–2.

16. Molaei M, Jones HE, Weiselberg T, *et al.* Effectiveness and safety of digoxin to induce fetal demise prior to second-trimester abortion. *Contraception* 2008;77:223–5.

17. Department of Health. *Abortion Statistics, England and Wales: Statistical Bulletin 2012/1*. London: Department of Health, July 2013. www.gov.uk/government/collections/abortion-statistics-for-england-and-wales (accessed 24 November 2013).

18. Graham RH, Robson SC, Rankin JH. Understanding feticide: an analytical review. *Social Science & Medicine* 2008;66:289–300.

19. Graham RH, Mason K, Rankin J, Robson SC. The role of feticide in the context of late termination of pregnancy: a qualitative study of health professionals' and parents' views. *Prenat Diagn* 2009;29:875–81.

20. Dommergues M, Cahen F, Garel M, *et al.* Feticide during second- and third-trimester termination of pregnancy: opinions of health care professionals. *Fetal Diagn Ther* 2003;18:91–7.

Fetal anomaly

Joanna Speedie, Richard Lyus and Stephen C. Robson

Introduction

In many developed countries antenatal screening for fetal anomalies is offered to all pregnant women. As antenatal screening tests and the use of ultrasound to detect fetal anomalies improve, more women/couples are discovering in early pregnancy that their unborn child has a structural or chromosomal anomaly [1,2]. This news is likely to be extremely distressing and is immediately followed by having to face difficult decisions regarding whether to continue with the pregnancy or not [1].

According to the British Abortion Act 1967, as amended by the Human Fertilisation and Embryology Act 1990, termination of pregnancy for fetal anomaly (TOPFA) can be legally performed either under section 1(1)(a) of the Act up to 24 weeks' gestation, or under section 1(1)(d) at any point in the pregnancy. Section 1(1)(a) can be used if two medical practitioners believe that as a result of the fetal anomaly 'the continuance of the pregnancy would involve risk, greater than if the pregnancy were terminated, of injury to the physical or mental health of the pregnant woman or any existing children or her family' [1]. Section 1(1)(d) can be used if 'there is a substantial risk that, if the child were born, it would suffer from such physical or mental abnormalities as to be severely handicapped'. At present there is no legal definition of what constitutes a 'substantial risk' or a 'serious handicap' [1]. Thus decisions around TOPFA after fetal viability are particularly challenging for both parents and health professionals. Fetal medicine specialists acknowledge the difficulties of ensuring they work within the law and within their own ethical frameworks [3]. Practice with respect to which abnormalities meet the legal criteria is governed largely by consensus between colleagues [3].

This chapter will focus on some of the considerations around care for women requesting TOPFA, specifically the implications around method of abortion.

Patterns and trends in termination for fetal abnormality

The World Health Organization estimates that 270,000 newborns worldwide die every year in the first month of life as a result of congenital anomalies. The prevalence of major congenital abnormalities, as estimated by the British Isles Network of Congenital Anomaly Registers (BINOCAR) [4], which cover 35% of births in England and Wales, is shown in Table 17.1. Prevalence figures are very similar to those reported across Europe by the European Surveillance of Congenital Anomalies (EUROCAT), where there has been a

Abortion Care, ed. Sam Rowlands. Published by Cambridge University Press. © Cambridge University Press 2014.

Table 17.1 Prevalence and termination of pregnancy for fetal anomaly (TOPFA) rates (per 10,000 total births) in 2010 for major congenital anomaly subgroups from BINOCAR registers (which cover 35% of births in England and Wales). Adapted from [4]

Congenital anomaly	Prevalence	TOPFA <20 weeks	TOPFA 20+ weeks	Total TOPFA
All anomalies	223.7	30.3	18.8	49.5
Nervous system	24.5	6.8	7.1	14.0
Congenital heart defects	59.2	1.8	5.2	7.0
Respiratory	8.3	0.8	1.2	2.0
Digestive system	18.0	1.0	1.7	2.7
Abdominal wall defects	9.5	2.5	0.3	2.8
Urinary system	26.3	2.1	3.3	5.3
Genital	19.0	0.3	0.6	1.0
Limb	34.3	1.4	3.3	4.8
Chromosomal	40.2	18.7	4.3	23.5

decline in the prevalence of non-chromosomal anomalies between 2001 and 2009 [5]; specifically the prevalence of severe congenital heart defects has fallen from 19.5 per 10,000 in 2000–1 to 16.7 in 2008–9 while the prevalence of neural tube defects has fallen from 10.8 per 10,000 to 9.7 per 10,000 over the same period. This may reflect improved folic acid supplementation. In contrast, EUROCAT reported an increase in the prevalence of the common trisomy syndromes with trisomy 21 increasing from 21.0 per 10,000 in 2000–1 to 22.2 per 10,000 in 2008–9, reflecting the increasing proportion of older mothers [5]. Rates of abortion for fetal anomaly vary (Table 17.1), reflecting variation in the prognosis and impact on quality of life with different anomalies. As one would expect, the severity of an anomaly correlates with abortion rates [6].

In England and Wales in 2012, 2,692 abortions were performed for fetal anomaly (i.e. under ground E of the Abortion Act); this represents 1.45% of the total of 185,122 abortions, a proportion which has remained reasonably stable over the past decade [7]. The main diagnostic groups are shown in Table 17.2. Chromosomal anomalies accounted for just over a third (38%) of cases; trisomy 21 was the most commonly reported chromosomal anomaly (20% of all cases) [7]. In England and Wales, approximately 90% of women given a prenatal diagnosis of trisomy 21 choose to have an abortion, and this figure has remained stable over recent years [8].

Most abortions for fetal anomaly take place in the second trimester. Of the 2,692 TOPFAs in England and Wales, 53% are performed between 13 and 19 weeks of pregnancy with only 14% below 13 weeks [7]. Abortions performed at more than 24 weeks' gestation make up 5.9% of TOPFA (0.1% of all abortions in England and Wales) [7]. This is very similar to the proportion reported by EUROCAT (6.6%) although the rate of TOPFA at 24 weeks or more varied from 0 to 2.65 per 1,000 births in the 12 countries studied [9]. The indications for TOPFA at over 24 weeks are shown in Table 17.2 and are fairly consistent with the types of anomaly reported in the European register-based study where central nervous system, cardiac and chromosomal anomalies made up 26%, 11% and 28% of the total anomalies undergoing abortion at 24 or more weeks respectively [9].

The relationship between gestational age at TOPFA and type of procedure is shown in Figure 17.1. At under 13 weeks of pregnancy 55% of abortions were performed surgically

Table 17.2 Termination of pregnancy for fetal anomaly in England and Wales 2012; principal medical conditions [7]

Congenital anomaly	Number (%)	Over 24 weeks, number (%)
All anomalies	2692 (100)	160 (100)
Nervous system	607 (23)	69 (43)
Cardiovascular system	191 (7)	12 (8)
Respiratory	16 (1)	1 (1)
Digestive system	6 (0)	1 (1)
Urinary system	104 (4)	7 (4)
Musculoskeletal system	174 (6)	11 (7)
Chromosomal	1012 (38)	32 (20)

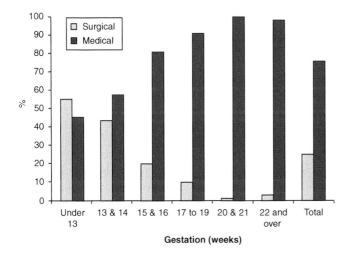

Figure 17.1 Termination of pregnancy for fetal anomaly in England and Wales 2012; relationship between gestational age of termination and type of procedure [7].

[7]. This proportion fell with increasing gestational age such that by 20 weeks and later less than 5% of TOPFA in England and Wales were performed surgically. The same pattern is seen in Europe.

Counselling following the diagnosis of fetal anomaly

When a fetal anomaly is detected antenatally women/couples should be given detailed information regarding their child's condition [10]. This should include written information explaining the nature of the anomaly and the outlook. The Fetal Anomaly Screening Programme (http://fetalanomaly.screening.nhs.uk/) in the UK has produced a series of useful leaflets for parents and health professionals for some of the more common anomalies. Many cases will require referral to a Fetal Medicine Unit for confirmation of diagnosis and more detailed counselling about prognosis, often from several members of the multidisciplinary team. It is important for the couple to have access to a member of the team who will provide support to them from the point of diagnosis to the end of the pregnancy and onwards [10]. Better quality information on the long-term outcome for children with specific prenatally detected anomalies will improve counselling at the point of diagnosis [1].

The decision as to whether to terminate an otherwise wanted pregnancy after a prenatal diagnosis of a fetal anomaly is complex. Factors that influence how different people choose to proceed are: their perception of how disabled their child will be and how they feel that they would cope with this; personal views on abortion; and levels of attachment towards their unborn baby [10]. In chromosomally normal pregnancies with an ultrasound diagnosis of structural anomaly, Pryde *et al.* [11] reported that the major predictor of the decision to abort was the severity of fetal prognosis – rates of TOPFA were 0%, 12% and 66% in the 'mild', 'uncertain' and 'severe' groups. The gestational age at diagnosis was not an important factor [11].

Methods of abortion

The methods available for termination of an anomalous fetus are identical to those for a non-anomalous fetus. Medical abortion in the second trimester entails administration of one dose of oral mifepristone (200 mg) followed 36–48 h later by 800 µg misoprostol given vaginally, then misoprostol 400 µg orally or vaginally every 3 h up to maximum of 4 more doses (see Chapter 9) [12]. If abortion does not occur, mifepristone can be repeated 3 h after the last dose of misoprostol and 12 h later misoprostol may be recommended [12]. An alternative to misoprostol is gemeprost, which should be administered as 1 mg vaginally every 6 h for 24 h followed by 1 mg every 3 h for 12 h if required [12]. There is no evidence that gemeprost is superior to misoprostol and it is considerably more costly. The average length of time from administration of the first dose of prostaglandin to abortion (~8 h) is unaltered by the presence of a fetal anomaly and overall around 95% of women deliver within 24 h [12].

Women should be offered regular analgesia throughout the procedure; paracetamol has been shown to have no effect (see Chapter 11). Regular NSAIDs should be used alongside opiate analgesia if required [12]. When opiates are required intravenous patient-controlled analgesia with fentanyl or morphine offers superior pain relief to intermittent injection. However, high-dose opiates slow gastric emptying and depress respiration [13]. Epidural analgesia provides high quality pain relief without these disadvantages but availability varies substantially, especially for TOPFA under 20 weeks of pregnancy [13].

At advanced gestations surgical abortion will always be done under general anaesthesia. Until 15 weeks' gestation this can usually be done by vacuum aspiration [12]. After this dilatation and evacuation (D&E) is necessary (see Chapter 10). Prior to a surgical procedure women should be given a cervical priming agent [12]. In the second trimester either vaginal misoprostol 400 µg or gemeprost 1 mg can be administered vaginally 3 h prior to surgery, or mifepristone 200 mg orally 36–48 h preoperatively [12]. The authors favour gemeprost 3 and 6 h prior to the anticipated time of the procedure for all nulliparous women over 13 weeks and multiparous women at 17 or more weeks [14]. Alternative agents are buccal misoprostol or overnight placement of osmotic dilators [12]. A recent retrospective review has suggested that vaginal misoprostol 400 µg and no more than three Dilapan-S® dilators 3–4 h prior to D&E up to 22 weeks' gestation provides effective same-day priming [15].

Choice of method in the context of TOPFA

Decision-making about method of TOPFA should be shared; women need to understand the risks and benefits of each option and clinicians need to be empathetic to their preferences. Several factors may influence decision-making in this context.

Complications and adverse effects

The risks of second trimester medical and surgical abortions are not influenced by the presence of a fetal anomaly and include haemorrhage, infection, retained products of conception, cervical trauma, uterine perforation and failure [13,16]. Department of Health data indicate that, for abortions at 13–19 weeks, serious complications (haemorrhage, uterine perforation and/or sepsis) occurred in 1 per 1,000 surgical abortions compared to 16 per 1,000 medical abortions [7]. Comparable figures for abortions at over 19 weeks were 3 per 1,000 and 29 per 1,000 respectively. This is consistent with the Cochrane review of surgical versus medical methods for second trimester abortion which found that complications were 2.6–7.9 times more common with medical abortion [17]. Rates of retained products of conception are much higher after medical procedures; in one study retained tissue was reported in 22% of women compared to 2% after D&E [18]. Similarly in a study of TOPFA at 13–24 weeks, Bryant *et al.* [19] reported retained tissue requiring D&C or manual removal of the placenta in 28/136 (21%) of cases having medical abortion compared to 2/263 (1%) having D&E. Studies on abortion for reasons other than fetal anomaly have found no evidence that method or gestational age influence the incidence of adverse future obstetric outcomes. A recent editorial identified several studies of subsequent pregnancy morbidity after D&E, none of which found a statistically significant association with adverse pregnancy outcomes [20].

Other less serious, but untoward, effects are also more common after second trimester medical abortion; apart from a higher incidence of fever and gastrointestinal side-effects (related to repeated doses of prostaglandin) women suffer more pain and bleeding during and after the procedure [12,14]. These, together with the higher incidence of unexpected overnight stay [14], may add to the distress experienced by women having TOPFA.

Preference and acceptability

Some women will express a strong preference for one method over the other. In the context of TOPFA women may prefer medical abortion because they wish to see and hold their baby, often wanting the opportunity to take photographs and hand- or footprints [1,10], or they may see medical induction and vaginal delivery as a more natural method of abortion. Other women express a preference for surgical abortion because they want to be asleep and have no awareness of the procedure, feeling this is psychologically less traumatic.

In the context of mid-trimester abortion for a non-anomalous fetus, more women express a preference for surgical abortion [14]; indeed one pilot randomized trial of medical versus surgical abortion for second trimester abortion from the USA was abandoned because so few women were willing to be randomized to the medical arm [21]. Women who express a preference for one method invariably report high rates of acceptability (as judged by whether they would choose the same method again). However, in randomized trials (where women were in equipoise over the method to have) surgical has been consistently shown to be more acceptable to women than medical abortion and this difference increases with increasing gestational age [1,14]. In the only randomized trial of abortion method using current regimens in women at 13–20 weeks' gestation, 100% of women randomized to surgical abortion stated that they would opt for the same procedure again compared with only 53% of women having medical abortion [14]. Reduced acceptability is related to the higher rate of untoward effects after medical abortion.

While these results are persuasive they cannot be extrapolated to women undergoing TOPFA where different factors are likely to influence both preference and acceptability. Very little research has been conducted into women's decision-making about choice of second trimester abortion method following diagnosis of fetal anomaly. Kerns *et al.* [22] conducted interviews in women terminating anomalous pregnancies at 14–24 weeks' gestation, most of which had a structural anomaly; 62% chose D&E over medical abortion. Women's preferences for a method were largely based on their individual emotional coping styles; those who chose a medical procedure sought to build upon their existing bond with their baby by actively creating new experiences and new emotional attachments. Women who chose D&E, while expressing equally intense sentiments of attachment and relationship to the baby, sought to preserve the existing bond rather than adding new dimensions to that bond. Women valued the ability to choose the method [22].

Availability

Access to surgical abortion and specifically D&E is limited in many countries including the UK where few gynaecologists have the necessary skills to perform the procedure [1]. While these skills are often available in the specialist independent sector, referral outside of the National Health Service is uncommon. A survey has recently been completed of 430 women resident in England who had undergone TOPFA at 7–24 weeks of pregnancy (Fisher J, personal communication); only 26% of surgical procedures were performed in the independent sector – a much lower proportion compared to surgical abortion without fetal anomaly. Critically only 14% of women overall were offered a choice of method – this figure fell to only 8% after 14 weeks' gestation. Even when surgical abortion is offered, this often requires travelling sometimes significant distances, invariably adding to procedural delays.

Post-mortem examination

A complete and detailed post-mortem examination requires an intact fetus. However, the value of post-mortem examination is dependent on the prenatal diagnosis; it is extremely unlikely to be of benefit in confirmed cases of common karyotypic anomalies such as trisomies and 45X which represent about one third of TOPFA [20]. Even in chromosomally normal fetuses with a structural anomaly diagnosed by a specialist fetal medicine unit, the proportion of TOPFA in which a post-mortem provides supplemental information is only 15–20% [23]. In these cases the information rarely alters counselling about future pregnancy management [23]. Diagnostic information can be successfully obtained from fetal parts examined after surgical abortion, especially if combined with genetic testing, even prior to 16 weeks' gestation. Thus, based on the prenatal diagnosis, it is important that women receive realistic advice about the likely value of post-mortem examination when deciding the method of TOPFA.

Feticide

When undertaking a TOPFA the intention is that the fetus should not survive and that the process of termination should achieve this [1]. Death may be induced by feticide or result from a compromised fetus being unable to tolerate induced labour. Death may also occur after birth either because of the severity of the abnormality or because of severe prematurity (or both) [1].

As mentioned in Chapter 16, the UK Royal College of Obstetricians and Gynaecologists recommends feticide for abortions at over 21+[6] weeks. The only exception is when the anomaly is so severe that early neonatal death is inevitable, irrespective of the gestation at delivery. However, it is clear from national abortion statistics in England and Wales that feticide is not performed for some TOPFA at over 21+[6] weeks [1]; in 2012, of the 1,312 abortions performed at 22 weeks and over, 71% were preceded by induced fetal demise [7]. It is unclear what proportion of this group were having TOPFA. In the context of TOPFA it is not known whether failure to induce fetal death relates to a decision not to offer the procedure on the part of the clinician or whether the procedure was offered but declined by the woman [1].

Feticide is an extremely stressful procedure; sympathetic and supportive counselling before and after the procedure is critical. Techniques for feticide are fully covered in Chapter 16. Feticide should be performed by an appropriately trained practitioner. Often this will require a further visit to a fetal medicine unit potentially adding to procedural delays.

Live birth can occur at gestations below 21+[6]; Wyldes and Tonks [24] reported that 3.5% of fetuses terminated for fetal anomaly at 20 weeks' gestation showed signs of life and this increased progressively to 9.7% of those delivered at 23 weeks. Thus it is important to discuss the possibility of signs of life, and how these will be managed, with all women undergoing medical abortion after 19 weeks' gestation.

Other considerations
Clinical setting
There is no current guidance regarding the optimal location for TOPFA. Above 20 weeks' gestation women are usually cared for on a delivery suite/labour ward as few nurses have the necessary experience to care for women at these advanced gestations. Prior to 20 weeks women are more often cared for on a gynaecology ward. This has the advantage that the woman will not be near to labouring and recently delivered women. Some centres have developed bespoke outpatient facilities for women undergoing TOPFA. Aside from having dedicated experienced staff, who can offer pre- and post-procedure counselling, such a facility ensures women will not link their experience with a maternity unit where, in the future, they may return to deliver a healthy baby.

Cremation and burial
Women/couples should be able to decide what to do with their baby's body. In the UK if they request that the abortion provider disposes of the fetus then this should be done in accordance with the Human Tissue Authority's Code of Practice 5: 'Disposal of human tissue for fetuses born dead at or before 24 weeks of gestation' [12]. If the couple wish to arrange disposal themselves then they should be supported throughout this process [12]. By law, if an abortion is performed at after 24 weeks' gestation, the fetus must be registered as a stillbirth and the body must be either cremated or buried [12].

Hospital follow-up visit
Follow-up after TOPFA is important but often the area of care that some women find lacking [1]. It is crucial that the woman's general practitioner and community midwife are informed of the pregnancy outcome so that support is available for her following her

discharge [1]. Hospital follow-up will usually be with the obstetric team but may be with a specialist centre if clinical genetics/fetal medicine input is required based on the prenatal diagnosis and, where relevant, the results of post-mortem examination. An appointment to discuss post-mortem results should be arranged as soon as possible and any unavoidable delays should be explained to women and their partners and the stress this causes acknowledged [1].

Psychological impact

While women and their partners grieve the loss of their baby they may experience feelings of guilt, failure and anger [10]. They may also become very anxious that they will not be able to conceive a 'normal' baby in the future. Although both parents find TOPFA to be a traumatic event, women tend to suffer more initial distress than men although levels become the same over time [2,12]. Korenromp and colleagues have performed detailed studies of the long-term psychological consequences of TOPFA; at 4 months after abortion 46% of women exhibited post-traumatic stress disorder, decreasing to 21% after 16 months. Rates of depression were 28% and 13% respectively. Importantly late onset of problematic adaptation was rare and psychological outcome at four months after abortion was the most important predictor of persistent impaired psychological outcome [25]. Other predictors were low self-efficacy, high level of doubt during decision-making, lack of partner support, being religious and advanced gestational age [25]. This is consistent with an earlier study by White-van Mourik et al., who reported long-term emotional consequences in 20% of women [26]. In a small number of cases couples divorced or underwent a temporary separation after the abortion. Couples need to be aware of these possible psychological impacts. However, it is important to recognize that very few regret their decision to terminate the pregnancy and most plan to conceive again [2].

In addition to medical follow-up, couples should have access to support services. They should be given relevant contact details of local services at the time of discharge after termination. Uptake varies although most couples who take up the offer derive benefit from supportive counselling. This is consistent with the results of one randomized trial of routine versus selective counselling by an experienced psychotherapist after bereavement for fetal anomaly; no differences were found in grief, anxiety or depression [27]. Sometimes couples derive benefit from a shared experience group [28].

Third trimester TOPFA

TOPFA is rare in the third trimester. The need usually arises when prenatal diagnosis has been delayed or women/couples have taken a long time to make a decision about TOPFA, usually because of initial uncertainties about prognosis – this typically arises with some nervous system anomalies [29]. The loss of a baby late in pregnancy is extremely distressing and, as discussed above, associated with a higher likelihood of adverse psychological outcome [25,29]. However, there appears to be no increased morbidity associated with third trimester abortion when compared with procedures performed in the second trimester [16,29].

Third trimester abortion can be achieved by labour induction or assisted fetal expulsion [16]. Cervical priming is essential for successful induction of labour and it may take several days for optimum results to be achieved prior to artificial rupture of the membranes and oxytocin infusion [16]. If assisted fetal expulsion is chosen, physicians may use forceps to control delivery of the fetus under ultrasound guidance [16].

Conclusions

An increasing number of pregnant women are offered screening and diagnosis for fetal anomaly. When people find out they have a fetus with a major anomaly they experience shock and distress and face challenging decisions about whether to continue the pregnancy. They need accurate information about the diagnosis and prognosis delivered in a sensitive manner. TOPFA can be performed by surgical or medical methods although there is accumulating evidence that, in experienced hands, a surgical procedure is safer and preferred by many women. Decision-making about the method should be shared and where appropriate both methods should be offered as there is good evidence that women favour choice. However, access to surgical abortion after 18 weeks is extremely limited in the UK and fetal medicine units need to work with external providers to ensure women are able to access this option.

References

1. Royal College of Obstetricians and Gynaecologists. *Termination of Pregnancy for Fetal Abnormality in England, Scotland and Wales: Report of a Working Party*. 2010. www.rcog.org.uk/termination-pregnancy-fetal-abnormality-england-scotland-and-wales (accessed 21 May 2013).

2. Korenromp MJ. Parental adaptation to termination of pregnancy for fetal anomalies. 2006. http://igitur-archive.library.uu.nl/dissertations/2006-0621-200023/full.pdf (accessed 21 May 2013).

3. Statham H, Solomou W, Green J. Late termination of pregnancy: law, policy and decision making in four English fetal medicine units. *BJOG* 2006;113:1402–11.

4. BINOCAR. Congenital Anomaly Statistics 2010, England and Wales. Published July 2012. www.binocar.org/content/Annual%20report%202010%20FINAL%2031_07_12%20v2.pdf (accessed 21 May 2013).

5. EUROCAT Statistical Monitoring Report – 2009. www.eurocat-network.eu/content/Stat-Mon-Executive-Summary-2009.pdf (accessed 21 May 2013).

6. Schechtman KB, Gray DL, Baty JD, Rothman SM . Decision-making for termination of pregnancies with fetal anomalies: analysis of 53,000 pregnancies. *Obstet Gynecol* 2002;99:216–22.

7. Department of Health. *Abortion Statistics, England and Wales: Statistical Bulletin 2012/1*. London: Department of Health, July 2013. www.gov.uk/government/collections/abortion-statistics-for-england-and-wales (accessed 18 November 2013).

8. Morris JK, Alberman E. Trends in Down's syndrome live births and antenatal diagnoses in England and Wales from 1989 to 2008: analysis of data from the National Down Syndrome Cytogenetic Register. *BMJ* 2009;339:b3794.

9. Garne E, Khoshnood B, Loane M, Boyd PA, Dolk H. The EUROCAT Working Group. Termination of pregnancy for fetal anomaly after 23 weeks of gestation: a European register-based study. *BJOG* 2010;117:660–6.

10. Brien J, Fairbairn I. *Pregnancy and Abortion Counselling*. London: Routledge, 1996.

11. Pryde PG, Isada NB, Hallak M, Johnson MP, Odgers AE, Evans MI. Determinants of parental decision to abort or continue after non-aneuploid ultrasound-detected fetal abnormalities. *Obstet Gynecol* 1992;80:52–6.

12. Royal College of Obstetricians and Gynaecologists. *The Care of Women Requesting Induced Abortion. Evidence-based Guideline 11*, 2011. www.rcog.org.uk/womens-health/clinical-guidance/care-women-requesting-induced-abortion (accessed 21 May 2013).

13. Benhamou D. Pain, epidural analgesia and late termination of pregnancy: a new challenge for obstetric anaesthesiologists. *Int J Obstet Anaesth* 2007;16:307–9.

14. Kelly T, Suddes J, Howel D, Hewison J, Robson S. Comparing medical versus surgical termination of pregnancy at 13–20 weeks of gestation: a randomised controlled trial. *BJOG* 2010;117:1512–20.

15. Lyus R, Lohr PA, Taylor J, Morroni C. Outcomes with same-day cervical preparation with Dilapan-S osmotic dilators and vaginal misoprostol before dilatation and evacuation at 18 to 21+6 weeks' gestation. *Contraception* 2013;87:71–5.

16. Hern WM. Outpatient abortion for fetal anomaly and fetal death from 15–34 menstrual weeks' gestation: techniques and clinical management. *Obstet Gynecol* 1993;81:301–6.

17. Lohr P. Surgical versus medical methods for second trimester induced abortion. *Cochrane Database of Systematic Reviews* 2008:CD06714.

18. Whitley KA, Trinchere K, Prutsman W, Quiñones JN, Rochon ML. Midtrimester dilation and evacuation versus prostaglandin induction: a comparison of composite outcomes. *Am J Obstet Gynecol* 2011;205:386. e1–e7.

19. Bryant AG, Grimes DA, Garrett JM, Stuart GS. Second-trimester abortion for fetal anomalies or fetal death: labor induction compared with dilation and evacuation. *Obstet Gynecol* 2011;117:788–92.

20. Lyus RJ, Robson S, Parsons J, Fisher J, Cameron M. Second trimester abortion for fetal abnormality. *BMJ* 2013;347:f4165.

21. Grimes DA, Smith MS, Witham AD. Mifepristone and misoprostol versus dilatation and evacuation for midtrimester abortion: a pilot randomised controlled trial. *BJOG* 2004;111:148–53.

22. Kerns J, Vanjani R, Freedman L, Meckstroth K, Drey EA, Steinauer J. Women's decision making regarding choice of second trimester termination method for pregnancy complications. *Int J Gynecol Obstet* 2012;116:244–8.

23. Vogt C, Blaas HG, Salvesen KÅ, Eik-Nes SH. Comparison between prenatal ultrasound and postmortem findings in fetuses and infants with developmental anomalies. *Ultrasound Obstet Gynecol* 2012;39:666–72.

24. Wyldes MP, Tonks AM. Termination of pregnancy for fetal anomaly: a population-based study 1995 to 2004. *BJOG* 2007;114:639–42.

25. Korenromp MJ, Page-Christiaens GCML, van den Bout J, Mulder EJH, Visser GHA. Adjustment to termination of pregnancy for fetal anomaly: a longitudinal study of women at 4, 8 and 16 months. *Am J Obstet Gynecol* 2009;201:160e1–7.

26. White-van Mourik MCA, Connor JM, Ferguson-Smith MA. The psychological sequelae of a second-trimester termination of pregnancy for fetal abnormality. *Prenat Diagn* 1992;12:189–204.

27. Lilford RJ, Stratton P, Godsil S, Prasad A. A randomised trial of routine versus selective counselling in perinatal bereavement from congenital disease. *Br J Obstet Gynaecol* 1994;101:291–6.

28. Gordon L, Thornton A, Lewis S, Wake S, Sahhar M. An evaluation of a shared experience group for women and their support persons following prenatal diagnosis and termination for a fetal abnormality. *Prenat Diagn* 2007;27:835–9.

29. Domergues M. The reasons for termination of pregnancy in the third trimester. *Br J Obstet Gynaecol* 1999;106:297–303.

Longer-term outcomes in women requesting abortion

Sam Rowlands

Introduction

In this chapter, the evidence for longer-term adverse health outcomes from abortion or from the restriction of access to abortion will be considered. The first part consists of physical and psychological health outcomes after abortion. The second part considers the effect on both the woman and the child born after abortion is denied. With respect to the first part, studies generally show that first trimester medical abortion, as compared to first trimester surgical abortion, is at least as safe with respect to the risks of ectopic pregnancy, miscarriage, pre-term delivery and low birth weight. This is important information in view of the increasing proportion of abortions being performed medically in many countries.

This chapter will not consider abortions carried out for medical and genetic reasons, which comprise only around 1.5% of total abortions and have their own particular associations; these are covered in Chapter 17. Neither will this chapter consider outcomes after unsafe abortion, which is dealt with in Chapter 14.

Association and causality

Before looking at the literature on this subject, it is useful to rehearse some epidemiological principles. There are no randomized clinical trials in this area of investigation. We have to rely solely on observational (cohort and case-control) studies. There are now many systematic reviews in the literature and these should be preferred over individual studies as they come higher in the hierarchy of evidence (see www.cebm.net/index.aspx?o=1025).

Association refers to the statistical dependence between two variables. Put another way, it is the degree to which the rate of a condition in people with a specific exposure (a drug, a toxic substance, a procedure) is either higher or lower than the rate of a condition among those without that exposure. The presence of an association, however, in no way implies that the observed relationship is one of cause and effect. The role of chance, bias (anything that erroneously influences the conclusions about groups and distorts comparisons) and confounding (mixing of effects between the exposure, the condition and a third factor that is associated with the exposure and independently affects the risk of developing the condition) are often at work: an account of these is beyond the scope of this chapter. So too is examination of the validity and generalizability of studies. Once a valid statistical relationship has been established between the exposure (abortion) and the condition, it is then necessary to consider whether this relationship is one of cause and effect. To help with this, we can examine some criteria put forward by Bradford Hill in 1965 [1]. It needs to be borne in mind that causal mechanisms usually have more than one component cause and that these different causes can interact with each other [1].

1. Is the association strong?

A strong association is much more likely to be causal. The risk of lung cancer in smokers is 9–10 times that in non-smokers. Many studies come up with weak associations (relative risks below 2); these are less likely to result from a causal relationship.

2. Is the association consistent from study to study?

Consistency is when a number of studies, conducted by different investigators at various times using alternative methodology in a variety of geographical or cultural settings and among different populations, all show similar results. Mere replication of a study by the same method will not be as convincing as the same results being obtained using different study designs, e.g. cohort and case control.

3. Is the association specific?

This is where a condition develops that appears to be specific to a particular exposure. Examples here are specific particles that cause typical occupational lung conditions.

4. Is the temporal relationship appropriate?

It should be clear that the exposure of interest preceded the outcome by a period of time consistent with any proposed biological mechanism. Induction times in the development of cancers can be lengthy; for example exposure of a female fetus to diethylstilbestrol and subsequent development of adenocarcinoma of the vagina takes more than 15 years.

5. Is there a dose-response effect?

A dose-response effect means that the risk of the condition increases with the degree of exposure; the greater the number of cigarettes smoked, the greater the risk of lung cancer. For abortion, this means that the condition under study will be more likely to develop the greater the number of abortions that the woman has.

6. Does the association make biological sense?

The belief in the existence of a cause and effect relationship is enhanced if there is a known or postulated biological mechanism by which the exposure might reasonably alter risk of developing a condition. For instance, the generally accepted causal association between combined oral contraceptive use and circulatory disease relates to a prothrombotic effect in users. However, a problem here is that science develops and reveals findings that were previously unknown. For example, before the advent of virology, fetuses affected by rubella were seen but the cause was unknown.

7. Does the association make epidemiological sense?

The cause and effect interpretation of an association should not seriously conflict with generally known facts about conditions being investigated. It should have coherence.

8. Is there evidence from true experiments in humans?

Here, it may be possible to take some preventive measure and see a reduction in the condition when exposure is stopped. This demonstrates reversibility.

Table 18.1 Prospective studies showing normal fertility after abortion

Study	Setting	Controls	Follow-up (months)	% conceived
WHO 1984 [3]	Obs/Gyn Hungary and South Korea	Postpartum family planning	30	>90% in both groups
MacKenzie and Fry 1988 [4]	Obs/Gyn UK	Self	24	97%
Frank et al. 1993 [5]	General practice UK	Deliveries of unplanned pregnancies	24	97% in both groups

9. Is the association analogous to a previously proven causal association?

Based on the known adverse effects of thalidomide and rubella on the fetus, another drug or another viral infection may be suspected of being teratogenic.

Physical and psychological health outcomes after abortion

Physical outcomes after abortion, apart from breast cancer, have been reviewed by Lowit and co-researchers in 2010 [2]. Physical outcomes studied cover future fertility and future pregnancy outcomes including early pregnancy loss, obstetric complications and perinatal complications.

Fertility

Genital tract infection is a recognized immediate complication of abortion; this is covered in Chapter 14. Pelvic inflammatory disease is the most severe form of genital tract infection. It is known that pelvic inflammatory disease is associated with subsequent infertility due to the Fallopian tubes becoming scarred and obstructed, so there is biological plausibility.

Early reports in the literature raised the possibility that abortion could adversely affect subsequent fertility. These reports from Eastern Europe and Japan were either unsupported by data or were lacking a control group for comparison. Some subsequent studies included women who had had illegal abortions, which negates their findings.

Three prospective studies [3–5] carried out during the 1980s and 1990s examining fertility after induced abortion consistently demonstrate no adverse effect of abortion on subsequent fertility (Table 18.1).

There are four case-control studies in the literature, three of which show no effect of abortion on subsequent fertility and one of which shows a negative association of borderline significance. Case-control studies should be interpreted cautiously as they are subject to bias and come lower down the list in the hierarchy of evidence than cohort studies.

In summary, there is no proven risk of an adverse effect on subsequent fertility when an abortion is carried out in proper, safe medical conditions and is not complicated by pelvic inflammatory disease.

Miscarriage

It is recognized that during surgical abortion the cervix may be damaged. It has been hypothesized that such injury could make it less competent in subsequent pregnancies and so less able to retain a pregnancy. Surgical abortions in which cervical preparation (priming) is carried out should make injury less likely. So there is biological plausibility.

The literature is inconsistent in this area. Two cohort and three case-control studies published prior to 1999 found no association [2]. Those that analysed data according to number of abortions could show no dose-response effect. However, two more recent studies have shown a weak positive association between abortion and subsequent miscarriage; one study showed this finding only if the pregnancy occurs within three months of the abortion. Neither of these studies could provide any information on cervical preparation prior to surgical abortion. One meta-analysis based on seven cohort studies found that the incidence of miscarriage is lower after medical abortion than after surgical abortion: odds ratio 0.48 (95% CI 0.25–0.92) [6].

In summary, the rather sparse literature on this subject is inconsistent and no clear conclusions can be drawn.

Ectopic pregnancy

Ectopic pregnancy is a known adverse outcome following pelvic inflammatory disease. It would be biologically plausible that the risk of having a subsequent ectopic pregnancy could be raised in women who have had induced abortions, as infection is a recognized complication of abortion.

Nine studies were reviewed by the UK Royal College of Obstetricians and Gynaecologists (RCOG) in 2011 [7]. Seven of these nine studies were of a case-control design and therefore prone to less reliable results. Two of the case-control studies reported a positive association; both were small studies relying on self-report of previous abortion. The other five case-control studies showed no association. The two large cohort studies that used medical records to define those who had had an abortion showed no such association.

In conclusion, all good quality evidence shows no association between abortion and subsequent ectopic pregnancy.

Placenta praevia

A large Danish cohort study based on record-linkage showed no association between abortion and subsequent placenta praevia [8]. Previous studies, some of poor quality, had showed variable results. Two meta-analyses by Ananth and co-workers examining the literature prior to 2000 showed differing results (cited in Lowit et al. [2]). The first included six studies, five of which were case-control design; pooled results showed a non-significant association between abortion and placenta praevia. The second identified eight case-control studies with an overall odds ratio of 1.5 (95% CI 1.3–1.9).

The literature on a possible association between abortion and subsequent placenta praevia is inconsistent, but one high quality study shows no association. The RCOG guideline concluded that there is no proven association between abortion and subsequent placenta praevia [7]. The evidence is insufficient to be able to provide a clear message to women undergoing abortion.

Placental abruption

There is little research on this outcome, but what there is shows no association between abortion and placental abruption in subsequent pregnancies [2].

Table 18.2 Meta-analyses showing the weak positive association between abortion and preterm delivery

Meta-analysis	No. of studies included	Adjusted odds ratio (95% CI)	
		1 abortion	2+ abortions
Shah and Zao 2009 [10]	37	1.27 (1.12–1.44)	1.62 (1.27–2.07)
Swingle et al. 2009 [11]	12	1.25 (1.03–1.48)	1.51 (1.21–1.75)

Pre-eclampsia

The feto-placental unit contains paternal antigenic tissue which is foreign to the maternal host. Immunological tolerance between fetus and maternal host is necessary for a successful pregnancy. It has been hypothesized that passage of trophoblast cells into the maternal circulation results in an immunological response which gives protection in a subsequent pregnancy through enhanced maternal-fetal tolerance.

The situation with a previous abortion in relation to pre-eclampsia is analogous to a previously proven causal negative association between a previous full-term pregnancy and pre-eclampsia. There are consistent findings from several studies [9] that the risk of pre-eclampsia is significantly reduced in those women at or near term who have had an abortion in the past, although the protective effect is not as strong as that conferred by a full-term pregnancy prior to a second pregnancy. This negative association is likely causal.

Preterm delivery

In the same way as for miscarriage, after fetal viability an incompetent cervix could increase the risk of preterm delivery in subsequent pregnancies. So there is biological plausibility.

There are two meta-analyses that have been done on the relationship between abortion and preterm delivery, defined as delivery before 37 weeks. Both of these were published in 2009. That of Shah and Zao [10] included 37 studies. That of Swingle et al. [11] had stricter quality criteria and included only 12 studies (8 cohort and 4 case-control). Three of the high quality cohort studies included in the Swingle meta-analysis showed no association.

The almost identical results of both meta-analyses are summarized in Table 18.2. They show a weak association with a dose-response effect. Many of the studies relied on maternal recall of abortion. The association could be explained by bias or confounding. Low socio-economic status, higher gravidity, high-risk sexual behaviours, smoking and drug misuse, prior adverse pregnancy outcomes, being single with poor social support and black ethnicity are all more common among women who have had prior abortions than among controls.

It must be borne in mind that for the subjects in most of the studies included in these meta-analyses the abortions were performed surgically (and the deliveries under scrutiny took place prior to 2000). In the few studies so far done on medical abortion, no association with preterm delivery has been shown.

A study of Scottish data from 1980 to 2008 showed a positive association between previous abortion(s) and preterm delivery, with a dose-response effect [12]. However, when the data were plotted over time, the association progressively weakened and disappeared after 2000. The authors draw attention to the fact that between 1992 and 2008, surgical abortions without cervical preparation decreased from 31% to 0.4% of the total and medical abortions increased from 18% to 68%. A record-linkage study is needed to confirm or refute this possible link between the two trends.

The preliminary conclusion must therefore be that there is evidence of a weak association between surgical abortion and subsequent preterm delivery, but causality has not been demonstrated. Final conclusions on this are not possible and further research is needed. The potential risk should be mentioned to women requesting abortion, as stated in Recommendation 5.12 of the RCOG guideline [7].

Breast cancer

This possible risk was mooted after research in rats. In a study by Russo and Russo in 1980, rats were given dimethyl-benzanthracene, a carcinogen [13]. In these rats, full-term pregnancy rendered the mammary gland less susceptible to carcinogenesis than virgin rats or those whose pregnancies were terminated. Some authors have made a big leap by extrapolating from rats to humans. It is postulated that nulligravidae have undifferentiated mammary gland cells and that parous women have fully differentiated cells, less vulnerable to carcinogens. It is further postulated that women having induced abortions may have partially differentiated cells. There is no evidence that these theories have any clinical applicability. Indeed, there are now alternative theories: human chorionic gonadotrophin produced by the placenta itself induces the production of inhibin, a tumour-suppressor factor which tends to protect the breast from carcinogenesis. So, biological plausibility is absent.

A meta-analysis by Brind in 1996 included 23 studies and chose not to include 19 other available studies. The study showed a weak positive association, with an odds ratio of 1.3 (95% CI 1.2–1.4) [14]. A systematic review by Wingo et al. in 1997 included 28 studies; the authors felt that a definitive conclusion on any association could not be reached because of inconsistent findings across studies [15].

A pooled analysis of 53 studies published in 2004 showed no association between induced abortion and breast cancer later in life (cited in Rowlands [16]). Taking the 13 studies with information on abortion recorded prospectively (before the diagnosis of breast cancer), the relative risk of breast cancer comparing women who had had one or more pregnancies that ended in induced abortion to women with no such record was 0.93 (95% CI 0.89–0.96).

More than 20 case-control studies have been published on this topic, some of which show a positive association. However, case-control studies are subject to recall bias, with more under-reporting of the potentially sensitive information about previous induced abortions in the healthy controls than in the breast cancer cases. This bias produces a spurious raised risk of breast cancer in the results of studies of this type.

There are also at least eight prospective cohort studies published up to 2003 which are more likely to give reliable results: these show no association or a negative association [16]. Recall bias does not occur in record-linkage studies in which study subject data are present in databases: at least seven such studies show no association. Five more recent cohort studies of high quality also show no association [17–21]: all relative risk confidence intervals include unity, even for multiple abortions (Table 18.3). High quality studies with consistent results continue to be published [22].

It can thus be stated in robust terms that no association exists between abortion and breast cancer. Bodies supporting this conclusion are the World Health Organization (2000), the American Congress of Obstetricians and Gynecologists (2009) and the RCOG (2004 and 2011).

Mental health

'Postabortion syndrome' was conceptualized in 1992 as a form of post-traumatic stress disorder, based on a small number of extreme reactions. The term is not recognized as

Table 18.3 Large cohort studies demonstrating no association between abortion and breast cancer

Publication	Cohort	Relative risk (95% CI) for one previous abortion	Relative risk (95% CI) for two or more previous abortions
Palmer *et al.* 2004 [17]	Black Women's Health Study	0.8 (0.4–1.5) for nulliparous women 1.0 (0.7–1.3) for multiparous women	1.0 (0.5–1.9) for nulliparous women 1.3 (0.9–1.8) for multiparous women
Reeves *et al.* 2006 [18]	EPIC study	0.93 (0.85–1.02)	0.99 (0.86–1.14)
Rosenblatt *et al.* 2006 [19]	Shanghai Textile Industry Bureau Study	1.06 (0.95–1.18)	0.87 (0.74–1.02) for 2 abortions 1.06 (0.80–1.42) for 3+ abortions
Michels *et al.* 2007 [20]	Nurses' Health Study II	1.02 (0.88–1.19)	0.95 (0.68–1.31)
Henderson *et al.* 2008 [21]	California Teachers Study	0.98 (0.77–1.25) for nulliparous women 1.08 (0.93–1.24) for multiparous women	0.86 (0.57–1.30) for nulliparous women 0.97 (0.76–1.24) for multiparous women

a diagnosis in the *Diagnostic and Statistical Manual of Mental Disorders*, nor by any professional group of psychiatrists or psychologists [23]. Unfortunately, this purported and disproven sequela is still being referred to by those campaigning against abortion (see Chapter 19).

It should be noted that women who seek abortion are not representative of the general population. They are more prone to mental health problems, social problems such as intimate partner violence and other factors mentioned in the section on preterm delivery. They do not necessarily have the same psychosocial characteristics as often-used comparator groups of women who choose to continue their pregnancies. Most studies, not surprisingly, cannot make comparisons with the women's psychological state before they became pregnant. Therefore these associations with mental health problems are not necessarily causal and probably reflect continuation of pre-existing conditions.

Many of the studies in the literature, even those selected for inclusion in systematic reviews, suffer from being of poor quality. There is a large variation in study design, measurement methods and outcomes reported. Sample sizes are often too small and there is a lack of adequate control for confounding variables including pregnancy intention and previous pregnancy history.

Study of the effect of abortion on mental health is difficult. The ideal study design would be that women with unwanted pregnancies are assigned to receive an abortion or to have their request denied without the possibility of having the procedure elsewhere. This, of course, would be an unethical study to perform. Second best to the ideal study design would be women with unwanted pregnancies who undergo abortion compared with women who have unwanted pregnancies but whose request for an abortion is denied. The small number of such studies are outlined in the second part of this chapter. Other comparator groups compared to women experiencing unwanted pregnancies who have abortions in decreasing order of appropriateness are:

- all women giving birth, some of whose births would be unwanted
- women who have not had a pregnancy

- women who got pregnant because they wanted to become mothers and went on to have a child.

An elegant record-linkage study in Denmark [24] has shown that for women with no prior history of mental health problems, the incidence of contact with mental health services was no different before and after an abortion.

The subject of abortion and mental health was reviewed by Cameron in 2010 [25]. Since then the detailed systematic review by the British Academy of Medical Royal Colleges has been published [26]. This put much weight on three reviews: the American Psychological Association's narrative review [27], the Charles systematic review [28] and a review of pooled data by Coleman. The Coleman review generated a large critical correspondence, some of it calling for retraction of the paper, and it was assessed as fatally flawed in a detailed analysis [29]. The authors of the AMRC and APA reviews concluded that the relative risk of mental health problems among adult women who have a single, legal, first trimester abortion of an unwanted pregnancy is no greater than the risk among women who deliver an unwanted pregnancy. For women who have a prior history of mental health problems, there is a higher likelihood of mental health problems following both abortion and birth.

The effect of denial of abortion on the woman and the child born

The effects of denial of abortion have been summarized by Potts and colleagues [30] and Rowlands [16]. It is important to understand the possible consequences of restrictive abortion laws, including the fact that many women are determined to control their fertility and will seek out a clandestine abortion rather than continue with the pregnancy.

Effect of denied abortion on the woman herself

Around 40% of women who are refused abortion will later obtain it elsewhere, some paying privately. The majority of women denied abortion who continue with the pregnancy raise the child themselves with relatively few children put up for adoption.

Höök studied 249 women whose applications for abortion were refused by the Swedish National Board of Health in 1948 under the terms of the Abortion Act 1938 as amended in 1946 (cited in Rowlands [16]). Follow-up was carried out at 7–11 years. Of these women, 46 attempted to procure an abortion illegally. Thirty had given up their child for adoption or permanent care by someone else. Sixty (24%) continued to display signs of mental illness and poor adjustment at follow-up; 131 (53%) had finally achieved adjustment after a lengthy period of mental disturbance and emotional strain.

In an English study by Pare and Raven around the time of the passage of the British Abortion Act 1967, 34% of women who were forced to continue with their pregnancy regretted that the pregnancy had not been terminated when interviewed one to three years later and admitted to frequent feelings of resentment towards the child [16]. A Scottish comparative study by McCance *et al.* carried out at around the same time found that the outcome at 15 months for women requesting abortion was better in those granted an abortion than in those refused [16].

There is not much recent data as laws and practices have been liberalized in many parts of the world. However, a study in Hong Kong by Yung *et al.* (cited in Rowlands [16]), in which appreciable numbers of women are considered not to have sufficient grounds for abortion, is a salutary reminder about the potential negative effects on women of denying them an abortion. Seventy-three women were asked how they would react if their abortion was refused. Most said they would seek abortion elsewhere, if necessary in the private sector or illegally. Only four women said they would continue with the pregnancy. Two women said they would commit suicide.

The research landscape is now changing with commencement of the prospective Turnaway study in the USA (www.ansirh.org/research/turnaway.php). Recruitment took place between 2008 and 2010 and five-year follow-up will be complete at the end of 2015. Two hundred and thirty-one women who were turned away because they presented to one of 30 facilities at over the gestational limit are being followed along with 725 women who had abortions in two comparator groups; all women are having six-monthly telephone interviews. Preliminary results presented at the Annual Meeting of the American Public Health Association in October 2012 (https://apha.confex.com/apha/140am/webprogram/Paper263858.html) showed no differences in levels of anxiety or depression between the groups at one year. Also at one year women denied abortion were more likely to be receiving public assistance and have household income below the federal poverty line than women who received an abortion.

Effect of denied abortion on the child born

There is a significant negative effect on children born after denied abortion which is long-lasting and involves diverse psychological and social components. In a classic study from Sweden by Forssman and Thuwe, 120 children born after abortion was refused in Göteborg between 1939 and 1941 were compared with matched controls followed up to age 21 (cited in Rowlands [16]). The researchers found that the cases had a more insecure childhood, being more likely to be placed in a foster home or a children's home. The cases also had more psychiatric care, more childhood delinquency, more early marriages and in the females more young motherhood than the controls. Fewer of the cases continued beyond secondary education.

Another Swedish study, by Blomberg, with even more rigorous matching of controls followed 90 such children born after refused abortion in 1960 until the age of 15 [16]. Cases had poorer school performance, more neurotic and psychosomatic symptoms and more likelihood of being registered with social services than the controls.

The Prague study is the most ambitious study of this type, conducted after Czechoslovak abortion law had been liberalized in 1957 (see Rowlands [16]). Two hundred and twenty children born in the years 1961 to 1963 to women twice denied abortion for the same pregnancy (appeal rejected) were followed until age 35. The cases were less likely to be breastfed, had more acute illness and had more behavioural problems and poorer school performance than the controls. When they had reached their 20s, the cases showed an ongoing propensity for social problems, more job dissatisfaction, fewer friends, more criminality and more registration for drug or alcohol problems.

Conclusions

Conclusions about women requesting abortion and possible longer-term outcomes can be grouped as follows.

First of all, the outcomes after abortion.

No effect:

- Large volume of high quality evidence:
  - breast cancer

- Large volume of reasonable quality evidence:
  - · mental health problems
- Substantial volume of high quality evidence:
  - · future fertility
  - · ectopic pregnancy
- Small volume of reasonable quality evidence:
  - · placental abruption

Beneficial effect:

- Small volume of reasonable quality evidence:
  - · pre-eclampsia

Adverse effect:

- Substantial volume of reasonable quality evidence showing a weak association:
  - · preterm delivery (surgical abortion only)

No conclusions can be reached:

- Substantial volume of inconsistent evidence:
  - · miscarriage
  - · placenta praevia.

Based on a substantial volume of reasonable evidence, denial of abortion has a negative psychosocial effect on both a woman and a child born.

When balancing the interests of women with unwanted pregnancies requesting abortion, account should always be taken of factors that might be operating which could dissuade a woman from going through with an abortion. Misinformation, covered in Chapter 19, can seriously interfere with a woman's decision-making. Care should be taken to ensure that accurate information has been given and that women are not pressured into continuing an unwanted pregnancy with the known adverse consequences on their mental health and on that of children born subsequently.

References

1. Rothman KJ. *Epidemiology: An Introduction*, 2nd edn. New York: Oxford University Press, 2012.

2. Lowit A, Bhattacharya S, Bhattacharya S. Obstetric performance following an induced abortion. *Best Practice & Research Clinical Obstetrics & Gynaecology* 2010;24:667–82.

3. World Health Organization Task Force. Secondary infertility following induced abortion. *Stud Fam Plann* 1984;15: 291–5.

4. MacKenzie IZ, Fry A. A prospective self-controlled study of fertility after second-trimester prostaglandin-induced abortion. *Am J Obstet Gynecol* 1988;158:1137–40.

5. Frank P, McNamee R, Hannaford PC, Kay CR, Hirsch S. The effect of induced abortion on subsequent fertility. *British Journal of Obstetrics & Gynaecology* 1993;100:575–80.

6. Gan C, Zou Y, Wu S, Li Y, Liu Q. The influence of medical abortion compared with surgical abortion on subsequent pregnancy outcome. *Int J Gynecol Obstet* 2008;101:231–8.

7. *The Care of Women Requesting Induced Abortion*, 3rd edn. London: Royal College of Obstetricians and Gynaecologists, 2011.

8. Zhou W, Nielsen GL, Larsen H, Olsen
    J. Induced abortion and placental
    complications in the subsequent
    pregnancy. *Acta Obstet Gynecol Scand*
    2001;80:1115–20.

9. Trogstad L, Magnus P, Skjærven R,
    Stoltenberg C. Previous abortions and
    risk of pre-eclampsia. *Int J Epidemiol*
    2008;37:1333–40.

10. Shah PS, Zao J. Induced termination
    of pregnancy and low birthweight and
    preterm birth: a systematic review and
    meta-analyses. *BJOG* 2009;116:1425–42.

11. Swingle HM, Colaizy TT, Zimmerman
    MB, Morriss FH. Abortion and the risk of
    subsequent preterm birth. *J Reprod Med*
    2009;54:95–108.

12. Oliver-Williams C, Fleming M, Monteath
    K, Wood AM, Smith GCS. Changes in
    association between previous therapeutic
    abortion and preterm birth in Scotland,
    1980 to 2008: a historical cohort study.
    PLoS Med 2013;10:e1001481. doi:10.1371/
    journal.pmed.1001481.

13. Russo J, Russo IH. Susceptibility of the
    mammary gland to carcinogenesis. II.
    Pregnancy interruption as a risk factor
    in tumor incidence. *American Journal of
    Pathology* 1980;100:497–512.

14. Brind J, Chinchilli VM, Severs WB,
    Summy-Long J. Induced abortion as an
    independent risk factor for breast cancer:
    a comprehensive review and meta-
    analysis. *J Epidemiol Community Health*
    1996;50:481–96.

15. Wingo PA, Newsome K, Marks JS, *et al.*
    The risk of breast cancer following
    spontaneous or induced abortion.
    Cancer Causes & Control 1997;8:93–
    108 [published erratum appears in *Cancer
    Causes & Control* 1997;8:260].

16. Rowlands S. Memorandum 25. In
    Science and Technology Committee
    (ed.) *Scientific Developments Relating to
    the Abortion Act 1967*, Volume II HC
    1045-II. London: The Stationery Office,
    2007: Ev 128–Ev 133. www.publications.
    parliament.uk/pa/cm200607/cmselect/
    cmsctech/1045/1045ii.pdf

17. Palmer JR, Wise LA, Adams-Campbell
    LL, Rosenberg L. A prospective study of
    induced abortion and breast cancer in
    African-American women. *Cancer Causes
    & Control* 2004;15:105–11.

18. Reeves GK, Kan S-W, Key T, Tjønneland
    A, Olsen A, Overvad K. Breast cancer
    risk in relation to abortion: results
    from the EPIC study. *Int J Cancer*
    2006;119:1741–5.

19. Rosenblatt KA, Gao DL, Ray RM, *et al.*
    Induced abortions and the risk of all
    cancers combined and site-specific cancers
    in Shanghai. *Cancer Causes & Control*
    2006;17:1275–80.

20. Michels KB, Xue F, Colditz GA, Willett
    WC. Induced and spontaneous abortion
    and incidence of breast cancer among
    young women: a prospective cohort
    study. *Arch Intern Med* 2007;167:
    814–20.

21. Henderson KD, Sullivan-Halley J,
    Reynolds P, *et al.* Incomplete pregnancy is
    not associated with breast cancer risk: the
    California Teachers Study. *Contraception*
    2008;77:391–6.

22. Braüner CM, Overvad K, Tjønneland A,
    Atterman J. Induced abortion and breast
    cancer among parous women: a Danish
    cohort study. *Acta Obstet Gynecol Scand*
    2013;92:700–5.

23. Robinson GE, Stotland NL, Russo NF,
    Occhiogrosso M. Is there an "abortion
    trauma syndrome"? Critiquing the
    evidence. *Harvard Rev Psychiatry*
    2009;17:268–90.

24. Munk-Olsen T, Laursen TM, Pedersen
    CB, Lidegaard Ø, Mortensen PB. Induced
    first-trimester abortion and risk of mental
    disorder. *N Engl J Med* 2011;364:
    332–9.

25. Cameron S. Induced abortion and
    psychological sequelae. *Best Practice &
    Research Clinical Obstetrics & Gynaecology*
    2010;24:657–65.

26. National Collaborating Centre for Mental
    Health. *Induced Abortion and Mental
    Health*. London: Academy of Medical
    Royal Colleges, 2011.

option of looking at more than 54 million web pages! Talk to a group of women or a group of health professionals and you will hear a diversity of views, thoughts and 'facts' – sometimes correct, but very often not. Helplines supporting people with reproductive health decisions regularly hear confused views, myths and misinformation about abortion.

Yet there is now recognized good, objective, evidence-guided information available on abortion from the World Health Organization (WHO) [1], UK Royal College of Obstetricians and Gynaecologists (RCOG) [2], UK Royal College of Psychiatrists [3], the American Psychological Association (APA) [4] and the American Congress of Obstetricians and Gynecologists (ACOG) [5]. These are *major* sources of information which clearly and systematically refute the misinformation and myths that surround abortion. The UK RCOG and US ACOG also produce excellent information for consumers and patients on reproductive health issues, including abortion. There are a large number of organizations dedicated to providing medically balanced and correct information on abortion such as the US National Abortion Federation (www.prochoice.org) that produces clinical guidelines and policy.

A major factor that magnifies myths and misinformation on abortion is in fact the silence that surrounds abortion – silence by women who have abortions – 'the best kept secret', silence by professionals who provide and perform abortions and silence by the press who have the power to remove stigma, myth and misinformation. The language we use to discuss sex and sexual health including abortion is archaic, unclear and confusing much of it is contradictory, obsolete, ambiguous and misleading. Terminology is important and words should convey meaning and preclude possible misinterpretation [6].

There are a very large number of myths around abortion. This chapter will address the main, common myths on abortion which result in misinformation and confusion for both the public, health professionals, policy makers and those who work in the media.

Addressing common myths
Myth – abortion is harmful

Legally induced abortion is a safe procedure rarely resulting in major complications or morbidity at any gestation (see Chapter 14). Procedures today are safe and simple. In the UK there were 107 direct maternal deaths between 2006 and 2008; of these only two were associated with abortion and they related to infection. This corresponds to a mortality rate of 0.32 per 100,000 procedures [7]. In the USA safe legal abortion results in 0.6 deaths per 100,000 procedures. Worldwide *unsafe* abortion accounts for a death rate that is 350 times higher. In sub-Saharan Africa the rate is 800 times higher. An estimated 215 million women in the developing world have an unmet need for modern contraceptives. If their needs were met this would prevent 54 million unintended pregnancies, 26 million abortions, 79,000 maternal deaths and 1.1 million infant deaths [8].

Myth – abortion causes infertility and problems with conception and pregnancy

Women need to be reassured that there is no proven association between legal induced abortion and subsequent problems with conceiving, miscarriage, ectopic pregnancy or infertility. Chapter 18 covers these longer-term outcomes in detail.

This myth is extremely widespread and is heard continually when talking with women. Hoggart and Phillips' research [9] addressing abortion and more than one abortion explores the factors that might lead to a greater understanding of what might reduce unintended and unwanted teenage pregnancy. The research highlights poor understanding of fertility amongst young women and shows how this results in poor and inconsistent contraceptive use. Their findings can be extrapolated to all women irrespective of age or country.

> Am I throwing away my chances of having children?
> You cannot have children after an abortion.

These are common questions/statements by women when talking about abortion. The same research [9] provides a view from an experienced family planning doctor:

> ... one of my key issues about repeat abortions is that if doctors and nurses and other people spent less time telling women they were risking their fertility by having an abortion there would be less second abortions.

This phenomenon relates to women 'testing' their fertility through unprotected sexual intercourse after an abortion believing they are now infertile.

Myth – abortion causes psychological and mental health problems

Women choosing to have an abortion should be informed that they are no more or less likely to suffer psychological problems whether they have an abortion or continue the pregnancy and have the baby (see Chapter 18).

The decision to have an abortion is *never* an easy one. Contrary to myth no woman uses abortion as a regular method of birth control. Rowlands' [10] comprehensive review on the reasons why women choose to have an abortion demonstrates a wealth of evidence relating to abortion decision-making, and notes how some common practices and service delivery practices are out of step with the evidence. Women's decision-making involves a number of processes from acknowledgement of the pregnancy to making the choice to have an abortion and being committed to that decision. For many women the decision is clear, but for some it is not. Women finding themselves unexpectedly pregnant often report feelings of disbelief, shock, anger or guilt. Such feelings relate to how well a woman is able to make a confident decision about her pregnancy. Good pregnancy decision-making support and/or counselling is important at this time (see Chapter 5). Whilst research is clear about psychological and mental health outcomes for most women, health professionals need to be aware of the need to provide more support for women:

- with a previous history of mental health issues
- who are ambivalent about the decision to have an abortion
- who are subject to coercion by a partner or family members
- who are very young (under 16)
- who hold religious views that do not support abortion.

Astbury-Ward's critique of the literature [11] concludes that emotional responses following abortion are multiple and profound and that feelings of relief, sadness, anger, guilt and regret are all normal reactions following an abortion. All major reviews addressing this aspect of abortion [1–4] show clearly that the 'postabortion syndrome' (PAS) does *not* exist. This is in contrast to the vast amount of incorrect literature, discussion and dedicated websites on the subject.

Myth – abortion causes breast cancer

There is widespread misinformation that abortion causes breast cancer. This is often called the ABC link. Women worry about breast cancer and, there is an enormous amount of following eloquent point: 'The myth that with effective contraception women will no longer need abortion is both dangerous and incorrect. Whilst there is a choice of safe and effective contraceptive methods in developed countries, the imperfections of contraception, the imperfections of human beings and the consequence of ambivalence about getting pregnant, the influence of alcohol and drugs, moments of passion and unplanned encounters can never be eliminated.' High quality care and good access to contraception is essential; the same holds for abortion. Contraception choices and efficacy have improved immeasurably in developed countries over the last couple of decades, but abortion will always be necessary.

Myth – there are too many abortions

A commonly held assumption – but what does too many mean? Who decides what number is too many? The media, politicians, the church, anti-choice groups and many clinicians believe there are too many abortions. Women who have an abortion may not agree and this stance also begs the question: is abortion a bad thing? In the UK one in three women will have an abortion at some point in their reproductive lifetime; in 2012, 37% of women undergoing abortion had had more than one abortion and, contrary to myth, these are not all teenagers [20]. Women in developed countries can be fertile for more than 30 years, there is no method of contraception that is 100% effective, sexual activity now starts earlier in life and so, with more partner changes resulting in probably more sex, it is amazing there are not more unintended pregnancies.

Abortion is a fact of life and there is no 'right' number of abortions. There is a need to recognize that women who choose to end a pregnancy by abortion are making a responsible reproductive health decision. What is important is that every woman with an unplanned pregnancy is able to make a choice about what is right for her and has access to the care she needs. Health policy should focus on reducing unwanted and unintended pregnancy through good sex and relationship education, evidence-guided accessible information, effective use of contraception and good access to sexual health services.

Myth – there is no need for second trimester abortion

There will always be a need to provide access to second trimester abortion; whilst today most women in developed countries have abortions at under 12 weeks' gestation, the reasons for having a second trimester abortion are often compelling. A variety of research studies illustrate the multifactorial elements as to why women present for second trimester abortion:

- Concealed pregnancy or inability to recognize pregnancy by teenagers
- Unrecognized pregnancy in peri-menopausal women
- Unrecognized pregnancy in women with irregular menstrual cycles, amenorrhoea or women using contraception
- Denial of pregnancy
- Late identification of problems in pregnancy, such as fetal abnormality
- Change of circumstances (abandonment of partner, violence by partner)
- Uncertainty about whether or not to have an abortion
- Fear/coercion by partner or family members
- Need to travel for an abortion.

Ingham and co-workers have written extensively about this and emphasize the need to improve education about pregnancy symptoms, improve information and discussion of abortion methods and safety issues, and the need to improve service provision to encourage women to seek help earlier (see Chapter 22).

In Britain anti-choice groups have constantly campaigned for lowering the upper gestational limit for abortion defined as 24 weeks in the Abortion Act 1967 (amended by the Human Fertilisation and Embryology Act 1990), arguing that as medical interventions and new technologies have improved fetal viability, allowing abortion up to this point is no longer acceptable. To address this concern, the UK Parliament's Science and Technology Committee carried out an enquiry considering all scientific developments (national and international) relating to abortion. Reporting in 2007 [21] the recommendation was clear: no change should be made to the upper gestation limit for abortion. The Committee's scientific conclusions were that while survival rates at 24 weeks and over have improved since 1990, survival rates (viability) have *not* done so below 24 weeks. This view is supported by many UK sexual and reproductive health organizations and medical organizations including the RCOG, the British Medical Association, the Royal College of Nursing and the British Association of Perinatal Medicine.

Harris [22] addresses the personal views and thoughts of clinicians providing second trimester abortions and how doctors decide whether or not to do second trimester abortions. Doing an early abortion and doing a second trimester procedure are very different. Harris argues that the pro-choice movement should have a more honest discussion about abortion procedures which addresses the realities of second trimester abortion. Abortion providers are caught between the anti-choice and pro-choice discourse which may reflect values but not necessarily experience.

Myth – banning legal abortion will remove abortion once and for all

This is false. Women have always and will always resort to ending an unwanted pregnancy either legally or illegally. Restrictive laws lead to more illegal, clandestine unsafe abortions. Where laws are less restrictive, abortion rates are lower. Studies and clinical experience continue to confirm that women who wish to terminate an unwanted pregnancy will seek abortion at any cost – even when it is illegal or involves risk to their own lives. Banning abortion will not end abortion – it will put women's lives at risk [23].

Myth – women are not able to take in advice on contraception at the time of an abortion

This is false. As with all information provision – it relates to *how* information is given. Women having an abortion are, mostly, very keen to prevent another unintended pregnancy. Ovulation after medical or surgical abortion occurs within one month of first trimester abortion in over 90% of women. More than 50% of women have been shown to resume sexual activity within two weeks of an abortion. Contraception, if required, should always be started as soon as possible after the abortion procedure (see Chapter 13). Hormonal methods can be started immediately after a medical or surgical abortion and their use does not affect the outcome of the abortion. Intrauterine contraceptives can be inserted soon after medical abortion or at the time of surgical abortion at all gestations. Contraceptive methods started up to and including day 5 postabortion do not need any additional contraceptive precautions. When contraception is started any later than day 5, it must be reasonably certain that the woman is not pregnant or at risk of pregnancy and additional precautions are needed for the first seven days in the case of combined hormonal methods, the implant, injectables and the intrauterine system and for 48 hours in the case of the progestogen-only pill. Sterilization can be safely performed at the time of an abortion, but may be associated with more regret and failure [2].

Conclusions

The subject of abortion creates passionate and very different views from people in all walks of life. Decisions about something that is intrinsically personal to women themselves can only be made when they are in receipt of accurate information. Myths and dishonest and deliberate misinformation around abortion result in misery, guilt and shame for many women who for whatever reason have made the decision to end a pregnancy. Health professionals supporting and enabling women to make confident reproductive health choices need to access the facts by using robust, objective, evidence-guided information that is now widely available; this improves their own knowledge which can in turn be imparted to women with honesty, empathy and compassion.

References

1. World Health Organization. *Safe Abortion: Technical and Policy Guidance for Health Systems*, 2nd edn. Geneva: WHO, 2012.

2. Royal College of Obstetricians and Gynaecologists. *Care of Women Requesting Induced Abortion. Evidence-Based Clinical Guideline No 7*. London: RCOG, 2011.

3. National Collaborating Centre for Mental Health. *Induced Abortion and Mental Health. A systematic review of mental health outcomes of induced abortion*. London: Academy of Royal Colleges, 2011.

4. American Psychological Association. Task Force on Mental Health and Abortion. *Report of the Task Force on Mental Health and Abortion*. Washington DC: APA, 2008.

5. American Congress of Obstetrics and Gynecology Committee Opinions. Committee Opinions 390 and 434. www.acog.org/Resources_And_Publications.

6. Belfield T. Words matter! *J Fam Plann Reprod Health Care* 2010;36:55–8.

7. CMACE. *Saving Mother's Lives. Reviewing maternal deaths to make motherhood safer. 2006–2008. The Eighth Report on the Confidential Enquiries into Maternal Death in the UK*. 2011.

8. Guttmacher Institute. Facts on Induced Abortion Worldwide 2012. www.guttmacher.org (accessed 18 September 2013).

9. Hoggart L, Phillips J. *Young People in London: Abortion and Repeat Abortion*. Research Report. London: Policy Studies Institute, 2010.

10. Rowlands S. The decision to opt for abortion. *J Fam Plann Reprod Health Care* 2008;34:175–80.

11. Astbury-Ward E. Emotional and psychological impact of abortion: a critique of the literature. *J Fam Plann Reprod Health Care* 2008;34:181–4.

12. RCOG. *Fetal Awareness. Review of Research and Recommendations for Practice. Report of a Working Party*. London: RCOG, 2010.

13. One Hundred Professors of Obstetrics and Gynecology. A statement on abortion by 100 Professors of Obstetrics: 40 years later. One Hundred Professors of Obstetrics and Gynecology. *Contraception* 2013;88:568–76.

14. Hallgarten L. *Decision-making Support within the Integrated Care Pathway for Women Considering or Seeking Abortion*. London: Brook and FPA, 2014. www.brook.org.uk.

15. Cannold L. Understanding and responding to anti-choice women centred strategies. *Reproductive Health Matters* 2002;10:171–9.

16. Education for Choice. *Crisis Pregnancy Centres*. London: EFC at Brook, 2014. www.brook.org.uk/images/brook/ professionals/documents/page_content/ EFC/CPCreport/crisis_preg_centres_ rept_10.2.14-2hiFINAL.pdf (accessed 9 March 2014).

17. Bryant AG, Levi EE. Abortion misinformation from Crisis Pregnancy Centres in North Carolina. *Contraception* 2012;86:752–6.

18. Department of Health. Judicial Review of Emergency Contraception. http:// webarchive.nationalarchives.gov.uk/+/ www.dh.gov.uk/en/Publichealth/ Healthimprovement/Sexualhealth/ SexualHealthGeneralInformation/ DH_4063853 (accessed 4 March 2014).

19. Berer M. Abortion: unfinished business. *Reproductive Health Matters* 1997;5:6–9.

20. Department of Health. *Abortion Statistics, England and Wales: 2012*. www.gov.uk/ government/uploads/system/uploads/ attachment_data/file/211790/2012_ Abortion_Statistics.pdf (accessed 9 March 2014).

21. House of Commons Science and Technology Committee. *Scientific Developments Relating to the Abortion Act 1967*. Twelfth Report of Session 2006–07, Vol 1 (HC 1045–1) September 2007.

22. Harris LH. Second trimester abortion provision: breaking the silence and changing the discourse. *Reproductive Health Matters (Supplement) Second trimester abortion: women's health and public policy* 2008;16:74–81.

23. Winikoff B, Sheldon WR. Abortion: what is the problem? *Lancet* 2012;379:594–6.

Chapter

20

Stigma and issues of conscience

Kelly R. Culwell and Caitlin Gerdts

Introduction

Abortion is a common experience for women of reproductive age around the world [1]. Just as common is the experience of abortion-related stigma. In different contexts, social, cultural and religious factors may all engender abortion stigma and may contribute to who is affected by abortion stigma and why and how [2,3]. Despite near universal stigma surrounding abortion [3], and most likely in response to the devastating public health consequences of unsafe abortion, the trend in recent decades has been toward liberalization of abortion laws in nearly all regions of the world [4]. With this progress has come an increased understanding of the role that abortion stigma plays as a barrier to safe services, in both legally restricted and legally permissive contexts. And in some countries, implementation of less restrictive abortion laws has been hindered by negative attitudes among healthcare workers leading to widespread, and often unregulated, conscientious objection [4]. In this chapter, the current theoretical understandings of these issues will be covered as well as the key research which has begun to explore how to measure abortion stigma as well as some early interventions to address stigma with the ultimate goal of improving access to safe abortion services. The potential links between abortion stigma and issues of conscience in abortion care will also be described along with the ways that professional organizations and health systems aim to balance refusals to provide abortion services based on conscience with women's right to access information and safe services. Finally, gaps in our current knowledge will be identified and recommendations made for future research in theory building, measurement and intervention.

Abortion stigma
Conceptualization

Over nearly half a century, and in multiple disciplines, the topic of stigma has received much theoretical and empirical consideration. In his seminal book, Erving Goffman offered a comprehensive description of the many manifestations of stigma and the mechanisms through which stigmas impact upon social interactions [5]. Goffman defined stigma as attributes that reduce an individual from a 'whole and usual person to a tainted, discounted one'. Throughout human history stigmas have been associated with myriad physical, behavioural and ideological differences that operate at the individual and group levels. Stigmas can be damaging to both individuals and to society [6]. Stigma-related research is necessary

Abortion Care, ed. Sam Rowlands. Published by Cambridge University Press. © Cambridge University Press 2014.

to improve understanding of the causes and consequences of stigmas and is important in mitigating the negative effects associated with stigmas.

Abortion stigma shares characteristics with other stigmas; however, it is a distinct manifestation and must be examined as such. One conceptual model establishes three categories of abortion stigma: internalized, felt, and enacted [7]. Internalized stigma can be understood as self-directed stigma or stigma directed at others. Felt stigma can best be understood as a stigmatized individual's understanding of others' beliefs and judgemental attitudes about abortion. Enacted stigma is the collection of negative interactions with others experienced by women who have had abortions. Another model of abortion stigma acknowledges that stigma can be experienced in multiple domains: 'personal interactions; families and communities; popular and medical discourses; government and political structures; and social institutions' [3]. Building upon these frameworks, it follows that abortion stigma contributes to punitive laws, weakens the infrastructure for safe abortion care and prevents women from seeking the involvement of others in their care or support. In many parts of the world abortion stigma also contributes to the incidence of unsafe abortion [1]. After an abortion, stigma may contribute to negative consequences in women's relationships, psychological wellbeing and even their physical health. Research also suggests that stigma may negatively affect the wellbeing and personal safety of abortion providers [8,9]. Across multiple cultural contexts, concealment of abortion experience from others is a common strategy employed by women and providers to manage stigma associated with abortion [10]. Secrecy has broad social consequences for the visibility of abortion (Chapter 4) and the needs of women who are considering abortion, accessing abortion care or who have had an abortion in the past.

Measurement

Valid and reliable measures of abortion stigma are critical to understanding the aetiology, actualization and outcomes of abortion stigma on specific populations that might be negatively affected. Well-designed measurement tools are fundamental to the assessment of interventions aimed at reducing abortion stigma or mediating the negative sequelae of abortion stigma and are necessary for the evaluation of programmes or policies that might exacerbate abortion stigma. As has been demonstrated by stigma research in other fields, the standardization of methodologies and instruments for the measurement of stigma is possible and can facilitate consistent evaluation of stigma in a specific population as well as the comparison of the effects of stigma across regions and populations.

The range of necessary tools and indicators for the measurement of abortion stigma is heavily dependent on the existing conceptual and theoretical constructs for abortion stigma, as well as the domains and levels within which abortion stigma is thought to operate. Standardized methodologies can be developed for both qualitative and quantitative assessment of abortion stigma.

Currently available methodologies

Existing mechanisms for the measurement of abortion stigma described in the literature can be categorized into qualitative methodologies and quantitative methodologies. Qualitative methodologies are driven by various theories and constructs and are primarily aimed at assessing the social and psychological elements of stigma on women who have sought and/or experienced abortions. Available quantitative methodologies for the measurement of abortion stigma are modified from instruments available in the psychiatric, psychological and demographic literatures and aim to measure a range of experiences with and outcomes of abortion stigma.

Qualitative tools

While many qualitative studies address the personal and societal issues surrounding abortion stigma, only one tool has been published which specifically addresses abortion stigma. This comprehensive guide to focus group questions was developed to explore the various domains of stigma among groups of women and men in communities, abortion providers, pharmacists and clinicians [11].

Quantitative tools

To date, only one validated quantitative tool exists in the peer-reviewed literature for the measurement of abortion stigma [12]. The Individual Level Abortion Stigma (ILAS) scale assesses four factors of individual-level abortion stigma: worries about judgement, isolation, self-judgement and community condemnation. The scale has been validated among women seeking abortions and is a valuable tool for the assessment of stigma experienced at the individual level. No validated methodology for other domains of stigma yet exists in the published literature. However, an additional quantitative scale is designed to measure abortion stigma at the community and individual level and was created for use in developing countries [13]. This work followed the development of the qualitative focus group guide noted above and has been tested in Zambia and Ghana. The scale, called the Stigmatizing Attitudes Beliefs and Actions Scale (SABAS), contains three subscales: negative stereotypes; discrimination and exclusion; and potential contagion. Other quantitative tools have been utilized to measure multiple aspects of stigma. Quantitative measures of race, ethnicity and sociodemographic, reproductive and situational characteristics as well as perceived and internalized stigma (but not experienced stigma) were studied among participants in the 2008 Guttmacher Abortion Patient Survey [14]. A quantitative tool, modified from a validated short instrument to measure stigmatized attitudes towards mental illness, was conducted among a nationally representative sample of 3,000 self-identified Catholics in Mexico and used to assess abortion stigma and its association with sociodemographic and political characteristics [15]. Finally, validated measures of stigma, secrecy, intrusive thoughts, thought suppression and emotional disclosure from the psychological literature were adapted to assess whether feelings of stigmatization from an abortion increase a woman's need to maintain secrecy about her abortion and, thus, increase more intrusive and stigmatized thoughts about her abortion [16].

Abortion stigma reduction interventions

Two articles appear in the literature describing interventions that have been implemented with the goal of reducing stigma related to abortion among a specific population.

The first, the Providers Share Workshop, was designed as a safe space for providers to discuss their experiences and ameliorate the burden of stigma for abortion providers [9]. Seventeen providers participated in a six-session intensive sharing and counselling intervention to reduce the burden of stigma among a team of abortion providers. The intervention was developed from the sociological literature that describes informal strategies used by clinicians for managing the burden of stigma. The framework of the intervention included six elements of sharing and community building among providers: (1) What abortion means to me; (2) Memorable stories; (3) Abortion and identity; (4) Abortion politics; (5) Future directions for self-care; (6) Reflections on the workshop. The intervention was designed as a small pilot study and, while participating providers reported feeling positively about the pilot intervention, the results are not meant for broader interpretation and are not generalizable.

The second intervention article describes a pilot test of an intervention that introduces women requesting abortion to a 'culture of support' by providing validating messages and information about groups and services that support women in their reproductive decision, addressing stigma and providing information to help women identify and avoid sources of abortion misinformation. The intervention was developed out of a hypothesis that elements of a 'negative cultural environment can contribute to women's perceptions of the socio-cultural factors associated with poor coping after abortion' [17]. Participating women were asked to comment on the materials developed in order to improve the intervention and while responses were, on the whole, positive the results of a scaled-up intervention have not yet been published.

Issues of conscience in abortion care

Abortion stigma and conscientious commitment

The right of conscience as it relates to abortion care has traditionally been understood as the right to refuse to participate in abortion procedures based on religious or moral beliefs. This common understanding illustrates how abortion stigma is embedded in our collective thinking. Commitment to provision of abortion and other reproductive healthcare services is and has historically been driven by conscience as well [18]. Doctors, nurses and advocates around the world have faced and, in some cases, continue to face prosecution and imprisonment for promoting contraception and providing safe abortion services prior to liberalization of abortion laws. Many doctors and nurses make the decision to provide safe abortion services in these contexts, despite their illegality, based on a conscientious commitment to the health of their patients after treating women who suffer from complications of unsafe abortion, often self-induced. Where providers have not personally encountered the devastating impact of unsafe abortion, most are still driven by core ethical beliefs, including women's right to autonomy and self-determination. In most countries where abortion laws have been liberalized, laws protect caregivers who are compelled by conscience to refuse to provide abortion or other reproductive healthcare services but do not recognize that conscience drives the provision of abortion care as well. The lack of acknowledgement of the role of conscience in provision of abortion care in both legal frameworks and public discourse contributes to the stigmatization of abortion providers. If these providers are not driven by conscience, it implies that they lack conscience altogether or are morally bankrupt. The International Federation of Gynecologists and Obstetricians (FIGO) addresses both sides of conscience regarding delivery of services in the *Ethical Guidelines on Conscientious Objection*: 'Practitioners have the right to respect for their conscientious convictions in respect *both not to undertake and to undertake* the delivery of lawful procedures' [19] (emphasis added).

The right to conscience

The right to conscience is grounded in international human rights principles, linked to freedom of religion, conscience and thought. Article 18 of the UN International Covenant on Civil and Political Rights states, 'Everyone shall have the right to freedom of thought, conscience and religion … [and] to manifest his religion or belief in worship, observance, practice and teaching' [21]. The right to conscience is so important because not acting in accordance with one's conscience is to betray oneself. This is different from refusals to provide care that stem from a discomfort with the abortion procedure, a concern regarding professional reputation or discriminatory attitudes against women needing abortion services.

Conscience is generally considered by ethicists and legal scholars to be an issue relating to an individual, meaning that institutions such as hospitals or health systems cannot object to provision of procedures based on issues of conscience. However, this limitation is not uniformly accepted. Some countries have laws defining the right to refuse to provide abortion services as an individual, not institutional right while others, such as Argentina and the United States, allow private institutions to opt out of providing these services, though in some cases require advance registration of this refusal or policies to ensure referrals to other institutions [22–24].

Abuses of conscience

The stigma surrounding abortion undoubtedly makes provision of abortion services less desirable for some healthcare workers, who in turn might invoke a right of conscience in refusing to provide such services, even if in fact the objection to participating in abortion services is not directly related to their conscience. Other documented abuses of invoking the right of conscience to refuse to provide abortion care include refusals by practitioners to provide abortion services in the public sector but who provide services for high fees in the private sector and those who refuse to participate in emergency care or postabortion care [20]. These abuses of invoking 'right of conscience' to refuse care are largely tolerated in society, probably due in part to the stigma surrounding abortion.

Refusals to provide abortion care by physicians and other healthcare providers have led to documented provider shortages [4]. These shortages are most likely to affect women with the fewest resources including poor, young, rural and less educated women. Provider shortages also impact on clinicians who are willing to provide abortion care, leading to increased stigma directed at these providers and provider burnout due to the stigma and high workload [9].

Limits of conscientious refusal of care

> Freedom to manifest one's religion or beliefs may be subject only to such limitations as are prescribed by law and are necessary to protect public safety, order, health or morals or the fundamental rights and freedoms of others. (International Covenant on Civil and Political Rights, Article 18(3) [22]).

Professional responsibilities

Professional organizations such as FIGO and the American Congress of Obstetricians and Gynecologists (ACOG) have developed ethical guidelines that delineate the professional responsibilities of healthcare providers who refuse to provide care based on deeply held religious or moral beliefs [19,25]. At a minimum, these professional bodies call for their members to provide care that is timely and evidence-based, including provision of accurate and unbiased information to women. Based on respect for an individual's autonomy, providers must ensure that the woman has access to a timely referral for the indicated service. In the updated safe abortion guidelines for health systems, the World Health Organization also emphasizes the duty of healthcare providers who refuse to provide abortion services based on conscientious objection to refer women, to personally provide services in cases of life or health endangerment if there are no other available providers and to treat women who arrive needing postabortion care in a timely manner and with respect and dignity [27]. Though not uniformly upheld in court cases on the matter, both FIGO and ACOG call for their members to provide information in advance to their patients and employers regarding services that they will not provide based on moral or religious beliefs. In addition, these organizations state that their members must provide indicated care in the case of an emergency when no other provider is available. ACOG goes further to state: 'In resource-poor areas, access to safe and legal reproductive services should be maintained. Conscientious refusals that undermine access should raise significant caution. Providers with moral or religious objections should either practice in proximity to individuals who do not share their views or ensure that referral processes are in place' [26].

The right to accurate and complete information in healthcare is declared in international and national laws and regulations. Denial of services necessary to make an informed decision about abortion has been found to be a violation of the right to be free from inhuman and degrading treatment by the European Court of Human Rights [28]. Many national legal frameworks require provision of information about the availability of abortion services, even by those who object to providing the services and who sanction delaying tactics or provision of false information.

Health system obligations

> … freedom of conscience does not confer a right to indiscriminate recourse to conscientious objection. When an asserted freedom turns into licence or becomes an excuse for limiting the rights of others, the State is obliged to protect, also by legal means, the inalienable rights of citizens against such abuses. (Pope John Paul II, Message for the 24th World Day of Peace, 1 January 1991)

In addition to the rights and responsibilities of individual providers, international courts and treaty monitoring bodies have consistently found that health systems have the responsibility to balance providers' rights to conscience with women's rights to have access to legal health services. The Committee on the Elimination of Discrimination against Women (CEDAW) has stated that 'it is discriminatory for a country to refuse to legally provide for the performance of certain reproductive health services for women' and that if healthcare providers refuse to provide such services based on issues of conscience, 'measures should be introduced to ensure that women are referred to alternative health providers' [29].

National systems have devised different ways to ensure access while also protecting the rights of conscience of individual providers [23]. Efforts to ensure adequate numbers of providers include establishment of criteria for designation as one who objects to provision of abortion care and requiring those who object to register in national systems and/or provide advance notice to employers and patients. Many health systems and national legal frameworks allow for inclusion of willingness to provide abortion care in job descriptions and for refusal to hire those who will not provide this care if adequate numbers of providers are not already available. Health systems also employ various efforts to ensure access to abortion services is not hampered by healthcare workers who refuse to participate in abortion care through efforts to ensure timely referrals. These efforts may include regulations that do not allow for refusal to provide advice and referral, establishment of criteria as to which types of healthcare workers can refuse to participate in care and which elements of care constitute participation. In general, most national regulations do not allow refusals of participation in auxiliary parts of care such as registration of patients or post-procedure care, though notable exceptions can be found in both legislative and judicial actions.

Discussion

In the developing world, abortion stigma is a known contributor to maternal mortality and morbidity, as women who feel the need to keep their abortions secret are more likely to seek unsafe procedures and fail to seek medical attention when necessary. In both developed and developing country contexts, abortion stigma is known to contribute to feelings of shame, social isolation and to diminished self-esteem. Refusal by healthcare providers to participate in abortion care, often seemingly based on conscientious objection to abortion, hinders access to safe abortion services, which is felt most by those who are vulnerable to lack of access including young, poor and rural women. Based on this knowledge, some progress has been made in raising the profile of abortion stigma and conscientious refusal of care by providers as key factors limiting women's ability to access safe, legal abortion services. Significant progress has been made in recent years in establishing a common framework for the definition or conceptualization of abortion stigma and establishing standardized tools for the measurement of abortion stigma but few pilot interventions have been developed to mitigate the negative impacts of abortion stigma and none has been rigorously evaluated. Addressing abortion stigma will continue to require a multidisciplinary approach including social scientists, advocates, researchers, healthcare providers, policy makers and women themselves to develop and rigorously evaluate interventions aimed at reducing stigma at the individual, community, institutional and societal levels. International legal precedent, opinions by treaty monitoring bodies, professional organization guidelines and many national regulations provide commonsense frameworks for protecting both the conscience of healthcare providers and the rights of women to obtain information and services. However, these legal standards and regulations are not uniformly implemented even in countries with progressive laws governing abortion. While targeting abortion stigma is likely to reduce some of the problems of widespread conscientious refusal of care by healthcare providers, additional legal and regulatory efforts based on innovative practices in many countries may still be needed to ensure women have timely access to high quality abortion care.

References

1. Sedgh G, Singh S, Henshaw SK, *et al.* Induced abortion: incidence and trends worldwide from 1995–2008. *Lancet* 2012;379:625–32.

2. Norris A, Bessett D, Steinberg JR, Kavanaugh ML, De Zordo S, Becker D. Abortion stigma: a reconceptualization of constituents, causes, and consequences. *Women's Health Issues* 2011;21:S49–54.

3. Kumar A, Hessini L, Mitchell EM. Conceptualising abortion stigma. *Culture Health & Sexuality* 2009;11:625–39.

4. Guttmacher Institute. Making abortion services accessible in the wake of legal reforms: A framework and six case studies. 2012. www.guttmacher.org/pubs/abortion-services-laws.pdf (accessed 30 September 2013).

5. Goffman E. *Stigma: Notes on the Management of Spoiled Identity*. Englewood Cliffs, NJ: Prentice-Hall, 1963.

6. Crocker J, Major B, Steele C. Social stigma. In D Gilbert, S Fiske, G Lindzey (eds.) *The Handbook of Social Psychology*. Boston: Oxford University Press, 1998: 504–53.

7. Cockrill K, Nack A. "I'm not that type of person": managing the stigma of having an abortion. *Deviant Behavior* 2013;34:973–90.

8. Joffe C. *Dispatches from the Abortion Wars: The Costs of Fanaticism to Doctors, Patients, and the Rest of Us.* Boston: Beacon Press, 2010.

9. Harris LH, Debbink M, Martin L, Hassinger J. Dynamics of stigma in abortion work: findings from a pilot study of the Providers Share Workshop. *Soc Sci Med* 2011;73:1062–70.

10. Shellenberg KM, Moore AM, Bankole A, *et al.* Social stigma and disclosure about induced abortion: results from an exploratory study. *Glob Public Health* 2011;6:S111–S25.

11. Billings D, Hessini L, Clark KA. *Focus Group Guide for Exploring Abortion-Related Stigma.* Chapel Hill, NC: Ipas, 2009.

12. Cockrill K, Upadhyay UD, Turan J, Greene Foster D. The stigma of having an abortion: development of a scale and characteristics of women experiencing abortion stigma. *Perspectives on Sexual and Reproductive Health* 2013;45: 79–88.

13. Shellenberg KM, Hessini L, Levandowski BA. Developing a scale to measure stigmatizing attitudes and beliefs about women who have abortions: results from Ghana and Zambia. *Stigma, Research and Action* 2013 (in press). Available at: www.ipas.org/~/media/Files/Ipas%20 Publications/SABASE13.ashx (accessed 30 September 2013).

14. Shellenberg KM, Tsui AO. Correlates of perceived and internalized stigma among abortion patients in the USA: an exploration by race and Hispanic ethnicity. *Int J Gynecol Obstet* 2012;118:S152–9.

15. McMurtrie SM, García SG, Wilson KS, Diaz-Olavarrieta C, Fawcett GM. Public opinion about abortion-related stigma among Mexican Catholics and implications for unsafe abortion. *Int J Gynecol Obstet* 2012;118:S160–6.

16. Major B, Gramzow RH. Abortion as stigma: cognitive and emotional implications of concealment. *J Pers Soc Psychol* 1999;77:735.

17. Littman LL, Zarcadoolas C, Jacobs AR. Introducing abortion patients to a culture of support: a pilot study. *Arch Womens Ment Health* 2009;12:419–31.

18. Dickens BM, Cook RJ. Conscientious commitment to women's health. *Int J Gynecol Obstet* 2011;113:163–6.

19. FIGO Committee for the Ethical Aspects of Human Reproduction and Women's Health. Ethical guidelines on conscientious objection. *Int J Gynecol Obstet* 2006;92:333–4.

20. De Zordo S, Mishtal J. Physicians and abortion: provision, political participation and conflicts on the ground – the cases of Brazil and Poland. *Women's Health Issues* 2011;21:S32–6.

21. International Covenant on Civil and Political Rights, adopted Dec. 16, 1966, G.A. Res. 2200A (XXI), U.N. GAOR, 21st Sess., Supp. No. 16, at 52, U.N. Doc. A/6316 (1966), 999 U.N.T.S. 171 (entered into force 23 March 1976).

22. Skuster P. *When a Health Professional Refuses: Legal and Regulatory Limits on Conscientious Objection to Provision of Abortion Care.* Chapel Hill, NC: Ipas, 2012.

23. Sonfeld A. Delineating the obligations that come with conscientious refusal: a question of balance. *Guttmacher Policy Review* 2009;12:6–10. www.guttmacher. org/pubs/gpr/12/3/gpr120306.html (accessed 31 October 2013).

24. Regulation to National Law No. 25.673, Art. 10 (Argentina). Ministerio de Salud de la Nación [National Health Ministry]. Guía Técnicapara la Atención Integral de los Abortos No Punibles [Technical Guide for Comprehensive Care for Legal Abortions] (2010) (Argentina).

25. ACOG Committee on Ethics. The limits of conscientious refusal in reproductive medicine. *Obstet Gynecol* 2007;110:1203–8.

26. World Health Organization. *Safe Abortion: Technical and Policy Guidance for Health Systems*, 2nd edn. 2012. http://apps.who.int/iris/ bitstream/10665/70914/1/9789241548434_ eng.pdf (accessed 30 September 2013).

27. Zampas C, Andión-Ibañez X. Conscientious objection to sexual and reproductive health services: international human rights standards and European law and practice. *Eur J Health Law* 2012;19:231–56.

28. Convention on the Elimination of All Forms of Discrimination against Women (CEDAW), adopted December 18, 1979, G.A. Res. 34/180, U.N. GAOR, 34th Sess., Supp. No. 46, at 193, U.N. Doc. A/34/46 (entered into force 3 September 1981).

Chapter

21

More than one abortion

Sam Rowlands, Kelly Cleland and James Trussell

Introduction

Many women experience more than one abortion throughout their reproductive years; although common, the fact of a woman experiencing more than one abortion is often quite stigmatized [1]. The terms 'repeat abortion' and 'repeat aborter' and even 'abortion recidivism' appear in the scientific literature from the early 1970s onwards. The initial concern appeared to be that women might be using abortion instead of contraception as a means of fertility control, with connotations of irresponsibility. There were also unfounded concerns about risk of morbidity and mortality for the woman from complications, psychiatric sequelae and cumulative adverse effects on future reproductive outcomes. These concerns are fully addressed in Chapter 18. The impact of postabortion contraception on subsequent abortion is dealt with in Chapter 13.

Women have been regarded by some clinicians as less deserving when they present for abortion with a history of having had a previous abortion. Doctors have felt for instance that to agree to a second abortion would only encourage immorality, or at least carelessness. Service providers have even placed limits on the number of abortions an individual woman will be allowed. In some countries doctors have threatened women with sterilization if they attend for subsequent abortions (cited in Rowlands [1]).

In countries that have good access to legal abortion, women typically use safe abortion as an adjunct to contraception. Even when more effective contraceptive methods are used, failures during typical use are substantial – for example, 8% in the first year of use for oral contraception [2]. It has been estimated that a fecund, sexually active woman relying only on abortion for fertility control would need to have 35 abortions during her lifetime if she wanted no children [3].

This chapter starts by illustrating the phenomenon of so-called 'repeat' abortion with statistics from several countries followed by outlining demographic factors affecting trends over time. Evidence of any differences between women having subsequent abortions and those having their first abortion is then summarized. Finally, evidence is presented of any differences in contraceptive behaviour between the two groups.

Terminology

Finding appropriate language to describe the experience of a woman who has several abortions in her lifetime is challenging. Labels such as 'recidivist', 'habitual aborter' and 'repeater'

Abortion Care, ed. Sam Rowlands. Published by Cambridge University Press. © Cambridge University Press 2014.

may introduce or reinforce stigma both for providers and for patients. Referring to multiple abortions unnecessarily labels women too, and may introduce confusion with multiple pregnancy (twins, triplets, etc.). Although describing women as having more than one abortion, having had a previous abortion or having subsequent abortions are cumbersome terms, we have chosen to use one or other of these throughout this chapter.

'More than one abortion' as a special category

No consistent definition of 'repeat' abortion was found in data sources which track statistics on demographic and reproductive health outcomes. Mostly it seems the term is used to describe more than one abortion ever. But is a second abortion 20 years after a first abortion really the same as two abortions within one year in terms of its antecedents? Qualitative research has shown that each abortion experience is a separate and distinct event with specific social circumstances [4].

When a history of previous abortion is obtained by asking women, substantial under-reporting occurs due to concerns about stigma [1]. Under-reporting at interviews is likely to approach 100% in the early days of liberalization of abortion law when most of the experience is of illegal abortion; women are unlikely to admit to an illegal act. This under-reporting means that data other than that from record-linkage systems are unlikely to be reliable and constitute a considerable underestimate of the true number. It must also be recognized that some statistics report only previous legal abortions. Statistics from England and Wales and from New Zealand report only legal abortions in their own jurisdiction; statistics from the USA and Canada report without qualification. How accurate reporting is for these statistics is not known.

Possible reasons for creating a distinct category for women who have had one or more previous abortions might include:

- monitoring of year-on-year trends in the proportions
- denial of further abortions by service providers after a certain number has been reached
- targeting by health professionals to promote use of a reliable method (preferably a long-acting method) of contraception in the future.

Worldwide statistics

Some countries produce abortion statistics; some countries do not. Of those that do, some are required to do this by law. Some countries are able to report in their abortion statistics procedures performed on women who report having had previous abortions and the number of these.

When examining abortion statistics, care needs to be taken to appreciate that the figures reflect the procedures that have been experienced by women; they do not represent women themselves. Take for example a woman who has two abortions in a particular year; her two procedures will generate two entries in that year's figures, but she is one woman in that population. If this woman is having her second and third abortions in her lifetime, these two episodes will be coded as 'one previous abortion' on the first occasion that year and as 'two previous abortions' on the second occasion.

In Sweden, the proportion of women having an abortion who had already experienced a previous abortion rose from 19% in 1975 to 38% in 2008 (www.sos.se). In New Zealand, the increase was from 23% in 1991 to 38% in 2011 (www.stats.govt.nz).

Table 21.1 Number (percentage) of previous abortions by selected age group, residents of England & Wales 2012

Previous abortions	All ages	Under 16	16 and 17	18 and 19	20–24	25–29	30 and over
0	117 166 (63)	2 836 (97)	9 118 (92)	15 015 (81)	35 966 (66)	23 405 (56)	30 826 (54)
1	50 454 (27)	84 (3)	779 (8)	3 054 (17)	14 658 (27)	13 265 (32)	18 614 (32)
2	12 974 (7)	4 (0)	48 (0)	392 (2)	3 152 (6)	3 818 (9)	5 560 (10)
3	3 194 (2)	1 (0)	3 (0)	44 (0)	577 (1)	999 (2)	1 570 (3)
4	914 (0)	0	0	2 (0)	153 (0)	281 (1)	478 (1)
5	267 (0)	0	0	0	36 (0)	75 (0)	156 (0)
6	91 (0)	0	0	0	10 (0)	28 (0)	53 (0)
7	29 (0)	0	0	0	5 (0)	5 (0)	19 (0)
8 or more	33 (0)	0	0	0	1 (0)	6 (0)	26 (0)
Total	185 122 (100)	2 925 (100)	9 948 (100)	18 507 (100)	54 558 (100)	41 882 (100)	57 302 (100)

Source: www.gov.uk/government/uploads/system/uploads/attachment_data/file/211790/2012_Abortion_Statistics.pdf.

In Canada in 1993, only 2% of abortions were obtained by women who had had more than two previous abortions, suggesting that abortion was not being widely used as a primary method of fertility control at that time [5]. A study from Hawaii has a similar finding [6]. This is in contrast to former Eastern Bloc countries where contraception was not freely available and women had large numbers of abortions: around six in their reproductive years in the former Soviet Union [7].

The proportion of English and Welsh abortions in which women reported undergoing a subsequent legal abortion has risen from 0.7% in 1969 (the first complete year in which abortion was legal) to 37% in 2012. During this same time period, in England and Wales there was a rise in age-standardized abortion rate per 1000 women aged 15–44 from 5.2 in 1969 to 18.6 in 2007, followed by a slight fall to 16.5 by 2012.

The proportion of abortions in which women reported having had one or more previous abortions in England and Wales is 37% for all ages, ranging from 8% in the under-18 age group to 46% in the 35 and over age group. A breakdown of the number of previous abortions from 2012 data for residents of England and Wales is shown in Table 21.1. The proportion of abortions in which women reported having had three or more previous abortions was 2%. Figures for England and Wales are similar to those for Finland, with a lower proportion of subsequent abortions than in New Zealand, Sweden and the USA.

Since 2005, the Department of Health in England has produced a 'repeat abortion indicator' for each local area in England and Wales. This is expressed as the percentage of abortion episodes in women aged under 25 in which a previous abortion was declared. It is unclear to the authors of this chapter how such data can be used to increase the quality of local services. Indeed, it would seem that the production of such statistics can be construed as stigmatizing (see Chapter 20).

Demographic aspects

As long ago as 1974, Tietze pointed out that for women who have already experienced an abortion, a substantial proportion of those who use highly effective contraception will experience a subsequent unplanned pregnancy within a few years; many of these women will opt for another abortion [8]. Tietze notes that, after abortion law is liberalized in a given country, it is typical that an increase in the proportion of those women having more than one abortion occurs over time. So, increasing age (and parity) correlates with a greater chance of having more than one abortion as the population of reproductive-aged women living in the context of legal abortion grows. This is probably the main factor responsible for increasing proportions of women having more than one abortion in most countries. A steady state, in which the proportion of women in the population having subsequent abortions stabilizes, is reached around 30 years after liberalization of abortion law, provided that the proportion of women having a first abortion stabilizes immediately after legalization [9]. It is important not to confuse denominators; the steady state refers to the proportion of women in the population belonging to the two groups, not to the proportion of abortions which are either first or subsequent. The significance of 30 years is that this is the time that it takes for a cohort of women to pass through the reproductive ages (15–44). If the proportion of women having a first abortion does not stabilize immediately, the proportion of women having subsequent abortions will not stabilize until about 30 years after the proportion of women having a first abortion stabilizes. Once the steady state is reached, the fraction of abortions which are subsequent will stabilize as well. This state of affairs appears to obtain in many countries.

It should be noted that there are very few statistics available on the proportions of women having first and subsequent abortions. Gathering such data requires repeated national surveys and is still subject to the vagaries of under-reporting. The British ten-yearly National Survey of Sexual Attitudes and Lifestyles has been used to study women having more than one abortion [10]. Identifying individual women in national abortion statistics can be done only in those countries that permit record-linkage between registries.

The ultimate proportion of women having subsequent abortions depends on a number of factors including the incidence of abortion (the abortion rate). A woman who has had a previous abortion is more likely to have another abortion in a given year than a woman who has had no previous abortions is to have a first. It is likely that women eligible for subsequent abortions are of higher fecundity than women potentially eligible for first abortions; some of the latter group will be infertile and some will not yet have reached their sexual debut.

A British study showed that the median time between first and second procedures, among women with experience of only two abortions, was 41 months with 17% of women undergoing a second abortion within one year of their first abortion and one-third within two years; 10% of these women experienced at least a 15-year time lapse between procedures [10].

In Hungary, where abortion on request became available in 1956, the number of abortions in which women had experienced previous abortions had almost stabilized by the early 1970s. The proportion of these subsequent abortions stabilized at the same time at around 60% and began to decrease from 1973 onwards [11]. In 1971, the interval between two successive abortions was less than two years in nearly half the cases; in 1981 this figure had declined to one-third.

Canadian abortion statistics reveal the proportion of subsequent abortions increasing from 8% in 1974 to 29% in 1993 (Canadian abortion law was liberalized in 1988; between 1969 and 1988, abortion was legal only with the approval of a three-doctor committee). US data show an increase from 18% in 1975 to 42% in 1987; the figure is now running at 47% [12]. In England and Wales, the proportion of subsequent abortions continues to rise gradually.

Policy makers and those responsible for service design and delivery should be cautious when interpreting and acting upon figures showing proportions of abortions obtained by women who have had previous abortions. Complex demographic factors dictate an in-built increase in subsequent abortions which can continue for some years. Such statistics do not necessarily indicate that contraceptive services are failing or that there is a simple fix by more forceful promotion of long-acting reversible contraception.

Comparative studies

Understanding the differences between women experiencing more than one abortion and those having first abortions is a complex area of research and few such studies have been done. An ideal study design is record-linkage, but this is precluded in many countries by data protection constraints. The methodology used in many studies to date has limitations. Some of the studies have small sample sizes which do not allow the significance of differences between subgroups to be estimated. There is reliance on self-reporting of sensitive issues which are potentially subject to response bias and could not be independently verified.

Responses immediately before an abortion may be influenced by anxiety about the forthcoming procedure. Also, the studies were performed in widely differing settings in terms of cultural attitudes and service provision.

Some of the studies show no differences between groups of women having first or subsequent abortions. Some differences between the groups have been shown; only those differences that have been replicated are mentioned here. Compared to women having first abortions, women having subsequent abortions are more likely to have had an earlier sexual debut, be poor users of contraception at sexual debut, have a higher coital frequency, be of lower socio-economic status, have left school at an earlier age, have suffered intimate partner (domestic) violence and be of black ethnicity [1,10].

It should be noted that there are inconsistencies between studies. So, some of the differences between the groups may be spurious. The above differences suggest that those women having subsequent abortions possibly display more vulnerability [13].

Psychosocial studies have shown a tendency for women who are undergoing subsequent abortions to have been neglected, to have had difficulties at school, had conflicts with their current partner and to be less mature, less independent and less stable individuals [1]. They are also more likely to have sexual problems. One study showed that women who had had two or more abortions were more likely to have been exposed to adverse events in childhood compared to women who had had no or only one abortion [14]. In this study there was a strong correlation between physical and sexual abuse at ages 0–12 and having had more than one abortion. An underlying adulthood outcome of childhood adversity is low self-esteem; women with such an attribute tend to lack confidence in their ability to exert control over their environment and are prone to such behaviours as sexual risk-taking. Further research is needed to elucidate such mechanisms.

In summary, although there is some evidence that women having more than one abortion tend to have characteristics that distinguish them from women having a first abortion, the overall impression remains that women having abortions, whatever the number, are generally similar.

Use of contraception

Many studies have shown no lesser use of contraception in those undergoing subsequent abortions compared to women having first abortions [1]. Several studies have shown that those having subsequent abortions had used contraception to a greater extent than women having first abortions [1], perhaps suggesting a higher level of underlying fecundity among these women. This higher use of contraception includes greater experience of using different methods of contraception and a greater likelihood that they used contraception at the time of the unwanted pregnancy in question. Three studies showed a greater use of coitus-independent contraceptive methods by women who had had previous abortions compared to women who had not [1,15]. A single study showed that women who had had previous abortions were more consistent in their use of contraception than women who had not. Use of emergency contraception has been shown to be equally low in both groups.

Women of lower socio-economic status are less likely to use highly effective contraception after abortion [16]. A postabortion contraception intervention reduces subsequent unintended pregnancy and the need for future abortions compared to receipt of no contraceptive advice at all [17]. Specialist contraceptive advice and enhanced provision compared to standard care has been shown in a randomized controlled trial to improve uptake of long-acting reversible contraception; however, the intervention had no effect on the likelihood of a woman returning for another abortion within two years [18].

Conclusions

Categorizing women by how many previous abortions they have had implies moral judgement on the part of the clinician and does nothing to improve service delivery. It compares with the situation where clinicians, before oral emergency contraception became available to buy as well as on prescription, put a limit on the number of times they would prescribe this to an individual woman. Every woman requesting abortion should be treated according to her individual circumstances, wishes and needs, and no assumptions should be made about a woman who has had more than one abortion or about the care that she needs.

There is no valid reason why women presenting for abortion who have had one or more previous abortions should be treated any differently from those who have not. All women requesting abortion should receive information and support; some need counselling (see Chapter 5). All women requesting abortion should be offered prophylaxis against pelvic infection and ideally screening for sexually transmitted infections. As all women seeking abortion, regardless of previous abortion history, are at higher risk of intimate partner violence, health professionals assessing such women should have an awareness of such an association and liaise with professional colleagues if there are concerns. In particular, clinicians should be aware that contraceptive sabotage may be a factor in unintended pregnancy for women experiencing intimate partner violence, and they should be prepared to suggest contraceptive methods that a woman can conceal if ongoing contraception is desired [19].

All women potentially have contraceptive needs and these should be met around the time of an abortion just as they should be at any other time. Periabortion contraceptive advice is important for all women; this should include offering and being able to provide long-acting reversible contraception for women who desire it. Clinicians should approach each woman as an individual, regardless of abortion history, and offer contraceptive options that suit her particular situation.

Improving access to contraception is an essential first step in helping women manage their fertility. Making long-acting reversible contraception more widely available is likely to have a general beneficial effect on unintended pregnancy rates. Provision of emergency contraception in advance of need may also facilitate uptake of oral emergency contraception; although studies of advance provision of emergency contraception have not shown an effect on abortion rates at the population level, it is an important option for individual women who have had unprotected sex. Future research should focus on further psychological factors for a whole population that detract from consistent use of contraception; from these possible effective interventions can be developed.

References

1. Rowlands S. More than one abortion. *J Fam Plann Reprod Health Care* 2007;33:155–8.

2. Trussell J. Contraceptive failure in the United States. *Contraception* 2011;83:397–404.

3. Harlap S, Kost K, Forrest JD. *Preventing Pregnancy, Protecting Health: A New Look at Birth Control in the United States.* New York: Guttmacher Institute, 1991.

4. Weitz TA, Kimport K. A need to expand our thinking about "repeat" abortions. *Contraception* 2012;85:408–12.

5. Millar WJ, Wadhera S, Henshaw SK. Repeat abortions in Canada, 1975–1993. *Family Planning Perspectives* 1997;29:20–4.

6. Steinhoff PG, Smith RG, Palmore JA, Diamond M, Chung CS. Women who obtain repeat abortions: a study based on record linkage. *Family Planning Perspectives* 1979;11:30–8.

7. Popov A. Family planning and induced abortion in the USSR: basic health and demographic characteristics. *Studies in Family Planning* 1991;22:368–77.

8. Tietze C. The 'problem' of repeat abortions. *Family Planning Perspectives* 1974;6:148–50.

9. Tietze C, Jain AK. The mathematics of repeat abortion: explaining the increase. *Studies in Family Planning* 1978;9:294–9.

10. Stone N, Ingham R. Who presents more than once? Repeat abortion among women in Britain. *J Fam Plann Reprod Health Care* 2011;37:209–15.

11. Klinger A. Hungary. In P Sachdev (ed.) *International Handbook on Abortion*. New York: Greenwood Press, 1988: 218–34.

12. Jones RK, Singh S, Finer LB, Frohwirth LF. *Repeat Abortion in the United States*. New York: Guttmacher Institute, 2006.

13. Makenzius M, Tydén T, Darj E, Larsson M. Repeat induced abortion – a matter of individual behaviour or societal factors? A cross-sectional study among Swedish women. *European Journal of Contraception & Reproductive Health Care* 2011;16:369–77.

14. Bleil ME, Adler NE, Pasch LA, Sternfeld B, Reijo-Pera RA, Cedars MI. Adverse childhood experiences and repeat induced abortion. *Am J Obstet Gynecol* 2011;204:122.e1–e6.

15. Scott R, Mann S, Douiri A, Kumar U. Factors associated with repeat abortion in a south London clinic population. Poster presented at the Faculty of Sexual & Reproductive Healthcare Annual Scientific Meeting, Warwick, UK, 18–19 April 2013.

16. Bajos N, Lamarche-Vadel A, Gilbert F, Ferrand M. Contraception at the time of abortion: high-risk time or high-risk women? *Hum Reprod* 2006;21:2862–7.

17. Johnson BR, Ndhlovu S, Farr SL, Chipato T. Reducing unplanned pregnancy and abortion in Zimbabwe through postabortion contraception. *Studies in Family Planning* 2002;33:195–202.

18. Schunmann C, Glasier A. Specialist contraceptive counselling and provision after termination of pregnancy improves uptake of long-acting methods but does not prevent repeat abortion: a randomized trial. *Hum Reprod* 2006;21:2296–303.

19. Miller E, Jordan B, Levenson R, Silverman JG. Pregnancy coercion: connecting the dots between partner violence and unintended pregnancy. *Contraception* 2010;81:457–459.

Chapter

22

Factors associated with second trimester abortion

Roger Ingham

Introduction and background

This chapter considers aspects of elective abortions that take place further along the gestation than the majority. These procedures are generally referred to as 'late' abortions, although the use of this term is not as simple as it may sound; some background to this concern is given below. Most researchers adopt the criterion of 12/13 weeks to mark the divide between early (first trimester) and late (second trimester) procedures, although it is not immediately clear why this dividing point was initially selected. Indeed, given the rapid increase in the use of early medical abortion in many countries there is an argument that nine weeks would be a more suitable – and clinically meaningful – criterion. Very few papers, however, have reported data using this particular dividing point. The term 'very late' abortions is sometimes used to describe procedures that occur towards the end of the second trimester, above 20 weeks or so.

Of course, researchers who have adopted the first/second trimester division are following the legal positions in many jurisdictions which make a distinction between the trimesters in relation to what is and is not permissible. But this begs the question as to why the various legislators in these countries adopted this criterion in the first place. Some similarity in countries' laws can be traced back to colonial influence, so such overlap is more than mere coincidence.

Of all medical interventions, abortion is one of the most contentious. Many (extremely) strongly held beliefs touch on every aspect of the procedures involved. A number of narratives run alongside each other competing for recognition, two of the main ones being the medical and the moral. The development of policies and laws governing what can and cannot be carried out and when and for what reason appears to be characterized by achieving an acceptable balance between these narratives. The resulting laws are often arrived at through a process of incremental reluctance. In other words, rather than starting from the principle of a woman's right to terminate a pregnancy and then develop what is required for this to be implemented successfully, a common compromise recognizes that there may be grounds for permitting availability, but these should not be too 'generous' or willingly granted. The end of the first trimester seems to provide a suitable 'moral' compromise.

It is within this socio-legal compromise that the seemingly simple term 'late' can take on high significance. Although it can be taken – at one level – as being a simple descriptive term of a relative point in time, within a more moral framework it can be taken as being negatively loaded. People are *late* for meetings or lectures or dates (through bad planning,

Abortion Care, ed. Sam Rowlands. Published by Cambridge University Press. © Cambridge University Press 2014.

irresponsibility, fecklessness, etc.), a train or a bus is *late* and this can cause inconvenience; *lateness* is often accompanied (at least in polite society) by an apology. To the extent that abortion itself (and women who undergo the procedure) are often stigmatized [1,2], so *late* abortion (and the women involved) are at risk of being stigmatized more strongly.

So, the use of the term 'late abortion' is not as simple as it may appear. In the light of the sensitivities of language in this area, many commentators prefer to use the more neutral clinical term of first trimester, second trimester, or be specific about the weeks of gestation that cover what they are describing. This is certainly not to imply that anyone 'innocently' using the term 'late abortion' is necessarily making a loaded judgement statement, but this brief discussion does serve to illustrate how certain phrases may inadvertently feed into, and imply adoption of, an unintended judgemental position.

Why does the timing of the abortion matter?

There are various reasons why delays in undergoing abortions should be avoided where possible; these will vary considerably between countries and contexts.

First, although properly conducted abortions at all stages are relatively low risk compared to the risk of giving birth, there is a higher risk of medical complications with each additional week of gestation (see Chapter 14). Estimates vary somewhat and will obviously be affected by context, but Lalitkumar *et al.* report that second trimester abortions constitute between 10 and 15% of all abortions worldwide but account for 65% of the major abortion-related complications [3].

Second, despite great advances in clinical techniques and increased awareness of, and communication about, abortion options in many countries, there seems to be a persistent pattern of around 10 to 15% of women who seek an abortion after 13 weeks' gestation; there is clearly high potential for improved safety.

Third, there are progressively fewer clinicians who are able and/or willing to carry out procedures as the gestation length increases.

Fourth, once a woman has made a decision to go ahead with an abortion, any subsequent delays are likely to be stressful and disconcerting.

Fifth, discovering more about why a substantial minority of procedures do not take place in the first trimester is of particular importance in those regimes where second trimester procedures are forbidden. Where women in these regimes fail to obtain a desired abortion during the first trimester, the alternatives are to continue with an unwanted birth (albeit their attitude may change as time passes), to give the baby up for adoption or to attempt an illegal (and almost certainly unsafe) procedure. None of these alternatives is ideal.

Sixth, some countries (and states in the USA) debate, from time to time, what the upper gestational limit to abortions should be, and whether changes are needed to their current legislation. For example, the UK Parliament debated lowering the upper limit in 2008, and successive motions were (unsuccessfully) voted upon to reduce this to 13, 16, 20 and 22 weeks from its current 24 weeks. In order to inform such debates in this and other countries, the implications of any changes need to be fully understood. An early paper from the Turnaway Study in the USA reports the negative outcomes for women who were denied abortions due to gestational age limits in different states; young and poor women were disproportionately affected [4].

Finally, to the extent that abortion may lead to negative reactions – such as guilt or shame – then these reactions are likely to be stronger the further into the pregnancy the woman is. A greater extent of close contact (fetal movement, more human attributes, and so on) is unlikely to have a neutral influence. The extent of any longer-term impact on the mental health of women is a hotly debated issue (see Chapters 18 and 19); however, even in the potentially highly distressing case of second trimester abortions due to fetal anomaly, evidence of widespread longer-term negative impact on mental health (as opposed to grief) is lacking [5].

The negative reactions of clinicians and, possibly, those of women, to abortions carried out at longer gestations is likely to be related to notions of personhood. Even before the feasibility of fetal viability enters the discussion, greater similarity in form to intact babies is likely to lead to stronger emotional responses.

Harris has written on this topic, and describes the need to conceal the details of some second trimester procedures from women so as to reduce possible trauma; she also describes the impact on staff. However, she argues that remaining silent on these topics is not helpful to the cause of the pro-choice movement, and that honesty and openness should be more strongly encouraged for a range of reasons [6].

Contextual issues to consider

In considering what is known about factors associated with second trimester abortions, a number of issues need to be considered that extend the realm of interest beyond the simple identification of antecedents.

As mentioned briefly above, there are vast variations in the legal positions between countries, as well as between states within the USA. Boland has recently summarized the legislation in 191 countries, and shows how seemingly quite minor changes in wording can have potentially profound effects on what is – or is not – legally permitted, as well as the ease of comprehension and interpretation. For example, some jurisdictions permit second trimester procedures where there is a risk or danger to the women's (physical and/or mental) health, whilst others specify that there needs to be a *serious* risk or danger. It is not clear quite where the differences lie [7].

Other stipulations that show variation across countries include risk to women's life, preservation of the physical and/or mental health of the women, fetal impairment, pregnancies resulting from a sexual offence and abortion on socio-economic grounds. The extent to which a simple request is granted also varies. Different combinations in first and second trimester may apply; for example, there is no distinction in UK (but not including Northern Ireland) law between first and second trimester procedures; both require two doctors to agree that certain conditions are met. On the other hand, the relatively recently introduced law in Nepal permits abortion on request during the first trimester, but imposes strict criteria in cases of second trimester requests.

Other degrees of variance – often beyond the formal legal framework – exist. These include who can carry out procedures, where they can be carried out, who needs to give permission in the case of minors (and, in some cases, wives), whether counselling and/or reflection periods are required and how strictly or liberally the laws are interpreted by clinicians and the courts. In some cases these regulations have been intended to create further barriers whereas in other cases they have been designed to protect women's health [7]. It would be an interesting analysis to ascertain what proportion of the reported 500 abortion-related laws passed in the USA between 1992 and 2008 were intended to service these alternative motivations. As well as variations in the legal position between states in the USA, variations in availability of funding add further complexities and confusions [8–10].

In other regimes where public and private facilities coexist, financial wherewithal may also have a large impact. In the UK (except Northern Ireland), for example, the majority of second trimester abortions are carried out in the specialist independent sector under contract to the National Health Service (NHS) free of charge. Some women may choose to pay to go to private facilities, rather than calling on NHS funding and its associated bureaucracy and perceived risk to confidentiality, or are required to do so by virtue of their non-resident status. Even when costs are covered by the NHS, the longer distances of travel to the facility still have financial implications that may affect the timing of access. Financial implications of accessing abortions at any stage vary in countries without a free health service and/or good insurance schemes, but saving up (or obtaining from elsewhere) the necessary funding will push procedures further into the gestation period.

Abortion is one of the few areas of clinical practice that permits conscientious objection to involvement amongst clinical staff (see Chapters 20 and 23). Although in some countries this can presumably be manifest through selecting not to work in a clinic that offers abortions, such a choice is not possible in some other countries. So, for example, in the UK (except Northern Ireland) the first port of call for many women will be their general practitioner. If he or she is anti-abortion then there is a professional obligation for this to be reported to the woman and for a rapid referral to be made to a colleague who feels able to provide advice and onward referral. From much anecdotal evidence, and some empirical data reported later, it is clear that some doctors and clinical staff influence the process in ways over and above just refusal and onward referral.

In other words, delays in dealing with the situation, negative attitudes being expressed, confusing (or plain wrong) advice regarding what is possible at different locations and at different gestation times, and other tactics, may all serve to add delays and possibly shift procedures from the first to the second trimester. It is simply not known how widespread these processes are, nor what impact they may have on the prevalence of delays in access to abortion or even abandonment of intentions and preferences to have an abortion. Indeed, research in many areas relating to abortion is fraught with difficulties, although space does not permit a detailed consideration of these.

What is known about antecedents of second trimester abortions?

A fairly small number of studies have identified factors that are associated with second trimester abortions; these are mainly from the USA and Europe.

A Finnish study [11] analysed data relating to all abortions occurring between 2000 and 2005 to identify risk factors for first-time and subsequent second trimester abortions; women also receiving sterilization or who had an abortion as a result of fetal anomaly were excluded. First abortions occurring in the second trimester accounted for 7% of all abortions and were associated with younger age; incidence of further abortions was higher amongst those whose initial abortion had been second trimester, and those further abortions that occurred in the second trimester (compared with the first) were associated with prior abortions in the second trimester, young age and previous deliveries. Because finance is not an issue in the Finnish healthcare system and clinics are encouraged – indeed, obliged – to act swiftly, the authors conclude that the women affected are 'displaced or have additional problems in life'.

Jones and Finer [12] used large-scale datasets from national surveys in the USA to identify characteristics of women most likely to have second trimester abortions. In sum, amongst the 10% of women receiving second trimester procedures, associated factors were age, black ethnic group, education and poverty status. A further finding related to 'potentially disruptive life events' (such as partner violence, physical or sexual abuse, falling behind on rent, partnership dissolution, moving house, and others); reporting three or more of these disruptive events was associated with a higher probability of second – as opposed to first – trimester abortions. A higher proportion of women who relied on health insurance (either private schemes or Medicaid) fell into the second trimester range than those who self-funded their procedures.

A different approach to assessing reasons for delays involves asking women to account for the various different stages in the process and how long each took. Drey *et al.* used audio computer-assisted interviews with almost 400 US women who had had abortions and compared first and second trimester time intervals for each stage. Half of the gestational time difference between first and second trimester procedures was accounted for by delayed suspicion of pregnancy and obtaining a test. Together, these accounted for over half of the women missing the opportunity to have a first trimester procedure. These women also experienced longer delays once they requested an abortion for a variety of reasons, including locating a provider, sorting out transport and obtaining state insurance; interestingly, regression revealed that prior second trimester abortion was a risk factor for a further one, as in the Finnish study mentioned earlier. Uncertainty regarding the time of the last menstrual period, and fewer signs of pregnancy (such as vomiting and nausea) were also independently associated with delays [13].

Finer *et al.* used self-completion questionnaires and qualitative interviews with over 1,000 women who had had an abortion and asked about the relative timings of the different stages of the process: the times from last menstrual period to suspecting pregnancy; from suspecting pregnancy to confirming by a test; from deciding to have an abortion to first contact; and from first contact to the actual procedure. Comparing women who had first and second trimester abortions, the authors report that delays were most likely associated with each of these steps in the process; no one stage was responsible for the additional time taken. However, practical issues like raising the money or getting insurance payments contributed significantly to delays amongst poorer women, and poorer women, black women and younger women reported longer times to realize that they were pregnant and/or how far into the pregnancy they were [14].

Foster *et al.* adopted a similar approach in San Francisco, exploring reported delays at three stages – first pregnancy test, calling a clinic and obtaining the abortion. Delays in the first stage were associated with obesity, lack of traditional symptoms and signs of pregnancy, being unsure of date of last period and emotional and behavioural factors such as being afraid and being in denial, use of drugs and alcohol and, again, having a prior second trimester abortion. Delays in the second stage were associated with difficulties in getting finance from Medicaid and difficulties with the decision to terminate the pregnancy. Delays during the final stage were associated with prior second trimester abortion, initial referral to another provider, an unsupportive partner and difficulty with finance [15].

The importance of partner support identified in the Foster *et al.* study above was reinforced in a study which compared abortions carried out at under nine weeks with those at longer gestations, albeit mostly still in the first trimester. The authors report that earlier procedures are more likely amongst women who report 'perceptions of supportive partner interactions and joint decision-making' [16].

One British study adopted a similar approach to that of Foster *et al.* (coincidentally at the same time) and obtained roughly similar results, despite the differences in financial and legal contexts. Ingham *et al.* analysed self-completed questionnaires from almost 900 women who had undergone second trimester abortions, mainly funded by the NHS. The study did not aim to compare characteristics of women who underwent first and second trimester abortions, but to explore reported reasons for delays. These were reported at all stages along the path from suspicion of pregnancy through to the actual procedure; the three major causes of delays were uncertainty about what to do about being pregnant (41%), not realizing they were pregnant (38%) and thinking the pregnancy was less advanced than it was (36%). Other key reasons included suspicion of pregnancy but not acting on this, lack of belief that they could be pregnant due to having used contraception or not doing anything that could have resulted in conception, relationship with partner breaking down and having to wait for appointments [17].

Amongst women who were under 18 years old, the main reported reasons were not acting on suspicions, not being sure what they would do if they were pregnant, concern about what was involved in an abortion and concerns about possible parental reactions. Separate analyses of abortions that occurred at gestations of 18 weeks or more revealed no clear and specific differences other than longer delays at each stage of the pathway, but especially the time taken to suspect and confirm that they were indeed pregnant [17]. These results mirror those reported in a qualitative study carried out on women having abortions at 19 to 24 weeks' gestation in London [18].

A few studies have explored aspects of second trimester abortion in non-western countries; for example, Lim *et al.* report that, in Singapore, they are more likely amongst young women, those of Malay ethnicity, single women, nulliparous women and those with 'no prior usage of contraception' [19]. Gallo and Nghia carried out qualitative interviews of women in Vietnam and reported barriers to access, failure to recognize pregnancy, needing time to decide and other events occurring in their lives. The authors reported high levels of ignorance and uncertainties amongst some of the women interviewed, as well as serious failures in the healthcare system. They also raised the possibility of sex selection accounting for some cases, but recognize the low likelihood of this being reported in research studies of this nature [20]. On this latter point, Belanger and Oanh estimate – based on study of patterns of family composition and abortion probability in Hanoi – that 14% of second trimester abortions to women with at least one living child are likely to be related to avoiding the birth of a female [21].

Although studies in the USA report that younger and less well-educated women are over-represented amongst second trimester abortions, a study from India reveals that this trend is not universal. Aggarwal and colleagues report that the 2% of second trimester procedures in their sample of over 4,000 cases contained a higher prevalence of women who were older, had higher educational status and higher parity. The authors point out that this sample may be biased due to the non-inclusion of women who access illegal facilities and that much further research is needed before this unusual pattern of results can be fully understood [22]. Their results also seem to be at odds with those reported by Kalyanwala *et al.* that older and better educated women generally report earlier for abortions [23].

Ganatra summarizes the legality and evidence surrounding abortion for sex selection in several Asian countries and highlights some of the difficulties in establishing its prevalence. However, she points out that some anti-choice organizations are exaggerating the use of abortions as a sex selection method in order to encourage further restrictions on the general availability of abortions. She argues that the issues of women's rights and the need to eradicate sex selection should not be confused but rather kept separate in policy developments [24].

Underpinning the statistics in this area, there are of course real stories concerning real women's lives. By way of illustrating some of these dynamics, a few quotes taken from qualitative studies are included in Box 22.1; in addition to adding the human voice, and despite the importance of cultural variation, these examples also illustrate that many aspects and concerns are universal.

Box 22.1 Selected quotes from qualitative studies on second trimester abortions

'I thought I wouldn't have my period anymore I didn't feel anything abnormal. In previous times [pregnancies], I did sometimes feel like eating this or that. This time I was still working very hard in the field, and I was still healthy. So I didn't have an examination until my pregnancy was big.' (35-year-old, married with four children) (a)

'I didn't know I was pregnant during those first few months, so I ate some peaches. You know, people told me that if ate dao diec ['undeveloped'] peaches, my baby would be dumb. I'm so anxious. I'm fearful for the future of my baby.' (25-year-old unmarried professional) (a)

'I had to wait until I got enough money. I had to wait for money sent from my family. This money is normally for my meals and studying fee in school. My boyfriend did so too. The total money for this time is more than one million [~US$63]. I think the abortion fee is too high.' (22-year-old unmarried student in Vietnam) (a)

'When I missed the first one, I was just happy, like "Yes!". Then I missed the second one, then I was just doubting a little bit. Like. Then I missed the third one; then it cut right through my head, like "Oh. My God!" Then I started getting scared and stuff.' (16-year-old, unmarried) (b)

'So we decided that it was too soon [to have a child together]. It just wasn't the right time for neither of us … it was like … sometimes [my partner] would say yes, and I would say no. I would convince him where I would think it's a bad decision and he'll say yes or no. Then [he'd] try to convince me … So, it was confusing at first, but we knew that it was going to be a decision that we would have to make.' (27-year-old, one child, 15 weeks pregnant at time of abortion) (b)

'I mean, when I first found out [that I was pregnant], I had it in my head to have [the abortion], but did not have the money. It was the money; I did not have no money to come down here and the money to do it … It is hard to take off work, you know, but it was really the money, because if I were to have it sooner, I would have come sooner, but I did not have it. And everybody was against [me having the abortion] so, there was nobody to help me, you know.' (22-year-old, three children, 13 weeks pregnant at time of abortion) (b)

'My partner is violent but when he found out I was pregnant he promised he would get help and change and for a few weeks he did but then he beat me with a baseball bat so I don't think it's right to involve a child in that.' (24-year-old, abortion at 19 plus weeks) (c)

'I had no symptoms of pregnancy, I did not gain weight. I did not experience nausea and until two weeks ago I didn't even notice a bump, considering I'm 20 weeks pregnant.' (22-year-old, abortion at 19 plus weeks) (c)

'Because I was in denial and scared about it.' (23-year-old, unmarried, Asian British, 18 weeks at time of abortion) (d)

'My pregnancy termination was delayed as the clinic I went to was a place that persuaded me not to have an abortion, and tried to put me off it. The clinic was actually for advice when I thought it was where the abortion took place.' (17-year-old unmarried, 16 weeks pregnant at time of abortion) (d)

'The hardest most difficult part of the process was seeing my GP and getting her to refer me from there. Once at the [young persons' specialist clinic] they were helpful and referred me to the right place – bpas – who are a very supportive organisation. I am currently 17 weeks; had my GP referred me straight away my decision would have been a lot easier to make – it's never an easy decision but when someone is inflicting their opinion on you it is even harder.' (22-year-old, cohabiting, 17 weeks pregnant at time of abortion) (d)

'The pregnancy was due to a sexual assault so pushed to the back of my mind and didn't want to tell anyone but I am pleased I did, when I did.' (25-year-old, separated, 23 weeks pregnant at time of abortion) (d)

Sources: (a) Gallo and Nghia, 2007 (Vietnam) [20]; (b) Finer *et al.*, 2006 (USA) [14]; (c) Marie Stopes International, undated (UK) [18]; (d) Ingham *et al.*, 2008 (UK) [17].

Conclusions and implications

Research has identified a range of factors that make abortions in the second trimester more likely. Some are factors that could not have been anticipated earlier, such as evidence of fetal anomalies; in these cases, the decision-making processes of parents are likely to be fundamentally different from most other life decisions (and were beyond the remit of this chapter). Similarly, second trimester abortions for reasons of sex selection represent a special case in terms of decision-making, as well as being very challenging to research on account of legality and stigma. The other major area that the chapter has not considered is the question of viability and associated intact dilatation and extraction (D&X) procedures (see Chapter 10); this again was felt to be outside the remit of this chapter, although policy discussions in this area should take account of the possible impact of reducing legal upper gestational limits.

For other cases, similar factors appear to operate in difference cultural settings, albeit the relative importance and prevalence of these will vary by contexts, including characteristics of the women (and partners, in some cases), the financial, attitudinal and logistical background to the procedures and other matters. In some cases – albeit not commonly, according to the research – there is a sense of concealment and/or denial on the part of the woman and this delays testing and seeking treatment. In the majority of cases, however, there are tangible (and addressable) reasons for delays.

Recurring themes involve a belief that pregnancy was not possible given contraceptive use or the activities engaged in, a lack of early enough recognition of the signs of pregnancy, delays in accessing pregnancy tests, delays in making appointments with relevant clinical or counselling staff, delays in obtaining finance to cover costs involved in travel and/or the procedures and others. In cases of delays in accessing clinicians, it is not always clear from studies if the delays are due to the women's prevarication or the clinician's busyness, or clinician reluctance to engage. Certainly there seems to be a universal shortage of clinicians (and associated facilities) willing and able to carry out second trimester abortions; the reasons for this are complex and challenging. Some of these other factors might respond to better education for young women about their own bodies, more available honest and open support facilities, reduction in stigma, greater recognition of a woman's right to choose and other developments.

What we do not know much about is the precise impact of different laws and policies on delays and impacts. So, for example, in countries or states in which second trimester abortions (or those over a certain number of weeks within the second trimester) are prohibited, do a greater proportion of women seek an earlier abortion (if possible), do they travel elsewhere, do they attempt a self-induced procedure or do they simply carry on with the pregnancy and birth (and with what consequences)? There are doubtless other crucially important issues with immense clinical, social and psychological implications.

What we do know, however, with great certainty, is that reducing the upper gestational limit for legal abortion, and/or placing more barriers in the way of access, will not make the demand and need for such provision disappear.

References

1. Kumar A, Hessini L, Mitchell EM. Conceptualising abortion stigma. *Cult Health Sex* 2009;11:625–39.

2. Cockrill K, Upadhyay UD, Turan J, Foster JG. The stigma of having an abortion: development of a scale and characteristics of women experiencing abortion stigma. *Perspect Sex Reprod Health* 2013;45:79–88.

3. Lalitkumar S, Bygdeman M, Gemzell-Danielsson K. Mid-trimester induced abortion: a review. *Hum Reprod Update* 2007;13:37–52.

4. Upadhyay UD, Weitz TA, Jones RK, Barar RE, Foster DG. Denial of abortion because of provider gestational age limits in the United States. *Am J Public Health* 2013;e1–e8. doi:10.2105/AJPH.2013.301378.

5. Steinberg JR. Later abortions and mental health: psychological experiences of women having later abortions – a critical review of the evidence. *Women's Health Issues* 2011;21(3 Suppl):S44–8.

6. Harris L. Second trimester abortion provision: breaking the silence and changing the discourse. *Reprod Health Matters* 2008;16:S74–81.

7. Boland R. Second trimester abortion laws globally: actuality, trends and recommendations. *Reprod Health Matters* 2010;18:67–89.

8. Jones BS, Weitz TA. Legal barriers to second-trimester abortion provision and public health consequences. *Am J Public Health* 2009;99: 623–30.

9. Guttmacher Institute. *State Policies in Brief (1 September 2013): An Overview of Abortion Laws.* www.guttmacher.org/sections/abortion.php (accessed 17 September 2013).

10. Guttmacher Institute. *State Policies in Brief (1 September 2013): State Policies on Later Abortions.* www.guttmacher.org/sections/abortion.php (accessed 17 September 2013).

11. Mentula MJ, Niinimäki M, Suhonen S, Hemminki E, Gissler M, Heikinheimo O. Young age and termination of pregnancy during the second trimester are risk factors for repeat second trimester abortions. *Am J Obstet Gynecol* 2010;107:e1–e7.

12. Jones RK, Finer LB. Who has second-trimester abortions in the United States? *Contraception* 2012;85:544–51.

13. Drey EA, Foster DG, Jackson RA, Lee SJ, Cardenas LH, Darney PD. Risk factors associated with presenting for abortion in the second trimester. *Obstet Gynecol* 2006;107:128–35.

14. Finer LB, Frohwirth LF, Dauphinee LA, Singh S, Moore AM. Timing of steps and reasons for delays in obtaining abortions in the United States. *Contraception* 2006;74:334–44.

15. Foster DG, Jackson RA, Cosby K, Weitz TA, Darney PD, Drey EA. Predictors of delay in each step leading to an abortion. *Contraception* 2008;77:289–93.

16. Kapadia F, Finer LB, Klukas E. Associations between perceived partner support and relationship dynamics with

timing of pregnancy termination. *Women's Health Issues* 2011;21(3 Suppl):S8–13.

17. Ingham R, Lee E, Clements SJ, Stone N. Reasons for second trimester abortions in England and Wales. *Reprod Health Matters* 2008;16:S18–29.

18. Marie Stopes International. *Late Abortion; a research study of women undergoing abortion between 19 and 24 weeks gestation*. London: Marie Stopes International, undated.

19. Lim L, Wong H, Yong E, Singh K. Profiles of women presenting for abortions in Singapore: focus on teenage abortions and late abortions. *Eur J Obstet Gynecol Reprod Biol* 2012;160:219–22.

20. Gallo MF, Nghia NC. Real life is different: a qualitative study of why women delay abortion until the second trimester in Vietnam. *Soc Sci Med* 2007;64:1812–23.

21. Belanger D, Oanh KTH. Second-trimester abortions and sex-selection of children in Hanoi, Vietnam. *Pop Stud* 2009;63:163–71.

22. Aggarwal P, Agarwal P, Zutshi V, Batra S. Do women presenting for first and second-trimester abortion differ socio-demographically? *Ann Med Health Sci Res* 2013;3:187–90.

23. Kalyanwala S, Francis Zavier AJ, Jejeebhoy S, Kumar R. Abortion experiences of unmarried young women in India: evidence from a facility-based study in Bihar and Jharkhand. *Int Perspect Sex Reprod Health* 2010;36:62–71.

24. Ganatra B. Maintaining access to safe abortion and reducing sex ratio imbalances in Asia. *Reprod Health Matters* 2008;16:S90–8.

Staff perspectives

Edna Astbury-Ward

Introduction

This chapter will focus on the medical, nursing and psychological care of the woman during the abortion process, in particular, from the perspective of staff caring for women undergoing induced abortion. The chapter will not discuss issues relating to the safety and welfare of staff who work in abortion services. However, the dedication and commitment of staff working in those parts of the world where the risk of violence and protest is part of the job is acknowledged.

Health professionals encounter women seeking abortion at all stages of women's abortion journey from the worried woman who attends requesting a pregnancy test to care and support after abortion. Caring for women undergoing induced abortion presents some challenges; the literature suggests that staff may experience abortion work as challenging in a number of ways. Some of the challenges encountered are practical (i.e. related to service delivery) but others could be described as personal (i.e. related to the emotional, social and psychological).

Personal challenges

The personal challenges encountered when delivering a service to women seeking abortion very much depend on the stage at which staff are involved in the clinical encounter. It would be reasonable to assume that the feelings and emotions evoked by onward referral to another clinician for abortion as opposed to conducting a dilatation and evacuation procedure of an 18-week fetus are significantly different. But this may not necessarily be so: therefore it is important that all staff who are involved in the care of women requesting abortion reflect on their own personal, moral and ethical position and consider their ability to commit to caring for the woman who requests abortion.

All staff involved in caring for women undergoing abortion are confronted by complex demands on many levels. It is undisputed that the woman's needs should remain central to the delivery of care and that her wishes remain paramount whilst delivering the necessary care. Caring for women through an abortion often means that the therapeutic bond between staff and patient has to be formed within a short timeframe. At times, caring for women through an abortion may often seem like a perfunctory process, especially given the large amount of paperwork that most jurisdictions require to be completed in order to comply with legislation. However, staff caring for women throughout this process must never forget

Abortion Care, ed. Sam Rowlands. Published by Cambridge University Press. © Cambridge University Press 2014.

that, whilst it may be a frequent occurrence for them, it is something a woman may only experience once in her lifetime, and for her to have arrived at this point has necessarily meant profound exploration of her own personal values and significant consideration of all her life circumstances which have contributed to her decision to undergo abortion. No woman *wants* to have an abortion; most make the decision after careful consideration of all the alternatives available to her at the time.

Based on the assumption that most women face an impending abortion with a complex set of emotions and a degree of fear, anxiety and sadness (sadness about *having* to make the decision, not about the reasons related *to* the decision), it would be reasonable to say that staff will be dealing with a complex and (temporarily) emotionally vulnerable patient group [1]. Indeed, many women's anxieties may be related to their specific concerns about how they are going to be treated by the staff. Perceived attitudes of staff are an important aspect of women's assessment of their abortion care. Women who have described the quality of care which they received favourably often refer to positive encounters with the staff. However, for staff, trying to maintain a positive outlook over time may well be difficult to achieve.

Length of service in the job has been highlighted as an important risk factor regarding development of judgemental attitudes in abortion care. A questionnaire survey carried out by Marshall *et al.* found that nurses who had worked longer than six years in abortion care demonstrated significantly more negative attitudes than those who had worked for two years or less in the same environment. The study also suggested that nurses who had previously held positive attitudes lost their objectivity when involved directly and continuously with abortion work [2]. This phenomenon has been described by social psychologists as 'inoculation theory' or difficulty maintaining original attitudes and beliefs in the face of persuasive attempts to do otherwise from those who do not share the same values or opinions.

Working in abortion care presents personal challenges associated with the work; in particular the psychological and emotional demands of the role may mean that remaining objective at all times can be difficult. The demands are twofold; dealing with the emotional needs of the woman whilst at the same time understanding and coping with one's own emotional and psychological responses to the process. Abortion work may be particularly challenging when personal views are at variance with the professional requirements of the job. This is of particular importance when considering the allocation of staff. Astbury-Ward *et al.* demonstrated that the issue of personal attitudes versus professional requirements was most apparent when staff had *not* elected to work in abortion care but instead had been deployed into this specialty out of necessity (i.e. staff shortages) [3]. These staff reported that, if given the choice, they would have chosen to work in another service and that it was preferable to have *elected* to work in abortion care rather than simply having this work allocated to them as part of their wider role. It was found that those staff who had not chosen to work in abortion care in particular exhibited aversion to some aspects of the role. Despite staff being aware of the conscientious objection clause, enshrined in the laws of most countries, some may find it difficult to invoke this at times.

Conscientious objection

As mentioned in Chapter 20, conscientious objection of doctors and nurses can present difficulties in providing the necessary staff in direct contact with women undergoing abortion procedures and in the division of relative workloads for staff; this may have the potential to lead to conflict between colleagues. UK professional guidance states that registered nurses and midwives must 'work cooperatively within teams' [4]. Failing to cover a clinical session could be interpreted as failure to adhere to these professional standards. For nurses with an objection there are specific practice guidelines. The Nursing and Midwifery Council (NMC) states that, if nurses or midwives raise a conscientious objection to being involved in certain aspects of care or treatment, they must do so at the earliest possible time, in order for managers to make alternative arrangements. The NMC recommends that:

> nurses and midwives should give careful consideration when deciding whether or not to accept employment in an area that carries out treatment or procedures to which they have a conscientious objection. [5]

This recommendation takes into account the needs of new staff entering into an area of employment but does not indicate how existing staff can navigate the issue. The General Medical Council makes the following statement about doctors who may wish to exercise conscientious objection [6]:

> You may choose to opt out of providing a particular procedure because of your personal beliefs and values, as long as this does not result in direct or indirect discrimination against, or harassment of, individual patients or groups of patients. This means you must not refuse to treat a particular patient or group of patients because of your personal beliefs or views about them.

The guidance continues:

> … you must do your best to make sure that patients who may consult you about it are aware of your objection in advance. You can do this by making sure that any printed material about your practice and the services you provide explains if there are any services you will not normally provide because of a conscientious objection.

In 2007 the UK Royal College of Obstetricians and Gynaecologists (RCOG) also issued a statement recognizing the growing problem of doctors refusing to train in abortion care [7]. The RCOG stated it is:

> aware of the slow but growing problem of trainees opting out of training in the termination of pregnancy and is therefore concerned about the abortion service of the future … The RCOG recognises that it is an important right for any doctors to object to performing an abortion. The future of the sexual healthcare services requires careful workforce planning in order for abortion services to be available to the women who need it most.

Furthermore, the RCOG has recognized the reduction in numbers of doctors recruited into the specialty in recent years and has stated 'unless recruitment improves there will be insufficient obstetricians to deliver the … service'. Strickland also warned of the 'looming crisis in abortion services in the coming years' as a direct consequence of large numbers of new medical students exercising their right to conscientiously object to abortion [8].

Interestingly, a 2011 US survey of obstetricians and gynaecologists' (OB/GYNs) attitudes towards conscientious objection and their willingness to provide abortion found that it was the *context* in which a woman sought abortion which mattered to many OB/GYNs, regarding both their judgements about the morality of abortion and whether they would help a woman obtain abortion [9]. This suggests not only are they implementing their own moral frame of reference by (in effect) categorizing the request for abortion as 'valid and justifiable' against those which they consider to be less easily justified, but that this approach is paternalistic in the extreme (a situation also found in the UK). According to Coulter:

> Paternalism is endemic in the National Health Service. Benign and well intentioned it may be, but it has the effect of creating and maintaining an unhealthy dependency ... making decisions on behalf of patients without involving them and feeling threatened when patients have access to alternative sources of medical information – these signs of paternalism should have no place in modern health care. [10]

Savage and Francome reported on how judgementalism (masquerading as paternalism) was very much still apparent in reproductive healthcare [11]. They bemoaned the fact that they found that doctors often declined to perform abortions after 12 weeks' gestation for 'social' reasons. They illustrated how women still face judgemental paternalism when requesting an abortion:

> I have always provided a 'social' service up to 13 weeks gestation, but only undertaken TOP for abnormality thereafter. In addition I will often refuse if it is the third or fourth abortion and there is no evidence of contraceptive responsibility. [11]

Savage and Francome continued that it 'cannot be right' to adopt such a position mainly because an individual doctor's opinion is that the woman has 'been careless' with her contraception.

Unpopular work

Staff may find that they can feel isolated from their other medical and nursing colleagues because of their decision to work in abortion care. This is a phenomenon referred to in psychosocial and psychiatric circles as 'stigma by association' [12]. It is not unusual for staff to say they work in gynaecology services rather than face a barrage of questions about their role (or more worryingly hostility) from others who do not work in the field. Staff may sometimes perceive abortion care work as unpopular among other staff working in different areas of healthcare. Because of the perceived complexity of patient needs, abortion work may be seen as unappealing to some other healthcare providers. For some the perceived unpopularity of abortion care work may engender a sense of isolation from other colleagues. Often this sense of isolation is linked to a lack of colleagues working in abortion services with whom staff can discuss their work. As well as feeling isolated from non-abortion care staff they may also become increasingly aware of anti-abortion attitudes among the general public (or even others in the health service with whom they work). These feelings in providers are discussed further in Chapter 20.

A particular challenge in abortion care work relates to the transfer of necessary information to the women. When information is not communicated effectively, or absorbed and retained, abortion may be experienced as traumatic by women undergoing the procedure. Provision of adequate and appropriate information is one of the strongest predictors of satisfaction with abortion care. Providing adequate information in order to gain valid consent may be problematic for staff, for several reasons. First, as the findings of previous studies have indicated, women may not necessarily either understand information communicated to them by health professionals or retain information which is communicated to them. Indeed, one of the difficulties of providing information to women is the sensitive, and potentially distressing, nature of the information to be transmitted. For those staff with personal reservations about abortion, and who in coping with conflict between professional role and personal attitudes focus upon more clinical aspects of the work, providing sensitive information may be particularly problematic. Staff who experience conflict between their professional role and personal views may find this aspect of abortion care work the most challenging.

Judgementalism in abortion care

It is acknowledged that for some women their experiences of contact with abortion services have left them feeling dissatisfied. Research tends to point towards women's dissatisfactions arising from psychological and emotional aspects rather than their experiences of the technical and clinical aspects of abortion. In particular women's dissatisfaction has centred on health professionals' attitudes and demeanour, which were perceived by some to be judgemental [1]. Four decades ago the British Lane Report highlighted evidence of judgemental attitudes in healthcare staff who provided abortion care [13]. Even today, there is much rhetoric written about non-judgemental care and the subject raises strong emotions. Koh [14] for example claimed, 'non-judgemental care is not just some sentiment expressed by a group of politically correct nurses'. Here Koh argued that non-judgemental care was not about ignoring the differences in others but involved awareness of personal prejudices. While a non-judgemental attitude is considered to be a core condition of person-centred care, it has been argued, for reasons discussed above, that this principle is not always evident in practice associated with abortion [11].

Judgemental attitudes surrounding abortion are not confined to nursing staff. There is also evidence of negative staff attitudes in the wider National Health Service (NHS) organization and these reportedly have implications for service provision. Attitudinal factors have been shown to impact on abortion service provision. For example, in 2000, Marie Stopes International funded the largest study undertaken to date (since a previous National Opinion Poll in 1973) on the attitudes of over 700 British general practitioners (GPs) toward abortion in order to understand how attitudes might affect abortion care provision. The findings indicated that the GPs generally demonstrated more favourable, and largely positive, attitudes towards the 1967 abortion law than suggested by the previous National Opinion Poll. Since then, Marie Stopes International commissioned a further study in 2007 of GPs' attitudes [15]. Broadly this study found that although there was little change in the GPs' position on abortion since the 2000 findings, increased ambivalence towards abortion and/or desire to restrict women's access to free abortion services on the NHS was evident. Findings of the 2007 survey also indicated that, compared with the 2000 study, fewer GPs believed doctors should be required to declare their moral position on abortion.

Finnie *et al.* in a UK survey [16] also found that some women were relatively dissatisfied with their GPs and, in particular, the manner in which primary care staff (not identified by occupation group) treated them. Finnie observed that judgemental attitudes of nurses appeared to negatively influence the woman's experience during the delivery of care and judgemental attitudes from GPs affected access into the service. Bajos *et al.*'s study [17] suggested that problems of access to abortion are not only confined to lack of awareness on the woman's part, but are also attributable to GPs' own positions on abortion and their perception of the legitimacy of the woman's request for an abortion and this may present personal challenges when GPs are faced with a woman requesting abortion. There also may be times in health professionals' private lives when they find working in abortion services especially difficult, for example if they are a bereaved parent, have recently had a miscarriage/stillbirth, are undergoing IVF or are currently pregnant. Harris poignantly reflects upon her own circumstances at the time of her pregnancy whilst also continuing to perform abortions [18]. It may be worth staff acknowledging and reflecting upon how their personal attitudes to abortion differ according to their life circumstances at the time.

Specific challenges (1): advanced gestation/fetal remains

According to the literature, overall, most healthcare professionals who choose to work in abortion care support the rights of women to choose abortion. However, it appears that even for the most committed of staff there are certain aspects of abortion care provision which cause particular consternation. These issues have been reported as, firstly, abortion at advanced gestations which may relate to the concept of increasing fetal viability and the legal gestational limit and, secondly, more than one abortion (see next section). Staff choosing to work in these areas need to bear in mind that these are some of the issues they may have difficulty in coming to terms with despite their commitment to and support of a woman's right to choose. The introduction of medical abortion constitutes a significant change in the way women's health services are provided, in that the role of the nurse is now extended and may include the additional responsibility of providing abortion care in out-patient clinics and wards which are now chiefly nurse-led. Increasing provision of medical abortion means that nurses who were initially employed to provide general gynaecology nursing care find themselves in the situation of having to provide pre- and postabortion nursing care for women choosing medical abortion. Gallagher *et al.*'s study of nursing in abortion services found that staff were comfortable being involved in caring for women at earlier gestations but their support became more 'tenuous' when the gestation of the pregnancy was more advanced [19].

Indeed, some staff may not be completely prepared for seeing a formed fetus for the first time following an abortion procedure, and this experience may be a shock for them. Nurse and midwives may develop their own coping mechanisms when handling the fetus [20]. Likewise, some staff may feel that responsibilities such as checking the products of conception (or fetus), thus ensuring that the abortion procedure is complete, are distressing. The Royal College of Nursing has produced guidelines for the correct disposal of all fetal remains [21]. The guidelines note that disposal of fetal remains should be sensitive and respectful, irrespective of how the pregnancy was lost. However, the guidelines say absolutely nothing about the feelings and/or needs of the staff who are called upon to do this. The Institute of Cemetery and Crematorium Management (ICCM) defines fetal remains as 'a human fetus of less than 24 weeks gestation that has at no time since delivery shown any visible sign of life'. The ICCM also stipulates that the hospital is required to maintain a register for the disposal of fetal remains. This and all other documentation relating to the disposal of fetuses has to be kept for a minimum of 50 years by the hospital in order that parents wishing to trace the disposal of their fetus may do so in the future [22].

Specific challenges (2): more than one abortion

Chapter 21 provides a review of more than one abortion. Doctors and nurses are not removed from the social forces that create and reinforce negative stereotypes of individuals and they are not immune to feelings or to prejudice. However, in the clinical setting, staff caring for women who seek abortion should put aside any prejudices if they are to provide objective, sensitive and non-judgemental care, and this includes those women who present for more than one abortion. That said, requests for subsequent abortions might generate negative feelings in the staff (particularly if they consider the woman to be somewhat 'culpable'). Negative feelings may include anger at the woman's seeming 'irresponsibility', frustration at her contraceptive choice (as seen in the 2011 Savage and Francome study [11]) or poor contraceptive adherence (or lack of use of any contraception), and distress, confusion and resentment for 'wasting time' [23]. Staff who accept abortion as a woman's right need to be cognizant that the nature of that right does not alter despite the number of times it has been exercised.

Conclusions

In jurisdictions in which the law does not permit abortion on request, clinicians' attitudes may have the potential for considerable influence over a woman's request for abortion. Harris and colleagues [9] commented that it often appears as if there are only two categories of healthcare providers: (1) those who support abortion and therefore assist women seeking abortion or (2) those who oppose abortion and do not provide abortion. These authors make the point that two other categories of abortion provider may coexist: (3) those who oppose abortion in general but still find it *acceptable* sometimes and (4) those who support abortion in general but still find it *unacceptable* sometimes. This concept is something worth debating, as not many health professionals work entirely within the boundaries of any of the four proposed categories. Which leaves the contentious issue of at what point does abortion become unacceptable to those who support abortion; or, acceptable to those who oppose it? Readers are reminded that abortion cannot be provided on a continuum based on personal ideologies of when a health professional judges it becomes more or less acceptable. It is not a case of personal decisions being made about 'granting' a woman her third, fourth or fifth abortion [11]; furthermore, it is not the function of individuals to exercise their judgement however many times a woman exercises her right to abortion at whatever stage of gestation. Nevertheless, it appears that for women, agreement to an abortion may depend more on the clinician she 'happens to see' rather than on an objective assessment of need.

Evidence suggests that for women the care related to the psychological and emotional aspects of their abortion experience is just as important in their evaluations of services as the clinical procedures. It is therefore vital that staff are encouraged and facilitated to address a range of dimensions relating to women's experiences of abortion. Supporting staff and encouraging doctors, nurses and other healthcare professionals to view abortion care as a rewarding specialty in which to work requires cohesive management, collaboration and proactive support from all senior staff. This may be encouraged among staff, through a system of staff peer support groups, clinical supervision, mentoring schemes for new staff and 'buddy' systems. Often regular staff meetings facilitate far more than updating staff on the latest clinical developments in the field; they also provide a safe place for sharing feelings, networking with like-minded staff and discussing the joys (and occasionally burdens) of working in abortion care.

References

1. Astbury-Ward E. Emotional and psychological impact of abortion: a critique of the literature. *J Fam Plann Reprod Health Care* 2009;34:181–4.

2. Marshall S, Gould D, Roberts J. Nurses' attitudes towards termination of pregnancy. *Journal of Advanced Nursing* 1994;20:567–76.

3. Astbury-Ward E, Parry O, Carnwell R. Stigma, abortion and disclosure – findings

from a qualitative study. *Journal of Sexual Medicine* 2012;9:3137–47.

4. Nursing and Midwifery Council. *The Code*, 2008; p. 5.

5. Nursing and Midwifery Council, Regulation in Practice, Conscientious Objection by nurses and midwives, 2013; www.nmc-uk.org/Nurses-and-midwives/Regulation-in-practice/Regulation-in-Practice-Topics/Conscientious-objection-by-nurses-and-midwives-/ (accessed 23 October 2013).

6. General Medical Council. *Personal Beliefs and Medical Practice* 2013: 1–7.

7. www.rcog.org.uk/what-we-do/campaigning-and-opinions/statement/rcog-statement-article-abortion-crisis-doctors-refuse- (accessed 31 May 2013).

8. Strickland S. Conscientious objection in medical students: a questionnaire survey. *Journal of Medical Ethics* 2012:38:22–5.

9. Harris L, Cooper A, Rasinski K, Curlin F, Drapkin-Lyerly A. Obstetrician-gynecologists' objections to and willingness to help patients obtain an abortion. *Obstetrics and Gynecology* 2011;118:905–12.

10. Coulter A. Paternalism or partnership? Patients have grown up and there's no going back. *BMJ* 1999;18:719–20.

11. Savage W, Francome C. British gynaecologists' attitudes in 2008 to the provision of legal abortion. *Journal of Obstetrics and Gynaecology* 2011;31:322–6.

12. Goldstein SB, Johnson VA. Stigma by association: perceptions of the dating partners of college students with physical disabilities. *Basic and Applied Social Psychology* 1997;19:495–504.

13. Lane J. *Report of the Committee on the Working of the Abortion Act*. Command 5579, paragraphs 500–509. London: Her Majesty's Stationery Office, 1974.

14. Koh A. Non-judgemental care as a professional obligation. *Nursing Standard* 1999;13:38–41.

15. Marie Stopes International, *General Practitioners: Attitudes to Abortion*. London: Marie Stopes International, 2007: 1.

16. Finnie S, Foy R, Mather J. The pathway to induced abortion: women's experiences and general practitioner attitudes. *J Fam Plann Reprod Health Care* 2006;32:15–18.

17. Bajos N, Moreau C, Ferrand M, Bouyer J. Access to health care for an induced abortion: qualitative and quantitative approaches. *Revue d'Épidémiologie et de Santé Publique* 2003;51:631–47.

18. Harris L. Second trimester abortion provision: breaking the silence and changing the discourse. *Reproductive Health Matters* 2008;16(31 supplement):74–81.

19. Gallagher K, Porock D, Edgeley A. The concept of 'nursing' in the abortion services. *Journal of Advanced Nursing* 2010;66:849–57.

20. Andersson I-M, Gemzell-Danielsson K, Christensson K. Caring for women undergoing second trimester medical termination of pregnancy. *Contraception* 2014;89:460–5.

21. Royal College of Nursing. *Sensitive Disposal of All Fetal Remains*. London: Royal College of Nursing, 2007.

22. Institute of Cemetery and Crematorium Management. *The Sensitive Disposal of Fetal Remains: Policy and Guidance for Burial and Cremation Authorities and Companies*. London: ICCM National Office, 2011. www.iccm-uk.com/iccm/library/FetalRemainsPolicyAug2011FINAL.pdf (accessed 4 March 2014).

23. Astbury-Ward, E. A reflective account of a consultation in abortion care. *Nursing Standard* 2009;23:35–9.

Chapter

24

Mid-level providers

Kristina Gemzell-Danielsson and Helena Kopp Kallner

Task shifting/sharing

Induced abortion is one of the most frequent interventions in medicine and also one of the main contributors to maternal mortality and morbidity. Nearly half of the abortions in the world are unsafe and 98% of unsafe abortions occur in the developing world where a shortage of physicians is common [1]. It is estimated that 13% of maternal mortality in the world, which amounts to approximately 47,000 women annually, is due to complications from induced abortions [2]. Any improvement in the treatment of abortion therefore has great impact on women's reproductive health, especially in developing countries.

Task shifting is defined as a process of delegating tasks, where/when appropriate, to less specialized healthcare providers and has been shown to increase productivity within health-care systems. Studies from an African setting show that training less specialized healthcare providers to perform tasks traditionally reserved for physicians, such as caesarean sections, can contribute to the building of sustainable, cost-effective and equitable healthcare serv-ices [3,4]. A shortage of human resources in the healthcare system is common in low-resource countries, especially in remote areas where maternal mortality is high. A task shift to nurses, midwives and other non-physician clinicians (so-called mid-level provid-ers) in providing women's healthcare is key to achieving Millennium Development Goal 5. It improves access by increasing the number of available providers and lowers cost, both of which are benefits especially in low-resource countries [5]. The World Health Organization (WHO) recommends task shifting in order to optimize the roles of healthcare workers [6] (see www.optimizemnh.org).

In many countries the provision of abortion is limited to medical practitioners or even gynaecologists according to national law. However, where allowed, a task shift to mid-level provision of induced abortion has been reported from many countries in mostly low-resource settings [7]. Furthermore, a task shift in providing treatment of incomplete abor-tion will increase women's access to postabortion care (PAC) [8] including postabortion contraception, a key activity in efforts to decrease maternal mortality. Focusing on health-care providers' skills and competence and how their capacity can be used in a cost-effective and evidence-based manner is thought to promote scientific and professional skills of pro-viders involved at all levels in the healthcare system.

Legal restrictions frequently subject women to unsafe abortions. In high-resource set-tings where abortion law has been liberalized it is generally a safe procedure. However, access to abortion may be limited by difficulties in finding a physician who is willing to perform

Abortion Care, ed. Sam Rowlands. Published by Cambridge University Press. © Cambridge University Press 2014.

the procedure. This could result in long waiting periods and delayed treatment especially in rural or remote areas.

Therefore, task shifting in women's healthcare should not be limited to low-resource settings. In some countries, such as Sweden, nurse-midwives monitor all normal pregnancies and are responsible for all vaginal deliveries in healthy women. They also deliver two thirds of all contraceptive advice and provision to healthy women and insert and remove intrauterine contraception and contraceptive implants. Nurse-midwives are therefore ideally placed to deliver abortion services.

Task sharing in abortion care involving both physicians and mid-level providers could potentially improve access to high standard care including contraceptive advice and supplies by reducing waiting times, demedicalizing services and increasing cost-effectiveness.

Legal restrictions to task shifting/sharing

Many European countries have abortion laws that date back to the 1970s. At that time the recommended technique for first trimester abortion was vacuum aspiration. To protect women from unsafe procedures by unskilled providers the laws frequently state that abortion should be performed in a hospital by a physician or even a gynaecologist. The combined regimen of mifepristone followed by a prostaglandin analogue is a Swedish invention from the mid-1980s [9]. In collaboration with WHO, the combined regimen has been developed into a safe and effective method for induced abortion. The development of medical abortion has also facilitated the involvement of mid-level providers in abortion care. Frequently information, support, administration of the drugs, pain management and care is provided by nurses or midwives. However, the physical examination, prescription of the drugs and the medical responsibility still rests with physicians.

Since the process of a medical abortion is similar to a miscarriage with a sometimes prolonged expulsion, and is very different from that of a surgical procedure, the legal requirement to perform the abortion in a hospital/clinic has become unnecessary. Some countries have therefore defined the medical abortion to legally occur when the woman swallows the mifepristone. This may not be the time of the actual expulsion or the medical definition of abortion but defines the woman's commitment to have the abortion. This allows administration of the prostaglandin analogue, misoprostol, and completion of the abortion to occur outside a clinical setting. Often the woman is given a telephone number to call if she has questions or needs advice. Most often a trained mid-level provider gives advice and answers questions. This so-called 'home abortion' or 'home administration' of misoprostol has become increasingly popular, where allowed. It increases women's choice and flexibility in abortion care. However, in some countries, including the UK, the legal interpretation of when the medical abortion occurs is different and home administration of misoprostol is still not permitted by law. In many countries where the abortion is defined as taking place at misoprostol administration the women are sent home from the clinic immediately after misoprostol administration and then have the expulsion at home. For the women this still means one extra visit to the clinic which is needed to receive the misoprostol.

Training of mid-level providers in abortion care

Many different training programmes have been designed for mid-level providers in abortion care. The nature of these depends on the degree of back-up by physicians in the unit and on the tasks the mid-level provider performs. The training must also be adjusted according to the pre-existing knowledge of the mid-level providers. Mid-level providers have varying backgrounds: they may be nurses, nurse-midwives, midwives, physician assistants or have a training completely separate from any of these. The training for abortion provision should include a theoretical module providing knowledge on the current abortion law and clinical guidelines as well as practical experience.

In many countries midwives may not necessarily be trained as nurses. They are trained to assist women in labour and delivery. They are also not trained to assist during termination of pregnancy. The 'Essential Competencies for Basic Midwifery Practices 2010' and the new International Confederation of Midwives (ICM) model for the midwifery curriculum, also include abortion care and contraception services [10,11]. However, healthcare providers in general and nurses and midwives in particular need emotional and technical training in comprehensive abortion care.

To perform a consultation for an abortion the mid-level provider should be able to perform an adequate examination and screening for genital infection. The mid-level provider should also be able to identify which women should have a consultation with a physician in the event of pre-existing conditions, allergies or pathological pregnancies or other possible issues. Women should be able to receive adequate advice and information about the available procedures.

In order to provide surgical abortion mid-level providers may need training in the options for and provision of analgesia such as intravenous sedation or paracervical block. Pre-treatment of the cervix with misoprostol before surgical abortion should be a prerequisite in order to reduce rates of immediate complications [12]. The actual training for vacuum aspiration can be done on live patients or on training models which may be advanced such as manikins or rudimentary, but adequate, such as watermelons or papayas. Vacuum aspiration may be performed manually (MVA) or electrically (EVA) – see Chapter 8. It may be beneficial to learn to assess the abortion material for the presence of products of conception.

Medical abortion (Chapter 7) is different in that no practical surgical skills are necessary for the mid-level provider. Rather, the mid-level provider needs experience in the natural course of a medical abortion and again it may be beneficial to be able to identify the presence of products of conception in the aborted material. Management of pain and provision of reassurance to the women undergoing medical abortion are important.

Experiences of mid-level provision of surgical abortion

Surgical abortion in the first trimester is generally a safe procedure with complication rates ranging from 0 to 5% depending on setting, type of analgesia and provider (see Chapter 8). In countries where abortion services may be provided by healthcare staff other than doctors, surgical abortion can be safely provided by mid-level providers with proper training. Surgical abortion provided by mid-level providers has been shown to be safe using either MVA or EVA. It has been evaluated using paracervical block, oral anaesthesia and intravenous sedation for pain relief [13,14].

Complications from surgical abortion may occur immediately in the form of cervical laceration, uterine perforation or bleeding (Chapter 14). These complications may be reduced by pre-treatment of the cervix with misoprostol or, although less effective, osmotic dilators [12]. Although pre-treatment of the cervix should always be performed, this is particularly important in the case of mid-level providers who may have problems handling the complications which may otherwise arise. In addition to immediate complications, there may be later complications such as delayed bleeding or infections due to retained products of conception or undiscovered perforations. Any study investigating the safety of mid-level provision in surgical abortion needs to evaluate both immediate and delayed complications.

Studies from the USA have shown that physician assistants can safely perform surgical abortions [15–17]. In a prospective, observational study from California evaluating the outcomes of 11,487 early aspiration abortions completed by physicians (n = 5,812) and newly-trained mid-level providers (nurse practitioners, nurse midwives and physician assistants) abortion complications were clinically equivalent between newly-trained mid-level providers and physicians [17]. However, these studies were not randomized. A large randomized multicentre equivalence trial aimed at evaluating the safety of mid-level provision of surgical abortion up to 12 weeks' gestation was performed in South Africa and Vietnam [12]. The trial was able to show that the difference in rates of complications between these specially-trained mid-level providers and physicians was well within the pre-set margin of equivalence of 4.5%. The rate of complications was low in both provider groups with overall complication rates as low as 0–1.4%. There was no difference in serious complications between the groups in any of the studies above.

Experiences of mid-level provision of medical abortion

Despite the fact that midwives and some nurses may already possess the required clinical skills to perform first trimester medical abortion or treatment of an incomplete abortion (spontaneous or induced), they are most commonly not permitted and/or formally trained to do so. Physical and pelvic examination, and when and where required ultrasound scanning, before an abortion is traditionally performed by a physician. Interestingly, several studies on attitudes, experiences and perceptions of mid-level providers involved with abortion care in Asia and Africa reveal that menstrual regulation (a procedure that uses MVA to safely establish non-pregnancy after a missed period) and medical abortion were frequently more accepted by them than MVA [18,19].

In a study from Nepal, including approximately 1,200 women, it was shown that the provision of medical abortion at up to nine weeks' gestation by mid-level providers and doctors was similar in safety and effectiveness [20]. Following training, mid-level providers could conduct safe, low-technology medical abortion services for women.

An important limitation of the above study is that randomization was undertaken after bimanual pelvic examination to estimate uterine size. Thus, the women were already partly examined before the randomization. Furthermore, in most high-resource settings, ultrasound dating of the pregnancy is part of the protocol and performed by a physician. Examination by a physician and support, treatment and care provided by a nurse or midwife is already standard practice in many European settings. Thus, the data from Nepal are not sufficient to show whether mid-level providers could independently provide medical abortion in a high-resource setting where ultrasound dating of pregnancy is part of the protocol. Another possible limitation of the study is that home administration of misoprostol was not allowed and all women were kept under observation in the clinic to monitor passage of the pregnancy.

Recently the Board of Health and Welfare in Sweden has stressed the need to increase the involvement of midwives in medical abortion. A randomized controlled study including more than 1,000 women has been performed to assess the feasibility and acceptability of medical abortion up to and including 63 days' gestation provided by either midwife or gynaecologist when used in clinical practice [21]. Healthy women were randomized to counselling and treatment by either a nurse-midwife or a gynaecologist. Importantly, women were self-referred and those who chose medical abortion and were estimated according to menstrual data to be eligible were randomized before any part of the consultation had been performed and without any prior examination.

The study showed that mid-level provision of medical abortion was as effective as that provided by physicians. Complication rates were low and did not differ between the groups. No significant differences were seen between the groups in the satisfaction with information about the abortion, contraceptive advice or feeling calm and safe before, during or after the abortion. Furthermore, there were no significant differences in perceived bleeding or pain between the two groups nor in the experience of the procedure as compared to that expected. Nurse-midwives consulted a physician in approximately 25% of cases for prescriptions, ultrasound queries or medical issues. However, the frequency of consultations by nurse-midwives for ultrasound queries went down as the study progressed, indicating a learning curve. Interestingly, more women randomized to care by a nurse-midwife chose to administer misoprostol in the clinic while home-use was more frequent in the group of women assigned to a physician.

Although a majority of women were indifferent as to whether the provider was a nurse-midwife or a physician, women who expressed a preference chose nurse-midwives to a larger extent in both groups. A possible explanation for this result may be the role of nurse-midwives in Sweden, where they oversee all medical abortions in healthy women and all uncomplicated vaginal deliveries. They prescribe contraception and insert intrauterine and implant contraception in all maternity clinics and youth clinics. Women have a high confidence in their professional capability.

The results of the study can be generalized to both low- and high-resource settings since ultrasound dating of the pregnancy was part of the protocol to confirm gestation. While it is well known that ultrasound dating is not necessary as a routine for medical abortion it is required by many local guidelines especially in high-resource settings.

Experiences of postabortion care

Emergency treatment of complications from unsafe abortion as well as from spontaneous abortion (postabortion care, PAC) is identified as an effective intervention to decrease maternal mortality globally [22,23]. Misoprostol has been shown to be effective in the treatment of incomplete abortion. Recently a Cochrane review studied medical treatments for incomplete miscarriage. There was a small but significant difference in effectiveness between medical treatment and the conventional surgical intervention with MVA for treatment of incomplete abortion [24]. International studies have revealed that trained mid-level providers are competent to conduct surgical treatment of incomplete abortion safely [25]. Ongoing programmes and studies are focusing on training and implementation of mid-level provision of misoprostol for treatment of incomplete abortion.

Provision of postabortion contraception to help women avoid another unwanted pregnancy is also a critical part of abortion care. Long-acting reversible contraceptives (LARCs) have been shown to decrease the rate of subsequent pregnancy and abortion [26–29] (see Chapter 13). In a Swedish study women treated by a nurse-midwife were significantly more likely to choose a LARC method postabortion compared to those who had been seen by a gynaecologist [21].

The future – teamwork and task sharing

Mid-level provision of medical abortion is being implemented in the developing world as well as in high-resource countries. It can be argued that one could accept a higher rate of complications with mid-level providers as mid-level provision benefits women in general by increasing access to safe abortion and by lowering cost. However, a higher rate of complications can only be accepted for mild complications; death or other serious complications must remain low. So far, no study has shown an increased risk of serious complications for mid-level provision of abortion services. It can therefore be considered safe.

The important role of mid-level providers in implementation of safe abortion services can be learned from experiences in Nepal. Training of mid-level providers has been identified as one of the factors that contributed to rapid, successful implementation of legal abortion in Nepal after liberalization of the restrictive abortion law in 2002 led by Nepal's Ministry of Health and Population [30]. Factors of importance in this successful model of scaling up safe legal abortion include the pre-existence of PAC services through which healthcare providers were already familiar with the main clinical technique for safe abortion, and embracing medical abortion and authorization of mid-level providers as key strategies for decentralizing care. Integration of abortion care into existing Safe Motherhood initiatives and the broader health system was essential for information about the new law to spread. Nepal's experience in making high-quality abortion care widely accessible in a short period of time offers important lessons for other countries seeking to reduce maternal mortality and morbidity from unsafe abortion and to achieve Millennium Development Goal 5.

Lack of clinicians willing to perform abortions in the USA has been attributed to the imbalance between incentives and disincentives. The single most powerful incentive has been reported to be altruism. On the other hand, disincentives include stigma, poor pay, frequent harassment, low prestige, suboptimal working conditions and tedium. Among the remedies suggested are increasing the integration of abortion training into mainstream residency education, improving the pay and work environments for clinicians and, where feasible, expanding the capacity of physician providers by task sharing with mid-level practitioners [31].

The demonstration that physician assistants and other mid-level providers can perform the entire surgical as well as medical abortion from examination including ultrasound to the actual performance of the abortion certainly opens up new possibilities in low- as well as high-resource countries. Having a physician present on site may be a prerequisite for adequate and prompt care and prevents women from having to make several visits if they need a physician consultation. However, the number of physicians in an abortion care facility may be limited. The future may consist of having larger abortion care facilities where mid-level providers perform the care and the physician merely remains as a consultant for pathological pregnancies or in the event of complications. Such care facilities should increase access to abortion services and still maintain the highest standard of care in low- as well as high-resource settings.

In addition it has been shown in Sweden that nurse-midwife provision of medical abortion with ultrasound as part of the examination process is highly acceptable to women. In South Africa and Vietnam women also find mid-level provision of surgical abortion highly acceptable. Thus, in addition to providing the highest standard of care, mid-level provision of abortion services is highly acceptable.

In the light of incentives and disincentives mid-level provision of abortion services may be the most effective way of increasing access to abortion services at a global level. Nurse or midwife provision of medical abortion can increase access to medical and surgical abortion where the number of physicians is limited. In countries where conscientious objection (see Chapter 20) to participation in abortion services by physicians denies women access to abortion services, increasing the number of possible providers may be the best solution to maintain the legal right to an abortion. The issue of legality is often raised in countries where abortions must be performed by registered doctors. In practice this issue can often be solved by mid-level providers acting on delegation from a physician as is the case in Sweden.

Acknowledgement

We are grateful to Monica Johansson, RNM and Eneli Salomonsson, RNM for their review of the manuscript.

References

1. Sedgh G, Singh S, Shah IH, Åhman E, Henshaw SK, Bankole A. Induced abortion: incidence and trends worldwide from 1995 to 2008. *Lancet* 2012;379:625–32.

2. WHO. *Unsafe Abortion: Global and Regional Estimates of the Incidence of Unsafe Abortion and Associated Mortality in 2008*, 6th edn. Geneva: World Health Organization, 2011.

3. Gessessew A, Barnabas GA, Prata N, Weidert K. Task shifting and sharing in Tigray, Ethiopia, to achieve comprehensive emergency obstetric care. *Int J Gynecol Obstet* 2011;113:28–31.

4. Pereira C, Bugalho A, Bergstrom S, Vaz F, Cotiro M. A comparative study of caesarean deliveries by assistant medical officers and obstetricians in Mozambique. *Br J Obstet Gynaecol* 1996;103:508–12.

5. Fulton BD, Scheffler RM, Sparkes SP, Auh EY, Vujicic M, Soucat A. Health workforce skill mix and task shifting in low income countries: a review of recent evidence. *Hum Resour Health* 2011;9:1.

6. WHO. *WHO recommendations: optimizing health worker roles to improve access to key maternal and newborn health interventions through task shifting.* Geneva: World Health Organization, 2012.

7. Yarnall J, Swica Y, Winikoff B. Non-physician clinicians can safely provide first trimester medical abortion. *Reprod Health Matters* 2009;17:61–9.

8. Fetters T, Tesfaye S, Clark KA. An assessment of postabortion care in three regions in Ethiopia, 2000 to 2004. *Int J Gynecol Obstet* 2008;101:100–6.

9. Fiala C, Gemzell-Danielsson K. Review of medical abortion using mifepristone in combination with a prostaglandin analogue. *Contraception* 2006;74: 66–86.

10. International Confederation of Midwives. Essential Competencies for Basic Midwifery Practice. 2010. www.internationalmidwives.org/ Portals/5/2011/DB%202011/Essential%20 Competencies%20ENG.pdf 2013 (accessed 1 February 2013).

11. International Confederation of Midwives. Model Midwifery Curriculum Outlines. www.internationalmidwives. org/Whatwedo/Policyandpractice/ ICMGlobalStandardsCompetencies andTools/ModelCurriculum Outlines/tabid/1116/Default.aspx (accessed 1 February 2013).

12. Warriner IK, Meirik O, Hoffman M, *et al.* Rates of complication in first-trimester manual vacuum aspiration abortion done by doctors and mid-level providers in South Africa and Vietnam: a randomised controlled equivalence trial. *Lancet* 2006;368:1965–72.

13. Ngo TD, Park MH, Free C. Safety and effectiveness of termination services

performed by doctors versus midlevel providers: a systematic review and analysis. *International Journal of Women's Health* 2013;5:9–17.

14. Renner RM, Brahmi D, Kapp N. Who can provide effective and safe termination of pregnancy care? A systematic review. *BJOG* 2013;120:23–31.

15. Freedman MA, Jillson DA, Coffin RR, Novick LF. Comparison of complication rates in first trimester abortions performed by physician assistants and physicians. *Am J Public Health* 1986;76:550–4.

16. Goldman MB, Occhiuto JS, Peterson LE, Zapka JG, Palmer RH. Physician assistants as providers of surgically induced abortion services. *Am J Public Health* 2004;94:1352–7.

17. Weitz TA, Taylor D, Desai S, *et al.* Safety of aspiration abortion performed by nurse practitioners, certified nurse midwives, and physician assistants under a California legal waiver. *Am J Public Health* 2013;103:454–61.

18. Cooper D, Dickson K, Blanchard K, *et al.* Medical abortion: the possibilities for introduction in the public sector in South Africa. *Reprod Health Matters* 2005;13:35–43.

19. Djohan E, Indrawasih R, Adenan M, *et al.* The attitudes of health providers towards abortion in Indonesia. *Reprod Health Matters* 1993;1:32–40.

20. Warriner IK, Wang D, My Huong NT, *et al.* Can midlevel health-care providers administer early medical abortion as safely and effectively as doctors? A randomised controlled equivalence trial in Nepal. *Lancet* 2011;377:1155–61.

21. Kopp Kallner H, Gomperts R, Salomonsson E, Johansson M, Marions L, Gemzell-Danielsson K. The efficacy, safety and acceptability of medical termination of pregnancy provided by standard care by physicians or by nurse-midwives – a randomized controlled equivalence trial. *BJOG* (in press).

22. Rasch V. Unsafe abortion and postabortion care – an overview. *Acta Obstet Gynecol Scand* 2011;90:692–700.

23. Faúndes A. Unsafe abortion – the current global scenario. *Best Pract Res Clin Obstet Gynaecol* 2010;24:467–77.

24. Neilson JP, Gyte GM, Hickey M, Vazquez JC, Dou L. Medical treatments for incomplete miscarriage. *Cochrane Database Syst Rev* 2013;3:CD007223.

25. Berer M. Provision of abortion by mid-level providers: international policy, practice and perspectives. *Bull World Health Organ* 2009;87:58–63.

26. Rose SB, Lawton BA. Impact of long-acting reversible contraception on return for repeat abortion. *Am J Obstet Gynecol* 2012;206:37.e31–6.

27. Winner B, Peipert JF, Zhao Q, *et al.* Effectiveness of long-acting reversible contraception. *N Engl J Med* 2012;366:1998–2007.

28. Cameron ST, Glasier A, Chen ZE, Johnstone A, Dunlop C, Heller R. Effect of contraception provided at termination of pregnancy and incidence of subsequent termination of pregnancy. *BJOG* 2012;119:1074–80.

29. Ames CM, Norman WV. Preventing repeat abortion in Canada: is the immediate insertion of intrauterine devices postabortion a cost-effective option associated with fewer repeat abortions? *Contraception* 2012;85: 51–5.

30. Samandari G, Wolf M, Basnett I, Hyman A, Andersen K. Implementation of legal abortion in Nepal: a model for rapid scale-up of high-quality care. *Reprod Health* 2012;9:7.

31. Grimes DA. Clinicians who provide abortions: the thinning ranks. *Obstet Gynecol* 1992;80:719–23.

Chapter 25

Telemedicine

Ellen Wiebe and Daniel Grossman

Introduction

Telemedicine involves the use of telecommunication and information technologies to provide a healthcare service at a distance. Telemedicine has been used for a variety of applications in almost every field of medicine, including providing consultation services by specialist physicians and providing care directly to patients [1–3]. The use of technology can improve access to medical services in both rural and urban environments where specialist care may be limited. In the area of reproductive health, telemedicine services have been used to provide hormonal contraception online to women who undergo medical screening via a website [4].

In recent years, telemedicine has also been extended to the provision of medical abortion. As the medical abortion procedure comprises mainly providing information and screening for eligibility and because confirmation of abortion completion may be determined using a variety of modalities, this service is particularly appropriate for telemedicine. Furthermore, telemedicine provision of medical abortion has the potential to greatly improve access to safe, early abortion in areas with limited access. This chapter reviews the different models of telemedicine abortion provision and the evidence in support of this innovative model of care.

Models of telemedicine abortion provision

There are four possible models when providing telemedicine abortions.

1. *Clinic-to-clinic* (Figure 25.1).
   This model has been used in several settings in the USA to extend the reach of physicians to be able to provide medical abortion, especially in states where non-physician clinicians such as certified nurse-midwives, physician assistants or nurse practitioners are prohibited from providing the service. The model developed by Planned Parenthood of the Heartland in Iowa has been extensively evaluated [5–7]. In this model, a woman presents to an outlying Planned Parenthood clinic that does not have a physician on site. A trained member of staff at the outlying clinic takes a medical history and performs an ultrasound scan, which is then uploaded to a secure server. The staff member also provides information about medical abortion, makes certain that the woman is sure of her decision to terminate, and obtains consent. The physician located at another clinic then reviews the medical history and ultrasound images remotely.

Abortion Care, ed. Sam Rowlands. Published by Cambridge University Press. © Cambridge University Press 2014.

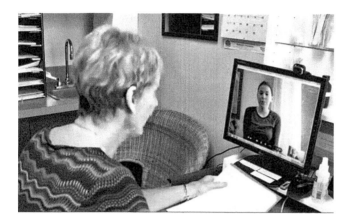

Figure 25.1 Model 1: clinic-to-clinic with video. Courtesy of Dr Ellen Wiebe.

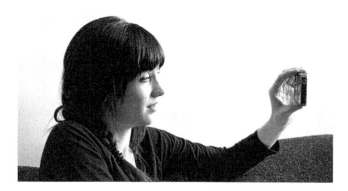

Figure 25.2 Model 2: clinician-to-woman with video. Courtesy of Dr Ellen Wiebe.

After this, the physician has a video conference with the woman using an encrypted internet connection, reviews all the information with her and determines if medical abortion is appropriate. In Iowa, Planned Parenthood used a telepharmacy system that allows a physician to enter a code to open a locked drawer in the remote clinic that has been preloaded with individual doses of mifepristone and misoprostol. In other settings, the medication is set out in front of the woman, and the physician instructs her to pick up the mifepristone and show it on video to confirm it is the correct drug. The physician then watches her take the mifepristone, reviews her final instructions and answers any questions. The woman returns for a follow-up visit one to two weeks later, and the physician is available for a remote consultation if necessary. If a surgical abortion is necessary, the woman is referred to a centre that is staffed by a physician or to a nearby emergency department in the rare case of an urgent need for aspiration or management of another complication.

2. *Clinic to woman at home* (Figure 25.2).

This model is used by a free-standing urban abortion clinic in Vancouver, Canada [8]. The clinic provides medical and surgical abortions in person and also uses video-conferencing for women who cannot easily travel to the clinic. Since mifepristone is not registered in Canada, medical abortions are provided with methotrexate and misopros-tol. To be eligible, the women must live in British Columbia (where the physicians are licensed), have access to a laboratory for timely serum hCG estimations and be able to

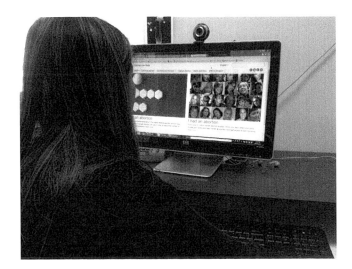

Figure 25.3 Model 3: clinician-to-woman with email. Courtesy of Dr Ellen Wiebe.

travel to the clinic or to another community for surgical completion, if necessary. They see a physician and counsellor by Skype video-conferencing for eligibility screening, information and consent. They go to a local laboratory for a baseline hCG test, then have repeat hCG tests on the day of the medication and one week later. If the initial hCG is greater than 5,000 mIU/mL, an ultrasound is booked at a local facility. The medicines are couriered or a prescription is faxed to a local pharmacy. In a follow-up visit by Skype, a physician discusses the woman's reaction to the medication and her blood test results. If the hCG level has fallen by 80% in one week, she is told that the abortion is complete, and she needs no further follow-up. If she needs more medication, surgery or further blood tests, these are arranged.

3. *Internet and email* (Figure 25.3).

   The online non-profit project Women on Web was set up in 2006 with the aim of increasing access to safe abortions [9–11]. The website (www.womenonweb.org) refers women to a doctor online who can provide them with a medical abortion using the combined regimen of mifepristone and misoprostol, provided they fill in the online consultation form and meet the specified eligibility criteria. Women who reside in countries without access to safe abortion, are up to nine weeks' pregnant, wish to terminate their pregnancy and have no contraindications receive the medication and a pregnancy test by mail or courier. Women are advised to have an ultrasound examination before treatment to determine gestational length. Three weeks following treatment, women are advised to do a urine pregnancy test, have an ultrasound examination performed or visit a doctor to confirm that the abortion is complete. In over 4,000 cases, the follow-up rate was 50–60%; 0.9% reported a continuing pregnancy (failure) and 12.3% reported a surgical aspiration.

4. *Internet website only*.

   In 2002, Ibis Reproductive Health and the Office of Population Research at Princeton University jointly developed a multilingual website dedicated to information about medical abortion: www.medicationabortion.com [12]. In a period of 12 months during 2004–5, the site received more than 78,000 visits and nearly 240,000 page requests in four languages. About one third of the Spanish language site visits included the misoprostol-only regimen, indicating that women in Latin American countries, where abortion is restricted and self-induced abortions using misoprostol are common, may be using this site to get the information they require. Other websites with accurate information on medical abortion are also available online, including www.womenon-web.com and www.medicalabortionconsortium.org.

Evaluation of telemedicine programmes

The use of information technology can certainly improve access to accurate information about medical abortion, but the real opportunity with telemedicine is to make services available to women who might otherwise face obstacles. In addition to understanding how telemedicine may improve access, it is important to know if medical abortion can be safely provided in this way without reducing effectiveness of the regimen. Information about acceptability is also crucial to knowing whether it will be used when scaled up. Similarly, it is important to know whether the model is feasible to offer and whether it might be cost saving.

The clinic-to-clinic programme in Iowa has been evaluated in several ways. Researchers performed a cohort study that recruited 223 women undergoing telemedicine medical abortion and compared them to a similar number of women undergoing medical abortion with an in-person consultation with a physician [5]. Among women who had a telemedicine consultation, 98.7% had a complete abortion without need for surgery, compared to 96.9% of women who had an in-person consultation with a physician. In multivariable analysis, the odds of having a successful abortion with telemedicine compared to an in-person consultation were not statistically different (odds ratio (OR) 2.34, 95% confidence interval (CI) 0.84–6.55).

In order to assess the safety of the Iowa programme, researchers analysed all of the adverse events associated with the medical abortion service over a 16-month period and compared the incidence between women receiving telemedicine and those with an in-person consultation [5]. Planned Parenthood is required to report certain adverse events to Danco Laboratories, the manufacturer of the mifepristone product used, including: continuing pregnancy, emergency room treatment, hospitalization, blood transfusion, unrecognized ectopic pregnancy, allergic reaction, infection requiring intravenous treatment and death. During this period, 1,172 women underwent a telemedicine abortion and 2,384 had a medical abortion with an in-person consultation. No deaths were reported during this period. The overall incidence of adverse events was 1.3% (95% CI 0.8–2.1%) for telemedicine and 1.3% (95% CI 0.9–1.8%) for in-person consultations. In multivariable analysis, the odds of having an adverse event among telemedicine compared to in-person subjects was not significantly different (OR 0.96, 95% CI 0.48–1.91).

Acceptability and satisfaction with the service were also assessed as part of the cohort study in Iowa [5]. Overall, satisfaction was high in both groups, with 94% of telemedicine subjects and 88% of in-person subjects reporting being very satisfied with the service. Telemedicine subjects were significantly more likely to report that they would recommend the service to a friend in a similar situation (OR 1.72, 95% CI 1.26–2.34). This higher level of satisfaction among telemedicine subjects was likely because they were able to obtain the abortion sooner or closer to home. However, 25% of telemedicine subjects reported that they would have preferred to be in the same room with the physician, and younger women (aged 18–25) and those without children or with less education (12 years or less) were significantly more likely to report this. In both this study and a follow-up qualitative study, it seemed that this was a relative preference [7]. In an ideal world, they would have liked to be in the room with the physician, but they were willing to compromise in order to obtain the abortion where and when they did.

The Planned Parenthood service delivery statistics in Iowa were also analysed to explore how they changed after telemedicine was introduced [6]. During the two years prior to launching the telemedicine programme, 46% of all abortions were medical; this increased to 54% in the two years after the launch. Interestingly, during this same period there was also a small but significant reduction in the proportion of abortions performed after 13 weeks' gestation from 3.9% to 3.5%. In multivariable analysis, women were significantly more likely to obtain a medical abortion (OR 1.51, 95% CI 1.41–1.61) and to have an abortion at or before 13 weeks after telemedicine was introduced (OR 1.46, 95% CI 1.22–1.75). The average distance women travelled to access abortion care decreased only slightly after telemedicine was introduced, from 33.2 to 30.7 miles. This reduction was possibly less than expected because some women travelled further in order to obtain an abortion sooner. Finally, the researchers also found that women living in more remote parts of the state were more likely to obtain an abortion – and particularly more likely to obtain a medical abortion – after telemedicine was introduced. Of note was that, after telemedicine was introduced, the abortion rate did not increase; instead, it continued a downward trend that preceded this period.

The physician-to-woman programme in British Columbia, Canada, was small and evaluated only in an observational report [8]. Of the ten women seen in the first year, one miscarried before taking her medication, one required a second dose of misoprostol, and the others aborted successfully during the first week with no complications. Two women did not have their second blood tests on time (were non-compliant with the protocol) but aborted uneventfully.

Women on Web reported on 4,325 women from 88 countries who used their telemedicine abortion service between February 2007 and September 2008 [11]. There were 2,585 women who provided follow-up information. Of these, 240 (9.3%) did not take the medication and 22 (0.9%) had continuing pregnancies. No blood transfusions or other serious complications were reported. Of the 2,323 women who self-administered the medicines and had no continuing pregnancy, 289 (12.4%) received a surgical intervention. This rate varied from over 14% in Eastern Europe to under 5% in the Middle East. Among the 1,983 women who answered the acceptability questions, 1,214 (64.1%) reported satisfaction and 426 (22.5%) women reported acceptable stress. More recently, Women on Web reported on 1,401 women in Brazil who completed an online consultation in 2011, of which 602 requested medical abortion. Of these women, 370 reported that they received and used the medication. At the time of taking the medication, 67% were at nine weeks' gestation or less, 23% were between 10 and 12 weeks and 10% were at 13 weeks or later. No serious complications were reported. The proportion of women reporting that they had had a surgical intervention was higher for women at 13 weeks or greater compared to those at nine weeks or less (45% versus 16%). However, 42% of women reported no symptoms at the time of the surgical procedure and the high rate of intervention may be more related to local practice than true failure of the method [13].

Websites providing information only have not been extensively evaluated. A recent study analysed the website use patterns of www.medicationabortion.com between 2005 and 2009 [12]. Over this period, the number of visits increased from 82,000 to over 400,000 annually, and 55% of the visits were by people from countries where abortion was legally

Table 25.1 Requirements for the four models for providing telemedicine abortions

	Clinic-to-clinic with video	Clinician-to-woman with video	Clinician-to-woman by email	Internet information to woman
Regulatory and licensing issues	Depends on state or local laws and regulations. At a minimum, the physician must be licensed in the jurisdiction where patient receives service	Clinician and patient within regulatory boundaries of jurisdiction	Anywhere	Anywhere
Information technology equipment	Owned and operated by clinics	Woman uses her own equipment, but must have audio and video	Woman uses her own equipment, no audio or video needed	Woman uses her own equipment, no audio or video needed
History-taking, gestational dating and investigations	In-clinic history, investigations and ultrasound	Use local lab or ultrasound and history by video	Email eligibility checklist	Self-screening
Consent/information/support	Witnessed written consent, in-clinic information and support	Witnessed written consent, video information and support	No written consent, information by email	No consent, written information
Follow-up – urine, blood, ultrasound scan	May use ultrasound or serum hCG	Usually blood or semi-quantitative urine hCG	Email follow-up, woman advised to use urine pregnancy test	No follow-up, woman advised to use urine pregnancy test

restricted. The English version was the most popular version of the website (accessed in 52% of all visits), followed by the Spanish (33%), Arabic (12%) and French (4%) versions. Both providers and women viewed information on the three methods of early pregnancy termination: mifepristone/misoprostol, methotrexate/misoprostol and misoprostol alone. Spanish-language visits were more likely to access the misoprostol-only section of the website.

Guidelines for establishing a telemedicine abortion service

Although requirements for setting up a telemedicine service may vary according to local laws and regulations, below are some suggested guidelines for initiating a service. They are summarized in Table 25.1.

1. *Regulatory and licensing issues.*

   In general, a physician providing medical care to a patient must be licensed in the jurisdiction in which the patient is located. However, depending on local laws or regulations, the physician may be located in another jurisdiction. When a physician is providing public information about evidence-based treatment, this is not necessary. Deciding when information becomes medical advice or care is not always easy. For the third model of care in which information is provided by internet, but email support and advice is given, there is some controversy. This includes whether the woman is committing a criminal offence by procuring her own abortion without the direct supervision of a physician. It is recommended that physicians considering setting up a telemedicine abortion service ensure that they are in compliance with all local laws and regulations.

2. *Hardware/software.*

With clinic-to-clinic telemedicine, the hardware and software is purchased, maintained and controlled by the clinician. Some health authorities have restrictions on using proprietary systems and this may increase costs. It is critical that the video-conferencing technology be encrypted in order to comply with regulations regarding the transfer of protected health information, such as the Health Insurance Portability and Accountability Act of 1996 (HIPAA) in the USA. Most commercially available video-conferencing systems, including Skype, are encrypted and HIPAA-compliant. With clinician-to-woman telemedicine using video, it is possible to use free video-conferencing systems, such as Skype or FaceTime, and the woman may use any smartphone or computer with video capability. There is less control by the clinician and this may affect the quality of audio and video. For the third and fourth models of care, the woman can use any method of accessing the internet and neither requires audio or video.

3. *Gestational dating and investigations.*

With clinic-to-clinic telemedicine, it is easier to use the more usual methods of ultrasound scanning and blood testing to screen for contraindications and date the pregnancy. With physician-to-woman telemedicine, a cut-off of 5,000 mIU/mL of hCG was used so that any undiagnosed ectopic pregnancy was small enough to respond to methotrexate. Above 5,000 mIU/mL, an ultrasound scan was required to rule out ectopic pregnancies and those over seven weeks' gestation. In the other models of care it may be difficult or impossible to use ultrasound and blood testing, but it should always be possible to use checklists for screening and to do urine testing.

4. *Consent/information/support.*

In the first two models of care, the same level of information and professional one-to-one support is available to those women using telemedicine as to those who are in-person. Good information is crucial to safe abortion care, but support could be considered a luxury and would not be possible with the third and fourth models.

5. *Follow-up.*

After medical abortion, it is important to identify continuing pregnancies. In North America, clinics frequently use ultrasound 1–2 weeks after mifepristone or serial hCG measurements showing a drop of 80% after 1 week [14–16]. In the UK, it is more common to use telephone follow-up with self-performed urine pregnancy test [17–19].

Delayed reactions, in which the pregnancy is non-viable but has not been expelled, are much more difficult to assess by hCG levels. Low-sensitivity urine hCG testing has been used successfully to monitor completion [17]. A study of 4,484 women found that, with the use of a self-administered questionnaire and a home-administered low-sensitivity pregnancy test, women themselves may be able to accurately and safely determine their need for a follow-up visit after early medical abortion. With the usual sensitive pregnancy tests, it may take three or four weeks before the test becomes negative. A study of 139 women used telephone follow-up and a high sensitivity urine pregnancy test done 30 days after the medication; 35 were evaluated clinically and all had completed abortions [20]. This protocol might delay diagnosis of a failed medical abortion, but is usually the only method available for the fourth model of care. Where available, semi-quantitative urine pregnancy tests may also be used and can confirm completion within one week [21].

Conclusion

Increasing access to abortion can improve women's health, and these four models of telemedicine abortions can increase access to abortion. Providers of telemedicine abortions need to use the best evidence available to ensure that women accessing abortions through their services receive the best information to make the best choices for themselves.

References

1. Jung SG, Kweon HJ, Kim ET, Kim SA, Choi JK, Cho DY. Preference and awareness of telemedicine in primary care patients. *Korean J Fam Med* 2012;33:25–33.

2. Kohl BA, Fortino-Mullen M, Praestgaard A, Hanson CW, Dimartino J, Ochroch EA. The effect of ICU telemedicine on mortality and length of stay. *J Telemed Telecare* 2012;18:282–6.

3. Gornall J. Does telemedicine deserve the green light? *BMJ* 2012;345:e4622.

4. Kaskowitz AP, Carlson N, Nichols M, Edelman A, Jensen J. Online availability of hormonal contraceptives without a health care examination: effect of knowledge and health care screening. *Contraception* 2007;76:273–7.

5. Grossman D, Grindlay K, Buchacker T, Lane K, Blanchard K. Effectiveness and acceptability of medical abortion provided through telemedicine. *Obstet Gynecol* 2011;118:296–303.

6. Grossman DA, Grindlay K, Buchacker T, Potter JE, Schmertmann CP. Changes in service delivery patterns after introduction of telemedicine provision of medical abortion in Iowa. *Am J Public Health* 2013;103:73–8.

7. Grindlay K, Grossman D, Lane K. Women's and providers' experiences with medical abortion provided through telemedicine: a qualitative study. *Women's Health Issues* 2013;23:e117–22.

8. Wiebe ER. Use of telemedicine for providing medical abortion. *International Journal of Gynecology and Obstetrics* 2014;124:177–8.

9. Gomperts R, Kleiverda G, Gemzell-Danielsson K, Davies S, Jelinska K. Using telemedicine for termination of pregnancy with mifepristone and misoprostol in settings where there is no access to safe services. *BJOG* 2008;115:1578–9.

10. Grindlay K, Yanow S, Jelinska K, Gomperts R, Grossman D. Abortion restrictions in the U.S. military: Voices from women deployed overseas. *Women's Health Issues* 2011;21:259–64.

11. Gomperts R, Petow SA, Jelinska K, Steen L, Gemzell-Danielsson K, Kleiverda G. Regional differences in surgical intervention following medical termination of pregnancy provided by telemedicine. *Acta Obstet Gynecol Scand* 2012;91:226–31.

12. Foster AM, Wynn LL, Trussell J. Evidence of global demand for medication abortion information: an analysis of www.medicationabortion.com. *Contraception* 2014;89:174–80.

13. Gomperts R, van der Vleuten K, Jelinska K, da Costa CV, Gemzell-Danielsson K, Kleiverda G. Provision of medical abortion using telemedicine in Brazil. *Contraception* 2014;89:129–33.

14. O'Connell K, Jones HE, Simon M, et al. First-trimester surgical abortion practices: a survey of National Abortion Federation members. *Contraception* 2009;79:385–92.

15. Fiala C, Safar P, Bygdeman M, Gemzell-Danielsson K. Verifying the effectiveness of medical abortion; ultrasound versus hCG testing. *Eur J Obstet Gynecol Reprod Biol* 2003;109:190–5.

16. Clark W, Panton T, Hann L, Gold M. Medication abortion employing routine sequential measurements of serum hCG and sonography only when indicated. *Contraception* 2007;75:131–5.

17. Clark W, Bracken H, Tanenhaus J, Schweikert S, Lichtenberg ES, Winikoff B. Alternatives to a routine follow-up visit

for early medical abortion. *Obstet Gynecol* 2010;115:264–72.

18. Cameron ST, Glasier A, Dewart H, *et al.* Telephone follow-up and self-performed urine pregnancy testing after early medical abortion: a service evaluation. *Contraception* 2012;86:67–73.

19. Grossman D, Grindlay K. Alternatives to ultrasound for follow-up after medical abortion: a systematic review. *Contraception* 2011;83:504–10.

20. Perriera LK, Reeves MF, Chen BA, Hohmann HL, Hayes J, Creinin MD. Feasibility of telephone follow-up after medical abortion. *Contraception* 2010;81:143–9.

21. Blum J, Shochet T, Lynd K, *et al.* Can at-home semi-quantitative pregnancy tests serve as a replacement for clinical follow-up of medical abortion? A US study. *Contraception* 2012;86:757–62.

Decriminalizing abortion – the Australian experience

Kerry Petersen

Introduction

The history of abortion in common law jurisdictions such as Australia and the UK has demonstrated that prohibitive abortion laws are unworkable, in part because 'they ignore pluralism and generate illegal practices' [1]. Abortion laws in Australia and the UK have been 'liberalized' by courts and parliaments since the 1960s; nevertheless most jurisdictions have retained the criminal provisions and given the control over decision-making to the medical practitioner rather than the unwillingly pregnant woman. Both women and doctors in these jurisdictions are exposed to legal risks and their status can be transformed from law-abiding citizens into criminals – if they are prosecuted and the laws are interpreted harshly [2]. The retention of criminal abortion laws encroaches upon a number of human rights (see Chapter 27), stigmatizes reproductive health practice and dissuades health professionals from training and practising in this area of women's health. In essence, criminal abortion laws are not acceptable in the twenty-first century and do not promote the health or wellbeing of women.

In Australia, the High Court has held that there is a negative right to reproductive autonomy or choice, but there is no fundamental right to reproduce which is independent of the right to personal inviolability [3]. The Australia Humans Rights Law Centre notes in a submission to the Parliamentary Committee reviewing the Reproductive Health (Access to Terminations) Bill 2013 (Tas) that criminal abortion laws engage a range of relevant human rights protected in key human rights treaties to which Australia is a party. The relevant rights include the right to non-discrimination, the right to the highest attainable standard of health, the right to privacy, the right to life, the right to liberty and security of the person, the right to freedom of religion and belief and the right to freedom of expression [4].

Since the late 1990s, the right to the 'highest standard of health' has underpinned four revised legal frameworks regulating abortion in Australian jurisdictions. Although Australia's abortion laws vary from state to state, there is a trend to classify abortion mainly as a health matter. The focus of this chapter is on the four jurisdictions where reform legislation has decriminalized or partially decriminalized abortion. These are: Western Australia; the Australian Capital Territory (ACT); Victoria; and Tasmania. These jurisdictions have adopted different pathways; however, all of them have struck down criminal laws which make it an offence for a pregnant woman to procure her own abortion at all stages of a pregnancy and abortion is now classified mainly as a health matter. Women in these jurisdictions

Abortion Care, ed. Sam Rowlands. Published by Cambridge University Press. © Cambridge University Press 2014.

do not risk going to jail for having an abortion. However, abortion remains an offence in Queensland, New South Wales, the Northern Territory and South Australia.

Evolution of abortion law in Australia

Throughout the nineteenth century Australia followed the English abortion laws: the first criminal abortion statute, Lord Ellenborough's Act, was passed in 1803 because the authorities believed that abortion would be more effectively controlled by statute law than the common law [5]. Six decades later the Offences Against the Person Act 1861 (OAP) was passed and it became an international model of criminal abortion legislation. In effect, the OAP makes it an offence: for a pregnant woman to attempt to self-abort unlawfully; for any person to attempt to procure a miscarriage unlawfully, even if the woman was not pregnant (and the woman could be charged with conspiring or aiding and abetting); and for a person to supply abortifacients or abortion instruments knowingly and unlawfully, even if the woman was not pregnant.

When Australia became a federation in 1901, the states and territories were given the power to regulate health and criminal matters. The early abortion laws passed in Australia's six states and two territories were based on the OAP Act. Medical practitioners who performed 'therapeutic' abortions worked in a realm of legal uncertainty and were advised to obtain a second professional opinion and written consent from the husband and the pregnant woman. In 1938, nearly eight decades after the OAP Act was passed, Mr Aleck Bourne, a gynaecologist in London, openly terminated the pregnancy of a 14-year-old girl who had become pregnant after being raped by two soldiers. He was charged with performing an unlawful abortion. In *R* v. *Bourne* [6] Judge Macnaghten's ruling provided some guidance on the concept of 'unlawful'. In his direction to the jury he stated that the presence of the word 'unlawful' in the legislation implied that in some circumstances an abortion could be lawful. He also said that the accused would not be guilty of performing an unlawful abortion if it was performed to save the pregnant woman's life; or if the accused believed on reasonable grounds that she was likely to become a physical or mental wreck if she continued with the pregnancy. Bourne was found not guilty

The English case *R* v. *Bourne* was not a binding legal precedent in Australia but it had a significant impact on abortion practice – even though abortion law was still unclear. Between the 1930s and 1960s, most abortions were performed by qualified and unqualified 'abortionists'. In the late 1960s some changes were made to the abortion laws in South Australia and Victoria. In South Australia, the Criminal Law Consolidation Act 1935 (SA) was passed. This Act, which was based on the Abortion Act (as amended) 1967 (Eng), prohibits unlawful abortion and has a specific provision in the legislation for therapeutic abortion. Around the same time as South Australian law was reformed there was a breakthrough in Victoria with the Supreme Court case *R* v. *Davidson* [7]. In this case, Dr Charles Davidson was charged under section 65 of the Crimes Act 1958 (Vic) with performing an unlawful abortion. Justice Menhennitt ruled that abortion was lawful in Victoria if the accused honestly believed on reasonable grounds that the abortion was *necessary* to save the woman from a serious danger to her life or her physical or mental health and it was *proportionate* to the danger. This ruling was not binding on other jurisdictions, but it was followed in the Australian Capital Territory, New South Wales, Tasmania and Queensland. As more doctors provided abortions under the protection of the Menhennitt ruling, the rates of morbidity and mortality decreased and abortion was no longer regarded as a high-risk procedure.

In contemporary Australia abortion is a politically sensitive as well as a common, safe and publicly subsidized medical procedure. There is no national reporting system, but it was accepted by the Victorian Law Reform Commission in 2008 that the number of abortions performed in Australia is between 80,000 and 85,000 per annum [8]. When compared to nine other developed countries, Australia has the third highest rate of abortion after the USA and New Zealand [9]. Most abortions carried out in Australia are surgical first trimester abortions. Early medical abortions (EMAs) (see Chapter 7) were virtually banned in Australia between 1996 and 2006 due to political interference with the role of the Therapeutic Goods Administration (TGA). After a long struggle, mifepristone was registered on the Australian Register of Therapeutic Goods (ARTG) in 2012 [10]. A year later the Australian Government made these drugs more affordable for EMAs by listing them on the Pharmaceutical Benefits Scheme (PBS). Unless there is further political interference in this area more women will be able to choose to have an affordable EMA and there should be no need for women to take the risky path of obtaining 'illegitimate' or unsafe abortifacient drugs via the internet or other sources – at least in jurisdictions where abortion is legal [11].

Before discussing the reform laws in Australia it is worth noting the following cases because they make it very clear that, while criminal abortion laws are retained, doctors and women in Australia and the UK are at risk of being treated as criminals. These sad cases speak for themselves and demonstrate that there is a need to find more enlightened ways of dealing with medical recklessness, desperate women with unwanted pregnancies and archaic laws.

In the New South Wales case *R* v. *Sood* (Ruling No 3) [12], Dr Suman Sood was convicted of performing an unlawful abortion on a woman who was nearly 24 weeks pregnant. Dr Sood not only committed an offence but was professionally careless and her mismanagement caused the woman to deliver a live baby into a toilet bowl at home. The baby died shortly after delivery. The jury found that the accused doctor did not act in good faith because she failed to form an honest belief about necessity and proportionality as required by the law in New South Wales. The accused was given a two-year behaviour bond and de-registered by the New South Wales Medical Board.

In the English case *R* v. *Catt (Sarah Louise)* [13] the defendant pleaded guilty in the Leeds Crown Court to self-administering misoprostol, with the intention of procuring a miscarriage, when she was at term. Sarah Catt obtained the misoprostol from India through the internet and delivered the baby which was induced by the misoprostol while she was alone at home. She told the police that the baby had been stillborn and this aroused suspicion when she refused to disclose the whereabouts of the body. When Mr Justice Cooke was sentencing the accused, he noted that abortion cases are rare in court these days but the critical element underlying this case was that Sarah Catt deliberately and unlawfully terminated her pregnancy after 24 weeks' gestation and very close to term with the full knowledge that it was an offence. Mr Justice Cooke sentenced her to eight years in jail. On appeal, this sentence was reduced to 3.5 years. This decision was very controversial and provoked a great deal of public debate. Barbara Hewson, a London barrister, points out that it is not an offence to give birth at home unattended nor is it an offence to have a stillbirth and that 'there's no evidence she sought to harm the baby before or during labour' [14].

In the Queensland case *R* v. *Brennan and Leach* [15] history was made when Tegan Leach was charged with one count of procuring her own abortion [16]. Her partner Sergie Brennan was charged with one count of supplying her with the drugs mifepristone and misoprostol to procure an unlawful abortion [17]. He obtained the mifepristone and misoprostol tablets from his sister in the Ukraine through the regular overseas postal service. The jury found Leach and Brennan were not guilty. The case turned on whether the drugs mifepristone and misoprostol were 'noxious things'. On the basis of evidence given by a medical expert witness, it was decided that these drugs were therapeutic not noxious [18]. It is not clear if a similar case would reach the same decision because *R v. Brennan and Leach* was decided on the particular facts of that case. Nevertheless, *R v. Brennan and Leach* demonstrates how vulnerable women and their partners are in states where abortion is still a criminal offence. The case was extensively covered by the media throughout Australia and was a shock to many Queenslanders who were unaware that women could go to jail in that state for having an abortion [19].

Western Australia

Western Australia was the first state to reform criminal abortion laws in Australia. The process was triggered by the arrest of two Perth doctors, Victor Chan and Ho Peng Lee, who were charged under Western Australia's abortion laws in 1998. They were the first charges to be laid against doctors in that state in 30 years and these events caused a crisis in abortion service delivery. The incident resulted in a widespread public debate on the regulation of abortion which led to the abortion laws being reformed in that state. The charges against the doctors were dropped by the Western Australia Director of Public Prosecutions shortly after the reform legislation was passed.

In Western Australia an abortion will be lawful if a medical practitioner performs an abortion in 'good faith and with reasonable care and skill' and it is justified under section 334 of the Health Act 1911 (WA). On the other hand, if a person who is not a medical practitioner performs an abortion it will be a crime [20].

An abortion will be justified only if:

- the woman has given an informed consent; or
- the woman will suffer personal, family or social consequences if the abortion is not performed; or
- the woman will suffer serious danger to her physical or mental health if the abortion is not performed; or
- the woman's pregnancy is causing serious danger to her physical or mental health.

These requirements are met where:

- a medical practitioner has provided the woman with counselling about the medical risk of an abortion and of carrying a pregnancy to term;
- a medical practitioner has offered the woman a referral for counselling before and after the abortion;
- a medical practitioner has informed the woman that counselling will be available for her if she has an abortion or carries the pregnancy to term.

A line is drawn at 20 weeks' gestation. From that time two medical practitioners from a panel of at least six medical practitioners appointed by the Minister must agree that the woman or a fetus has a severe medical condition that justifies an abortion. Advanced gestation procedures must be performed in an approved facility. Very few advanced gestation abortions are performed in Western Australia and 'congenital anomalies were reported as the reason for 95.5, 93.6 and 90.4% of all induced abortions at 20 weeks' gestation or more occurring during 2010, 2011 and 2012 respectively' [21].

The Australian Capital Territory

The Australian Capital Territory (ACT) decriminalized abortion in 2002. This is the most minimal legal model regulating abortion in Australia. Under section 80 of the Health Act 1993 the term abortion includes surgical and medical abortions. Abortions are no longer regulated by the Crimes Act 1900 (ACT) and the few rules dealing with abortion in the ACT have been transferred to the Health Act 1993 (ACT). It is an offence for anyone other than a medical practitioner to perform an abortion and all abortions, including early medical abortions induced by mifepristone and misoprostol, must be carried out in approved medical facilities. There is no legal duty for anyone to assist or perform in the carrying out of an abortion and a person may refuse to assist in abortions. There are no time limits in the ACT and although there is still a child destruction provision in section 42 of the Crimes Act 1900 (ACT) this section is primarily concerned with causing or contributing to the death of a child during childbirth rather than whether or not the child is capable of being born alive.

Victoria

The Abortion Law Reform Act 2008 (Vic) which decriminalized abortion in Victoria was passed after the Victorian Law Reform Commission conducted an inquiry into the abortion laws and published a report recommending reforms [8]. The provisions in sections 65 and 66 of the Crimes Act 1958 (Vic) relating to abortions and sections 15–17 of the Crimes Act 1958 (Vic) relating to the grey area of child destruction laws were repealed. A new offence of an abortion being carried out by an unqualified person has been created and a woman who consents to, or assists in, the performance of an abortion on herself is not guilty of an offence.

Under section 4 of the Abortion Law Reform Act 2008 (Vic) 'A registered medical practitioner may perform an abortion on a woman who is not more than 24 weeks pregnant'. This provision excludes state interference with a woman's decision to have an abortion when it is made in consultation with her medical practitioner within the prescribed gestational limits. However, if a woman is more than 24 weeks' pregnant, section 5 of the Act permits a medical practitioner to perform a lawful abortion only where:

- a registered medical practitioner reasonably believes that it is appropriate in all the circumstances; and
- has consulted at least one other registered medical practitioner who also believes that the abortion is reasonable in all the circumstances.

When considering whether the abortion is appropriate, a registered medical practitioner *must* take into account all relevant medical circumstances and the woman's current and future physical, psychological and social circumstances. As there is no specific reference to a fetus, it can be assumed that the Act includes the medical circumstances of a fetus and therefore the Act legitimates cases of fetal anomaly if a medical practitioner reasonably believes it is appropriate to carry out an abortion. This is a very sensitive area of medicine as most 'women will request abortion after the diagnosis of a major fetal abnormality – 95% do so after the diagnosis of Down syndrome in Victoria [moreover] clinical experience shows that even women who consider themselves to be antichoice commonly re-evaluate their in-principle opposition to abortion' [22]. In practice, hospital policies and the views of medical practitioners and administrators continue to influence the provision of abortion services, particularly higher gestation abortions in public hospitals.

Sections 6 and 7 of the Abortion Law Reform Act 2008 (Vic) are concerned with the role of other registered health practitioners who are permitted to supply and administer abortifacient drugs in some circumstances. A registered pharmacist or registered nurse may supply abortifacient drug(s) to a woman who is not more than 24 weeks pregnant. When a woman is more than 24 weeks pregnant, a registered medical practitioner may give a written direction to a registered pharmacist or registered nurse employed or engaged by a hospital to supply or administer a drug for the purpose of causing an abortion but only if the medical practitioner reasonably believes an abortion is appropriate in all the circumstances and has consulted at least one other registered medical practitioner who also reasonably believes an abortion is appropriate in all the circumstances.

Section 8 of the Act addresses the obligations of a registered health practitioner who has a conscientious objection to abortion [23]. If a woman requests a registered health practitioner for advice on a proposed abortion, and the health practitioner has a conscientious objection, the practitioner must inform the woman that he or she has a conscientious objection. The practitioner must also refer the woman to another registered health practitioner who he or she knows does not hold a conscientious objection. Despite a conscientious objection, a medical practitioner has a duty to perform an abortion in an emergency where it is necessary to save the pregnant woman's life. Similarly, a registered nurse has to assist a medical practitioner in these circumstances. These sections in the Act are seen by some as a restriction on clinical freedom; and by others as an expansion of reproductive autonomy. The intention is to stop the practice of anti-choice medical practitioners from placing obstacles in the path of a woman seeking an abortion which can be detrimental to her health. The Act does not prescribe penalties for breaches, but non-compliance with the Act could attract professional sanctions.

Tasmania

Tasmania is the latest state to reform abortion laws in Australia. The Reproductive Health (Access to Terminations) Act 2013 (Tas) became law in November 2013. Under this Act access to abortion services is more restrictive and less respectful of personal autonomy than it is in Victoria. The Act establishes a health framework for the provision of abortion and a woman is not guilty of a crime or any other offence if she consents to, or performs an abortion on herself. In the Second Reading Speech, the Minister emphasized that the word 'termination' is used in the Tasmanian legislation because the term abortion 'is the name given to a crime in our current laws. It has been used by certain groups throughout history in a derogatory manner, to demean and stigmatise women for making their own decisions about their reproductive health' [24].

A medical practitioner is permitted to perform an abortion, at or before 16 weeks' gestation if the woman gives her consent. The Minister also addressed the issue of consent in the Second Reading Speech and noted that:

> Consent takes its usual meaning within the medical context; that is, voluntary consent by a patient, after receiving proper and adequate information about the proposed treatment, including potential risks and benefits and alternative options. These requirements exist for all medical procedures and are imposed by professional medical standards. [24]

However, after a woman has been pregnant for more than 16 weeks conditions have been imposed on the availability of an abortion. Interestingly, this line is drawn before many pregnant women undergo prenatal testing. Two medical practitioners, one of whom must be a specialist in obstetrics and gynaecology, must reasonably believe that the woman's physical or mental health would involve greater risk of injury from continuing the pregnancy than from terminating it and that the woman has given her consent. When assessing the risk of injury to a woman's physical or mental health each medical practitioner is required to take into account the woman's physical, psychological, economic and social circumstances. If medical practitioners fail to follow the 16-week framework laid out in the legislation, professional sanctions may apply.

It is an offence under section 178D of the Criminal Code Act 1924 (Tas) for a person who is not a medical practitioner to perform an abortion. It is also an offence under section 178E of the Criminal Code Act 1924 (Tas) if a person 'intentionally or recklessly' terminates the pregnancy of a woman without her consent, for example as a result of an assault. However, no prosecution will be instituted against a medical practitioner who performs an abortion when the woman is incapable of giving consent if the abortion is performed in good faith for the woman's benefit and the termination was reasonable in the circumstances.

Section 7 of the Reproductive Health (Access to Terminations) Act 2013 stipulates that if a pregnant woman requesting abortion consults a medical practitioner who has a conscientious objection to abortion, or if she seeks advice about all of the pregnancy options, the practitioner must give her a list of relevant prescribed health services offering counselling and information. However, where an abortion is necessary to save a woman's life or to prevent her serious injury the practitioner has a duty to perform an abortion.

Medical practitioners and counsellors in Tasmania who have a conscientious objection to abortion are obliged to refer women seeking advice about abortion or pregnancy options to another service provider who the medical practitioner knows does not hold such an objection. The penalty for non-compliance is a fine and possibly professional sanctions.

Finally, the Reproductive Health (Access to Terminations) Act 2013 (Tas) follows North America [25,26] and establishes buffer zones around premises where abortion services are provided to protect women and clinical staff. Section 9(1) states that any person who engages in prohibited behaviour in an access zone may face a fine or imprisonment, or both.

Conclusions

The abortion reform laws that have been passed in these four Australian jurisdictions reflect reproductive autonomy principles as well as the concept of clinical freedom. Furthermore, and most importantly, the laws are clear in these jurisdictions and the majority of abortions are performed in the first trimester. These reform laws represent a significant socio-legal shift insofar as they no longer criminalize abortion. Under these laws the personal autonomy of the unwillingly pregnant woman is respected in varying degrees; autonomy rights diminish as the pregnancy advances unless there is a serious threat to her health or life. The Australian Capital Territory is the only jurisdiction which does not impose specific gestational limits and there have been no reported repercussions.

References

1. Petersen K. Classifying abortion as a health matter: the case for de-criminalising abortion laws in Australia. In S McLean (ed.) *First Do No Harm: Law, Ethics and Healthcare*. Cambridge University Press, 2006.

2. de Crespigny L, Savulescu J. Abortion: time to clarify Australia's confusing laws. *Medical Journal of Australia* 2004;181:201–3.

3. *Secretary, Department of Health and Community Services* v. *JWB and SMB* (1992) 175 CLR 218.

4. Zampas C, Gher JM. Abortion as a human right – International and Regional standards. *Human Rights Law Review* 2008;8:249.

5. Petersen K. *Abortion Regimes*. Aldershot: Dartmouth, 1993.

6. *R* v. *Bourne* [1939] 1 KB 687.

7. *R* v. *Davidson* [1969] VR 667.

8. Victorian Law Reform Commission: Law of abortion: final report www. lawreform.vic.gov.au/home/completed+projects/abortion/lawreform+-+law+of+abortion_+final+report. Melbourne, VLRC, 2008 (accessed 24 December 2011).

9. Chan A, Sage LC. Estimating Australia's abortion rates 1985–2003. *Medical Journal of Australia* 2005;182:447–52.

10. Registration of Medicines for The Medical Termination of Early Pregnancy. Therapeutic Goods Administration, Department of Health, Australian Government, 30 August 2012. www. tga.gov.au/hp/information-medicines-mifepristone-gymiso.htm#.Uxq2-4UZOYI (accessed 24 November 2013).

11. Petersen KA. Early medical abortion: legal and medical developments in Australia. *Medical Journal of Australia* 2010;193:26–9.

12. *R* v. *Sood (Ruling No 3)* [2006] NSWC 762.

13. *R* v. *Catt (Sarah Louise)* [2013] EWCA Crim 1187.

14. Hewson B. Abortion should be removed from the criminal law. *Solicitors' Journal* 2012;156. www.solicitorsjournal.com/comment/abortion-should-be-removed-criminal-law (accessed 4 March 2014).

15. *R* v. *Brennan and Leach* (2010) (unreported Dist Ct, Qld, Criminal Jurisdiction, Indictment 74 of 2010. DIS-000000610/10).

16. Criminal Code (Qld) 1899 as amended 2009, s 225.

17. Criminal Code (Qld) 1899 as amended 2009, s 226.

18. Petersen K. Abortion laws and medical developments: a medico-legal anomaly in Queensland. *Journal of Law and Medicine* 2011;18:594–600.

19. de Costa CM, Russell DB, Carrette M. Abortion in Australia: still to emerge from the 19th century. *Lancet* 2010;375:804–5.

20. Criminal Code Compilation Act 1913 (WA), s 199.

21. Hutchinson M, Joyce A, Cheong M. *Induced Abortions in Western Australia 2010–2012. 4th Report of the Western Australian Abortion Notification System*. Department of Health, Western Australia, 2013.

22. de Crespigny LJ. Pregnant with fetal abnormalities: the forgotten people in the abortion debate. *Medical Journal of Australia* 2008;188:100–3.

23. O'Rourke AO, de Crespigny L, Pyman A. Abortion and conscientious objection: the new battleground. *Monash University Law Review* 2012;38:87–119.

24. Parliament of Tasmania. Reproductive Health (Access to Terminations) Bill 24 of 2013. Second Reading Speech. www. parliament.tas.gov.au/bills/24_of_2013. htm (accessed 9 March 2014).

25. Access to Abortion Services Act 1995 (British Columbia, Canada).

26. Freedom of Access to Clinic Entrances Act (FACE), 18 United States Congress § 248: 2013.

Abortion in international human rights law

Joanna N. Erdman

Public health and political consensus

Abortion and human rights in the global context owes much to the United Nations (UN) conferences of the 1990s, particularly the Cairo *International Conference on Population and Development* (ICPD) [1]. Participating governments agreed to a shift in conceptual approach on population and development, moving from controlling fertility to promoting *reproductive rights* – bringing this term into the global lexicon, and the concept into the global consciousness. Reproductive rights recognize a 'basic right to decide freely and responsibly the number, spacing and timing of ... children and to have the information and means to do so. It also includes the right of all to make decisions concerning reproduction free of discrimination, coercion and violence' (para 7.3) [1]. Political endorsement of reproductive rights – that reproductive health is a legitimate subject of human rights – was crucial to the evolution of abortion rights. This was not because access to abortion was obviously a reproductive right of women, but on the contrary, because abortion has always lain imperfectly within the concept.

At the ICPD, several governments joined a Vatican-led opposition to any suggestion that abortion be included within reproductive rights, or otherwise regarded as a health service or method of fertility regulation [2]. These governments framed abortion as a threat to national values, religious and cultural, and succeeded in isolating abortion as a subject of national sovereignty, beyond international reach. To the extent that abortion was a legitimate subject of reproductive health, let alone reproductive rights, it was only with respect to the devastating public health impacts of unsafe abortion. As early as 1967 the World Health Assembly identified unsafe abortion as a serious public health issue, but it was the safe motherhood initiatives of the 1980s that brought the burden of maternal mortality, of which unsafe abortion was a significant cause, to international attention [3]. A maternal mortality frame averts social conflict over abortion based on the status of human embryos and women as moral subjects. By focusing on its health-related risks and harms, abortion is addressed not on its moral or legal status but only as a descriptive cause of reproductive death and disability. The values of protecting life and preventing death, being widely shared, allow consensus to be found amidst ideological conflict.

At ICPD, governments thus agreed 'to deal with the health impact of unsafe abortion as a major public health concern and to reduce the recourse to abortion through ... family-planning services' (para 8.25). Prevention of abortion was given the highest priority. Women with unwanted pregnancies were to have access to reliable information and support, and in all cases, access to postabortion care. Where the ICPD agreement addressed abortion,

Abortion Care, ed. Sam Rowlands. Published by Cambridge University Press. © Cambridge University Press 2014.

it spoke of prevention, avoidance of risk and reduction of harm. Abortion was otherwise a matter 'only [to] be determined at the national or local level according to the national legislative process' (para 8.25). This position was softened one year later, at the *Fourth World Conference on Women* in Beijing, China, where governments agreed not to reform, but to 'review laws containing punitive measures against women who have undergone illegal abortions' (para 106(k)) [4].

The consensus on abortion and human rights was thus: To the extent of the law, abortion should be safe and accessible. Beyond the law, women should not suffer or die from unsafe abortion. Governments made no commitment on access to abortion as a mainstream reproductive health service. This consensus came to be known as the *Cairo compromise*, and would influence the development of abortion rights for years to come.

From political commitments to legal rights

The UN agreements reflected the political commitments, not legal obligations of governments. Reproductive rights, however, were defined as embracing certain human rights already recognized in binding instruments of law. Realization of the limited abortion rights of the ICPD compromise therefore required that existing human rights, like rights to life and health, be interpreted and applied to the prevention of unsafe abortion, the provision of information, support and postabortion care and the guarantee of safe and accessible abortion services to the extent of the law [5]. That is, abortion rights needed to be transformed from political commitments to legal rights. This was primarily the work of women's health advocates who filed cases before regional human rights courts and made submissions to UN treaty bodies in an effort to translate political rhetoric into legal obligation [6]. The public health consensus on unsafe abortion proved crucial to this work.

International human rights law is a form of consent-based governance. Sovereign states bind themselves to human rights treaties, which then become legal obligations of the state. Human rights treaties as legal text, however, require interpretation. Human rights to life and health, for example, are written in broad and open language and rarely if ever make specific textual reference to abortion, or even reproduction. What any of these rights mean in the context of abortion requires an act of interpretation. This is the work of advocates and expert treaty bodies, including courts and committees. Human rights are applied to issues of abortion and this interpretation is then legitimated by states changing their practices [7]. State acceptance is an essential part of international human rights law, because it has no enforcement machinery of its own, and must work through rather than against states. States, in other words, have the primary obligation to protect and promote human rights and within the UN system, for example, assume obligations to report on the measures they have undertaken in this respect.

The role of state acceptance in international law suggests why the Cairo consensus was valuable to the continued evolution of abortion rights. The consensus on unsafe abortion provided a strong basis for the elaboration and acceptance of abortion rights as enforceable state obligations. UN treaty bodies could and did use the ICPD and Beijing recommendations to elaborate legal obligations on state parties to prevent unsafe abortion, and to provide information and services to protect against public health harms.

Among its more valuable aspects, a public health perspective shifted attention away from explaining the causes of unsafe abortion in individual pathology, as moral failing, and reoriented the analysis towards broader social factors that render women vulnerable to unsafe abortion, or that otherwise influence their decisions to terminate a pregnancy. It thereby shifted responsibility for unsafe abortion away from the woman herself towards others with the capacity, if not the obligation, to act – namely state governments. As parties to international treaties, states have positive obligations to address avoidable suffering and death. This is the moral and legal claim of human rights.

In its general comment on the equality of rights between men and women, for example, the UN Human Rights Committee asks states to report on measures taken to help women prevent unwanted pregnancy and to avoid life-threatening clandestine abortions [8]. The assumption of the request is that such measures are required to protect the right to life of women on a basis of equality with men. In its concluding observations on country reports, the Committee has specifically called on governments to increase access to family planning services and education, and to ensure accessible emergency postabortion care [9]. Both the UN Committee on Social, Economic and Cultural Rights and the UN Committee on the Elimination of Discrimination against Women have also interpreted rights to life, health and non-discrimination as requiring states to increase access to education and contraception to reduce women's recourse to unsafe abortion [9]. In its General Comment on adolescent health and development, the UN Committee on the Rights of the Child has focused not merely on prevention through access to contraception, but has also urged governments to provide safe abortion services where not against the law [10].

The public health influence on the treaty bodies' interpretive work can be seen on two levels. Unsafe abortion is conceptualized as a public health problem, but also the favoured mechanisms of its redress are within the health system: the provision of health information and services; the training of health providers; and the equipping of health facilities. Abortion rights, in other words, entail government obligations not merely of restraint, but positive obligations to protect life and health through health and social programmes and services. Under a public health approach, human rights interventions focus on the environment that structures women's vulnerability and constrains their available choices, and for this reason, abortion rights in the global context have fared better on a measure of reproductive justice. Though the UN treaty bodies have never recognized abortion on request as a human right, or more broadly a woman's right to decide, this attentiveness to the structural conditions of women's vulnerability and capacity for choice suggests a more profound understanding of the relationship between reproductive rights and social justice.

The public health framing of abortion has also proven advantageous to advocates, who have used international human rights law to support safe abortion interventions in the field. Of recent note are initiatives that provide women with access to safer-use information on medical abortion, especially the off-label use of misoprostol in clandestine settings [11]. The information is designed to prevent the use of more dangerous methods and to ensure the safer use of drugs, both with the intention to reduce abortion-related harm. Safer-use information in this respect is described as preabortion care and justified as a human rights intervention on the same harm reduction rationale as postabortion care. The right to health requires governments to refrain from censoring or withholding health-related information, and on a more progressive interpretation, to facilitate the provision of health information that will allow women to survive unwanted or unsustainable pregnancy.

Law reform as a public health intervention

A public health and human rights approach that asks why women are vulnerable to unsafe abortion inevitably leads to the criminal law (see Chapter 26), and in so doing, tests the limits of the Cairo compromise. Historical and comparative social science research reveals that legal restrictions do not result in fewer abortions. On the contrary, legal restrictions have a strong association with both a higher incidence of abortion and related mortality. In Romania, for example, after contraception and abortion were made illegal under the Ceausescu pronatalist regime, abortion-related mortality increased to rates ten times higher than in other European countries [5] (Figure 3.2). Today the overwhelming majority of unsafe abortions occur in developing countries, most with restrictive legislation. In contrast, where safe and legal abortion is accessible on broad social grounds or at a woman's request, abortion incidence and mortality decrease to a minimum (see Chapter 3). In Tunisia and South Africa, abortion law reform accompanied by trained providers, equipped facilities and available medicines have dramatically reduced unsafe abortion and its harms [12]. Together public health and human rights have built a near irrefutable case against criminal prohibition on grounds of its dysfunction – both that it does not achieve its intended effect, but more so, that it creates its own order of harm. Law reform is thus supported as a public health intervention.

Using this rationale, UN treaty bodies have routinely called on governments to amend their laws by introducing or broadening legal grounds for abortion to protect a woman's life and health, and in cases of pregnancy resulting from rape [9]. In a General Recommendation, the UN Committee on the Elimination of Discrimination against Women declared that '[i]t is discriminatory for a State party to refuse to provide legally for the performance of certain reproductive health services for women' (para 11) [13]. The committee advised that when possible, criminal legislation be amended to withdraw punitive measures imposed on women who undergo abortion. This statement directly contradicts the ICPD compromise, which limited the scope of reproductive rights to methods of fertility not against the law. National law no longer circumscribes abortion rights, rather international human rights recognizes safe and legal abortion as a mainstream reproductive health service – at least in a minimum set of circumstances. In an unprecedented letter condemning a government for regressive legal reform, the Rapporteur on Women's Rights in the Inter-American system expressly named therapeutic abortion as a necessary health service for women, the denial of which constitutes a violation of human rights [14]. Moreover, given that the public health harms of unsafe abortion are almost always inequitably distributed, UN treaty bodies have also challenged restrictive criminal laws for reason of their discriminatory impact on poor, rural and adolescent women [9].

The breakthrough of international human rights law beyond the Cairo compromise is perhaps best shown in the *Protocol to the African Charter on Human and Peoples' Rights on the Rights of Women in Africa* [15]. The text of this human rights treaty calls on 'States Parties to … protect the reproductive rights of women by authorising medical abortion in cases of sexual assault, rape, incest, and where the continued pregnancy endangers the mental and physical health of the mother or the life of the mother or the foetus' (Art. 14(2)(c)). The Protocol remains the only binding treaty that explicitly addresses abortion, and more so, entails a right of access on a prescribed set of grounds. Its very text inscribes the health and human rights of women into abortion law [16].

Women's health interests in pregnancy and its termination have also served as an effective defence against challenges to liberal abortion laws based on the right to life of the unborn. In the interpretation of the right to life under international law, both the European Court of Human Rights and the Inter-American Court of Human Rights have affirmed that women's rights to life and health necessarily limit any application of the right to life before birth, even if the extent of that limit is undefined [17,18]. Otherwise, to treat the protection of the right to life as absolute would prohibit all abortion and many other reproductive health services, with the consequence that unborn life would be regarded as of higher value than the life and health of pregnant women.

The limits of public health in abortion rights

The tethering of abortion rights to public health has its limitations. Most directly, it may simply render abortion rights obsolete with greater access to safe services in liberal jurisdictions and the increasing availability, and use, of safer clandestine methods. In these changing circumstances the principal harm of criminal laws will be social inequality. Women are vulnerable to economic exploitation in seeking services in informal settings and, when forced to travel, women face additional barriers of cost and isolation. These barriers can be insurmountable for socially disadvantaged women, creating gross inequities. Even where women can access safe services, the banishment and hardships of being forced to seek services away or underground constitutes a dignity-based harm of social exile. This harm, however, cannot register in a public health frame. Where abortion rights are too closely linked to the protection of life and limb, dignity-based harms are too easily ignored or neglected. The European Court of Human Rights, for example, recently held that because women had the right to lawfully travel abroad for abortion services, with access to information and postabortion services, a criminal ban on abortion save where necessary to protect a woman's life did not violate human rights [19]. Where criminal laws do not lead to death or disability, public health affords no protection.

While marrying abortion rights to public health may once have been necessary for their realization, it now threatens their relevance and limits their use. Moreover, it does so precisely by obscuring the ideological stakes in abortion, namely feminist claims grounded not in rights of life and health, but rights of dignity and equality. The challenge is thus to expand human rights on abortion to capture the substantive core of reproductive rights, that is, the basic right to decide the number, spacing and timing of children and to have the information and means to do so. In the UN system, the Special Rapporteur on the Right to Health took an important step in this direction in recommending the decriminalization of abortion on grounds of more than public health harm [20]. His report explained that criminal prohibition violates human rights by restricting a woman's control over her body, and requiring her to continue pregnancy when it is not her choice to do so. The injustice of criminal abortion lies in the state substituting its will for that of the individual. There are yet other stirrings in international human rights law that intimate a similar shift in the nature of abortion rights.

Abortion rights of access, equality and citizenship

Across human rights systems, there have been significant legal developments on access to abortion under legal grounds: that is, rights of access to the extent permitted by law. The trend in liberalization over the past three decades has shown that changing the legal status of abortion often provides little guarantee of effective access to services [21]. This is sometimes the consequence of laws written in vague terms, breeding both uncertainty and conflict among women and providers on what the law does or does not allow. In most cases authority for the determination resides with doctors alone, leaving women no opportunity to appeal or otherwise challenge a refusal. Sometimes doctors refuse on a cautious interpretation of the law, legitimately fearing prosecution under its uncertain standards. Too often, however, doctors and hospital administrators deny services in bad faith, with the deliberate intention to frustrate women's exercise of their legal rights. This includes circumstances where services are denied for reason of conscientious refusal (see Chapter 20).

A transnational litigation strategy has thus emerged, premised on the human rights obligations of the state to implement abortion laws through clear standards and procedural safeguards, and to curb arbitrary exercises of discretion that deny women access to lawful services. The strategy has found success in the UN [22,23], Inter-American [24,25] and European human rights systems [26]. Collectively this case law elaborates a standard whereby once a state lawfully allows for abortion, it must structure the regulatory framework to ensure that women can access these services. This includes: clear legal grounds; written reasons for decisions; and a timely mechanism of appeal and review with an opportunity for the woman to be heard and her views considered. The widespread endorsement of access rights likely reflects their justification in widely shared values, such as equal treatment under the law, which again allows consensus amidst ideological conflict.

These features of access rights – that they extend only to the limits of the law and are rooted in consensus values – has raised concern of a retreat to the ICPD compromise. A careful reading, however, cannot support this claim. The significance of this case law lies in the linking of abortion rights to dignity-based harm. The UN Human Rights Committee and the European Court of Human Rights have both interpreted the infliction of suffering in the denial or obstruction of lawful abortion as a violation of the right to be free from inhuman and degrading treatment [22,27]. On this interpretation, human rights entitle women to more than safe services to the extent permitted by law. These rights entitle women to be treated with respect, dignity and worth including while pregnant. This commitment is most strongly reflected in the right of a woman to be heard and to have her view considered when seeking abortion services. This right challenges a basic normative premise underlying criminal regulation, namely that a woman and her body may be used instrumentally in the service of the state. That a woman must be heard and her views considered reflect minimum conditions of respect for her dignity and worth as a person. This shift in international human rights law on abortion is strongly reflected in the revised edition of the World Health Organization's *Safe Abortion: Technical and Policy Guidance* [28]. The guidance references the growing body of human rights standards on abortion, among them, that women are to be treated as rights bearers within the health system, entitled not merely to access safe and lawful services, but to do so in a manner that respects women's dignity, and reflects their needs and perspectives [29].

Despite a general reluctance in international human rights law to speak of any right to abortion, with these new commitments the law gestures to a conception of abortion rights that pre-dates the ICPD compromise. These are the ideas of transnational feminist movements that claimed the right to abortion as an aspect of women's full and equal citizenship. These are also the ideas that compel many human rights advocates today to campaign for abortion rights in international law.

References

1. United Nations. *Programme of Action of the United Nations International Conference on Population and Development.* New York: United Nations, 1994.

2. Johnson S. *The Politics of Population: The International Conference on Population and Development.* London: Earthscan Publications, 1995.

3. Cook RJ, Dickens BM. Human rights dynamics of abortion law reform. *Hum Rights Q* 2003;25:1–59.

4. United Nations. *Beijing Declaration and Platform for Action. Fourth World Conference on Women.* New York: United Nations, 1995.

5. Shaw D. Abortion and human rights. *Best Pract Res Clin Obstet Gynaecol* 2010;24:633–46.

6. Hessini L. Global progress in abortion advocacy and policy: an assessment of the decade since ICPD. *Reprod Health Matters* 2005;13:88–100.

7. Roseman MJ, Miller AM. Sexual and reproductive rights at the United Nations: frustration or fulfillment? *Reprod Health Matters* 2011;19:102–18.

8. UN Human Rights Committee. General Comment No. 28: Equality of rights between men and women, UN Doc. CCPR/C/21rev.1/Add.10 (2000).

9. Zampas C, Gher JM. Abortion as a human right – international and regional standards. *Hum Rights Law Rev* 2008;8:249–94.

10. UN Committee on the Rights of the Child. General Comment No. 4: Adolescent health and development, UN Doc. CRC/GC/2003/4 (2003).

11. Erdman JN. Harm reduction, human rights and access to information on safer abortion. *Int J Gynecol Obstet* 2012;118:83–6.

12. Ngwena C. State obligations to implement African abortion laws: employing human rights in a changing legal landscape. *Int J Gynecol Obstet* 2012;119:198–202.

13. UN Committee on the Elimination of all Forms of Discrimination against Women. General Recommendation No. 24: Women and Health, UN Doc. A/54/38/Rev.1 (1999).

14. Letter dated 10 November 2006, from Victor Abramovich of the Inter-American Commission on Human Rights, and Santiago A. Canton to Norman Calderas Cardenal, Nicaraguan Minister of Foreign Affairs.

15. *Protocol to the African Charter on Human and Peoples' Rights on the Rights of Women in Africa.* AHG/Res, 240 (XXXI), adopted 11 July 2003, entered into force 25 November 2005.

16. Ngwena CG. Protocol to the African Charter on the Rights of Women: implications for access to abortion at the regional level. *Int J Gynecol Obstet* 2010;110:163–6.

17. *Vo v. France*, Application No. 53924/00, (2005) 40 E.H.R.R. 12, Eur. Ct. H.R. (2004).

18. *Artavia-Murillo et al. ("in vitro fertilization") v. Costa Rica*, Preliminary Objections, Merits, Reparations and Costs, Judgment, Inter-Am. Ct. H.R. (series C) No. 257 (November 28, 2012).

19. *A, B, and C v. Ireland*, [2010] E.C.H.R. 2032.

20. UN Special Rapporteur on the Right to Health. Interim report to the General Assembly. UN Doc. A/66/150 (2011).

21. Guttmacher Institute. *Making Abortion Services Accessible in the Wake of Legal Reforms: A Framework and Six Case Studies.* New York: Guttmacher Institute, 2012.

22. *K.L. v. Peru*, Communication no. 1153/2003, UN Doc. CCPR/C/85/D/1153/2003 (Human Rights Committee) (2005).

23. *L.M.R. v. Argentina*, Communication no. 1608/2007, UN Doc. CCPR/C/101/D/1608/2007 (Human Rights Committee) (2011).

24. *X and XX v. Colombia*, MC-270/09, Inter-Am. C.H.R. (2011).

25. *Paulina Ramirez v. Mexico*, Case 161–02, Report no. 21/07, Inter-Am. C.H.R., Friendly Settlement (2007).

26. Erdman JN. The procedural turn: abortion at the European Court of Human Rights. In RJ Cook, JN Erdman, BM Dickens (eds.) *Rethinking Abortion and the Law: A Transnational Perspective.* Pennsylvania Press, 2014.

27. *R.R. v. Poland*, Application no. 27617/04, Eur. Ct. H.R. (2011).

28. World Health Organization. *Safe Abortion: Technical and Policy Guidance for Health Systems*, 2nd edn. Geneva: WHO, 2012.

29. Erdman JN, DePiñeres T, Kismödi E. Updated WHO guidance on safe abortion: health and human rights. *Int J Gynecol Obstet* 2013;120:200–3.

Appendix: List of useful organizations

Advancing New Standards in Reproductive Health

www.ansirh.org

ANSIRH works to ensure that reproductive health care and policy are grounded in evidence. ANSIRH's multidisciplinary team includes clinicians, researchers and scholars in the fields of sociology, demography, anthropology, medicine, nursing, public health, and law. ANSIRH is a programme of the Bixby Center for Global Reproductive Health, University of California San Francisco.

ANSIRH is conducting the highly acclaimed Turnaway Study.

American Congress of Obstetricians and Gynecologists

www.acog.org

ACOG represents American gynaecologists. Its website provides information regarding women's health, including practice guidelines, patient education materials, and policy updates. ACOG Committee Opinions are an excellent resource.

Association of Reproductive Health Professionals

www.arhp.org

ARHP is a membership association for experts in reproductive health. Its website provides information on medical abortion and reproductive health. The site offers an abortion resource centre, including patient information, clinical information and health provider training materials.

Center for Reproductive Rights

www.reproductiverights.org

The Center for Reproductive Rights uses the law to advance reproductive freedom as a fundamental right that all governments are legally obliged to protect, respect and fulfil. Its website provides information on legal issues surrounding abortion, reproductive health and women's rights worldwide.

Concept Foundation

www.conceptfoundation.org

An international not-for-profit organization which supports work on the quality of reproductive health medicines and the introduction and promotion of essential healthcare products around the world. With a pharmaceutical partner, Concept has registered Medabon®, the first product to package mifepristone and misoprostol in the same pack, in more than 40 countries.

Education for Choice

www.brook.org.uk

Education for Choice is a project of Brook dedicated to enabling young people to make informed decisions about pregnancy and abortion. Its website provides youth-friendly information about abortion, as well as information for parents and professionals. Training materials for healthcare professionals are also available.

Exhale

www.4exhale.org

Exhale creates a social climate where each person's unique experience with abortion is supported, respected and free from stigma. Exhale provides services, training and education to empower individuals, families and communities to achieve postabortion health and wellbeing.

FIAPAC

www.fiapac.org

FIAPAC is an international organization of professionals working in abortion care and contraception. It holds biennial Congresses in different countries, with downloads of the presentations available. Its website has good links to not-for-profit organizations, abortion providers, statistics of different countries and world abortions laws.

FIGO: International Federation of Gynecology and Obstetrics

www.figo.org

FIGO is an international organization of obstetricians and gynaecologists. FIGO has a Prevention of Unsafe Abortion initiative involving 54 countries. FIGO's journal, the *International Journal of Gynecology & Obstetrics* (www.ijgo.org), has an excellent track record of publishing articles on medical and human rights aspects of abortion.

Guttmacher Institute

www.guttmacher.org

The Guttmacher Institute is a non-profit organization focused on sexual and reproductive health research, policy analysis and public education. The Guttmacher Institute publishes *Perspectives on Sexual and Reproductive Health, International Family Planning Perspectives, The Guttmacher Policy Review* and special reports on topics relating to sexual and reproductive health and rights. Its website is an excellent source of worldwide abortion statistics.

Gynuity Health Projects

www.gynuity.org

Gynuity Health Projects is a research and technical assistance organization dedicated to the idea that all people should have access to the fruits of medical science and

technology development. Its website provides information on medical abortion, including misoprostol-only use.

Ibis Reproductive Health

www.ibisreproductivehealth.org

Ibis Reproductive Health aims to improve women's reproductive autonomy, choices and health worldwide. Ibis accomplishes its mission by conducting clinical and social science research, leveraging existing research, producing educational materials and promoting policies and practices that support sexual and reproductive rights and health.

International Consortium for Medical Abortion

www.medicalabortionconsortium.org

Founded in 2002, ICMA has brought together key players in the field from all regions of the world, to promote medical abortion within the framework of support for safe abortion worldwide, focusing on the needs of women in developing countries including those countries where abortion is unsafe or not accessible.

International Network for the Reduction of Abortion Discrimination and Stigma (inroads)

www.endabortionstigma.org

Inroads is a global network of advocates, scholars, health providers and donors with the goal of shifting the global conversation on abortion to reimagine a world free of abortion stigma. Its website offers a detailed reference list on abortion stigma and webinars on the subject.

International Planned Parenthood Federation

www.ippf.org

IPPF's work is grounded in the belief that access to quality, sexual and reproductive health, information and services is a basic human right. By making these services available, IPPF helps to empower individuals to make decisions about their fertility and thus contributes to improving health and well-being, national development and environmental quality. The IPPF website contains information, educational materials and publications related to abortion and reproductive health.

Ipas

www.ipas.org

Ipas has worked for three decades to increase women's ability to exercise their sexual and reproductive rights and to reduce deaths and injuries of women from unsafe abortion. Ipas manufactures and distributes manual vacuum aspiration equipment and trains providers in early abortion techniques worldwide. The website also provides information for health service providers, policy makers and the public on four abortion procedures: vacuum aspiration, medication regimens, sharp curettage and dilatation and evacuation.

Marie Stopes International

www.mariestopes.org.uk

MSI is committed to reducing maternal mortality due to unsafe abortion through improved access to reproductive health services to prevent unwanted pregnancy, advocacy initiatives to stress the importance of safe, legal abortion and the provision of quality abortion services in countries where the procedure is legal, including postabortion care, training in manual vacuum aspiration and postabortion family planning.

Misoprostol in Obstetrics and Gynecology

www.misoprostol.org

This site provides information about the obstetric and gynaecological uses of misoprostol, including dosing regimens.

National Abortion Federation

www.prochoice.org

NAF is an association of abortion providers in the USA and Canada. NAF has developed high quality educational resources for health service providers, researchers and counsellors including its Clinical Policy Guidelines.

Planned Parenthood Federation of America

www.plannedparenthood.org

This website provides information and resources on medical and aspiration abortion. Planned Parenthood's affiliates operate almost 750 centres throughout the USA.

Population Council

www.popcouncil.org

The Population Council is an international, non-profit institution that conducts research on three fronts: biomedical, social science, and public health, ultimately seeking to affect thinking about reproductive health and population growth. The Population Council provides information on reproductive health issues worldwide, including publications on medical abortion methods and acceptability among diverse populations.

Postabortion Care Consortium

www.pac-consortium.org

The PAC Consortium works to inform the reproductive health community about health concerns related to unsafe abortion and to promote postabortion care as an effective strategy for addressing this global problem. The website includes an extensive list of postabortion care resources.

Royal College of Obstetricians and Gynaecologists

www.rcog.org.uk

The professional body of obstetricians and gynaecologists in the UK. The RCOG has produced evidenced-based guidelines on abortion care since 2000. The latest edition is that of 2011. As medical abortion becomes widely delivered in the community, sexual and reproductive health specialists are extensively involved in abortion care. The Faculty of Sexual & Reproductive Healthcare (www.fsrh.org) has the RCOG as its parent College.

United Nations

www.un.org
The UN website includes complete texts of the international human rights treaties and accompanying documents:
www.ohchr.org/EN/HRBodies/Pages/HumanRightsBodies.aspx
Also full details of the Millennium Development Goals:
www.un.org/millenniumgoals/

Women on Web

www.womenonweb.org
WoW is supported by a loose and growing network of independent organizations and individuals that have no legal affiliation.

This website provides women with information on how to perform an abortion themselves if they do not live in a country that provides safe, legal abortions. On the 'I need an abortion' part of this site women in need of abortions can find more information on how to obtain a medical abortion, even in legally restrictive settings. On the 'I had an abortion' part of this site, people can upload their portraits and share their stories to break the taboo surrounding abortion.

World Health Organization

www.who.int
WHO set up a special programme of research in human reproduction in 1972, widely known as HRP. WHO's Department of Reproductive Health and Research produced the important publication *Safe Abortion: Technical and Policy Guidance for Health Systems* in 2003; this has been revised in 2012. WHO also produces a document on the incidence of unsafe abortion, which is now in its sixth edition.

Index